# THIAMINE DEFICIENCY DISEASE, DYSAUTONOMIA, AND HIGH CALORIE MALNUTRITION

# THIAMINE DEFICIENCY DISEASE, DYSAUTONOMIA, AND HIGH CALORIE MALNUTRITION

DERRICK LONSDALE

CHANDLER MARRS

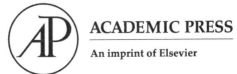

Academic Press is an imprint of Elsevier
125 London Wall, London EC2Y 5AS, United Kingdom
525 B Street, Suite 1800, San Diego, CA 92101-4495, United States
50 Hampshire Street, 5th Floor, Cambridge, MA 02139, United States
The Boulevard, Langford Lane, Kidlington, Oxford OX5 1GB, United Kingdom

Copyright © 2017 Elsevier Inc. All rights reserved.

No part of this publication may be reproduced or transmitted in any form or by any means, electronic or mechanical, including photocopying, recording, or any information storage and retrieval system, without permission in writing from the publisher. Details on how to seek permission, further information about the Publisher's permissions policies and our arrangements with organizations such as the Copyright Clearance Center and the Copyright Licensing Agency, can be found at our website: www.elsevier.com/permissions.

This book and the individual contributions contained in it are protected under copyright by the Publisher (other than as may be noted herein).

**Notices**
Knowledge and best practice in this field are constantly changing. As new research and experience broaden our understanding, changes in research methods, professional practices, or medical treatment may become necessary.

Practitioners and researchers must always rely on their own experience and knowledge in evaluating and using any information, methods, compounds, or experiments described herein. In using such information or methods they should be mindful of their own safety and the safety of others, including parties for whom they have a professional responsibility.

To the fullest extent of the law, neither the Publisher nor the authors, contributors, or editors, assume any liability for any injury and/or damage to persons or property as a matter of products liability, negligence or otherwise, or from any use or operation of any methods, products, instructions, or ideas contained in the material herein.

**Library of Congress Cataloging-in-Publication Data**
A catalog record for this book is available from the Library of Congress

**British Library Cataloguing-in-Publication Data**
A catalogue record for this book is available from the British Library

ISBN: 978-0-12-810387-6

For information on all Academic Press publications visit our website at
https://www.elsevier.com/books-and-journals

 Working together to grow libraries in developing countries

www.elsevier.com • www.bookaid.org

*Publisher:* Andre Gerhard Wolff
*Acquisition Editor:* Megan R. Ball
*Editorial Project Manager:* Jaclyn A. Truesdell
*Production Project Manager:* Lisa M. Jones
*Designer:* Matthew Limbert

Typeset by TNQ Books and Journals

*In memory of my daughter Susan M. Foley*

**Derrick Lonsdale**

# CONTENTS

*Introduction: Why Thiamine? Why Now?*     xi

**1. The History of Thiamine and Beriberi**     1

    From Kakke to Beriberi     1
    Beriberi in Children     6
    Wet and Dry Beriberi and Wernicke's Encephalopathy     7
    Beriberi: The Great Imitator     8
    From Beriberi to Dysautonomia     13
    Underlying Mechanisms of Autonomic Dysfunction: Thiamine,
        the Mitochondria, and Oxidative Metabolism     15
    Therapeutic Nutrition for Autonomic Balance     17
    References     23

**2. The Autonomic Nervous System and Its Functions**     27

    The Autonomic Nervous System: General Arrangement and Function     28
    Autonomic Signaling: Layered Control     29
    Autonomic Chemistry and Neurotransmission     35
    The Myths of Linearity and Symmetry     41
    Autonomic Dysfunction: Clinical Patterns and Clues to Sympathetic
        Dominance     44
    Autonomic Imbalance     52
    References     53

**3. Mitochondria, Thiamine, and Autonomic Dysfunction**     59

    Understanding Mitochondrial Disorders: Moving Beyond Genetics     60
    Mitochondrial Basics of Macro- and Micronutrients     64
    From Diet to ATP: The Essential Nutrients in Mitochondrial Functioning     67
    Thiamine Chemistry and Mitochondrial Function     70
    From Diet to Mitochondria: Understanding Thiamine Transporters     77
    Modern Thiamine Deficiency and Mitochondrial Damage     79
    Nutrient Deficiency, Mitochondria, and the Autonomic System     90
    Rethinking Nutrition     93
    References     93

## 4. Evaluation and Treatment of Thiamine Metabolism in Clinical Practice — 105

When to Consider Thiamine Deficiency — 107
How to Evaluate Thiamine Status in Clinical Care — 108
Laboratory Measures to Evaluate Thiamine — 110
Measuring Thiamine Functionally — 111
Alternative Observations That Point to Thiamine Deficiency — 114
Nonlaboratory Methods to Evaluate Thiamine Deficiency and Autonomic Function — 126
Thiamine Therapy: Beyond the Recommended Daily Allowance — 130
IV Thiamine for Acute and Chronic Cases — 137
Thiamine in Clinical Care: Treating Functional and Genetic Disturbances — 139
Nutrient Interactions — 146
Conclusion — 152
References — 152

## 5. Thiamine-Deficient Dysautonomias: Case Insights and Clinical Clues — 161

Beriberi, Dysautonomia, and Thiamine Deficiency: Symptoms and Time Course — 163
Functional Dysautonomia: Family Studies With Case Details — 165
Pediatric Cases of Thiamine Responsive Dysautonomias — 172
Thiamine-Responsive Dysautonomias in Adults — 200
Familial Dysautonomia and Epigenetics — 205
Conclusion — 207
References — 208

## 6. High-Calorie Malnutrition and Its Impact on Health — 213

High-Calorie Malnutrition: A Different Kind of Mitochondrial Stress — 215
From the Obvious to Not so Obvious Signs of High-Calorie Malnutrition — 216
High-Calorie Malnutrition and Thiamine: Clinical Cases — 241
Conclusion — 253
References — 254

## 7. The Three Circles of Health — 263

Of Stress and Stressors — 265
Energy Metabolism Mediates the Stress Response — 268
Reconsidering Stress and Stressors: Metabolic Mismatches and Autonomic Adaptations — 274

| | |
|---|---|
| Genetic Stressors | 276 |
| Conclusion | 297 |
| References | 299 |

## 8. Energy Metabolism in a Revised Medical Model — 305

| | |
|---|---|
| Malnutrition in the Face of Obesity: Economics Versus Chemistry | 307 |
| Medically Unexplained Symptoms | 309 |
| Chemistry, Energy, and Metabolism | 311 |
| Beyond Cartesian Dualism | 313 |
| Iatrogenesis and Medically Unexplained Symptoms: Two Sides of the Same Question? | 314 |
| Return of the Case Study and N-of-1 in Clinical Care and Research | 316 |
| Next Time the Labs are Negative | 317 |
| Why Thiamine? Why Now? | 318 |
| Those Who Have the Privilege to Know Have the Duty to Act | 320 |
| References | 321 |

*Index* — *327*

# INTRODUCTION: WHY THIAMINE? WHY NOW?

Thiamine, also known as vitamin B1, plays a fundamental role in energy metabolism. It is the rate-limiting cofactor for no less than five enzymes involved in the initial steps of mitochondrial ATP production via the glucose, fatty acid, and amino acid pathways.[1] As a rate-limiting cofactor, one that occurs at the entry points of oxidative metabolism, it is easy to imagine how thiamine deficits, even slight ones, would derail mitochondrial function and initiate complex compensatory cascades that then affect cellular function broadly and diversely. Despite the critical and accepted role of thiamine in oxidative metabolism, however, the downstream effects of its deficiency are still poorly recognized, especially in clinical care.

Experimentally, thiamine deficiency produces reversible damage to the mitochondria[2] and clinically, when the deficit is identified early enough, symptom resolution can be expected.[3] Unfortunately, beyond its accepted role in alcohol-induced beriberi and Wernicke's encephalopathy,[4] thiamine deficiency syndromes in clinical care are rarely considered in modern medicine. Thiamine deficiency appears to have been relegated to the annals of history, a disorder that once plagued populations. Now, however, it is generally believed that it is no longer a relevant issue, thanks to modern nutrition. We will provide evidence that this presumption is simply not true. In fact, it is precisely because of modern nutritional practices that thiamine deficiency is latent across populations.[5]

## UNTANGLING CLINICAL ANOMALIES

This book represents the life's work of the senior author Dr. Derrick Lonsdale and a recent collaboration with his coauthor Dr. Chandler Marrs. Dr. Lonsdale was educated in England, graduated from London University with the degree MB BS. After National Service in the RAF as a medical officer he became a family physician under the National Health Service. Tiring of the bureaucratic interference he immigrated to Canada by joining the RCAF as a medical officer for a short service commission. On completion he was accepted as a pediatric resident at Cleveland Clinic and in 1962 was invited to join the pediatric staff.

For 6 years Dr. Lonsdale was a pediatric oncologist but switched his interest to studying the clinical and biochemical aspects of uncommon diseases known as inborn errors of metabolism. A number of these diseases, if not all, cause severe mental retardation if they are not spotted at birth and this gave rise to the screening tests for newborn infants that are applied to every state in the United States. In some of them, the mental retardation can be forestalled by giving the infant a special diet. One of the rarest of these diseases is known as maple syrup urine disease (branched-chain ketoaciduria), caused by an abnormal recessive gene. The disease gets its name because there is a substance that occurs in the urine that smells exactly like maple syrup. Estimated to occur once in 100,000 births, the enzyme is a dehydrogenase that processes the branched-chain amino acids leucine, isoleucine, and valine. This enzyme has the same construction as pyruvic and alpha ketoglutarate dehydrogenases. The decarboxylating component in each of these enzymes requires thiamine and magnesium as cofactors. The binding of the cofactors to the enzyme, like its gene, is also under genetic control. It is therefore sometimes possible to treat the corresponding disease by the epigenetic use of pharmacological doses of the respective cofactor. Epigenetics is a relatively new science that studies the effect of nutritional elements on the action of genes. Although epigenetics had not yet been discovered when the research reported here had been conducted, the clinical results from using thiamine and magnesium in megadoses tended to foretell its inception.

An initial diagnosis of maple syrup urine disease (branched-chain ketoaciduria) having been made, an epigenetic trial would be the first attempt at treatment. If this should fail, the special diet required to prevent mental retardation would have to provide the infant with an exact amount of the branched-chain amino acids that are essential to life. This was the introduction to the value of thiamine for Dr. Lonsdale but it also introduced him to the extraordinary power of nutrition if tailored to the genetic needs of a given individual. From that point forward Dr. Lonsdale was committed to uncovering the connections between thiamine and metabolic health.

The experience of Dr. Marrs is a bit more diverse. She received a BA in Philosophy and then spent many years in the tech industry before returning to academia for an MS in Clinical Psychology and an MA and PhD in Experimental Psychology with an emphasis in neuroendocrinology. Her research career reflects a relentless pursuit of the root mechanisms and pathways that initiate disease, unbridled by conventional barriers. Drawing from her early entrepreneurial ventures in the technology sector, as a graduate student, she founded and directed the UNLV Maternal Health Lab to conduct clinical and Internet-based research on maternal health and mental health. Her lab research identified a pattern of aberrant late pregnancy adrenal androgen concentrations that would predict postpartum psychiatric disturbances, while her clinical research suggested a necessary reorganization of clinical symptomology within that diagnostic paradigm.

Recognizing the lack of women's health and hormone research, Dr. Marrs founded Lucine Health Sciences, a health research and media company that publishes the online journal *Hormones Matter* and conducts postmarket, direct-to-patient medication safety and efficacy studies. Currently, she has six ongoing safety and efficacy studies, with thousands of participants on the following drugs/procedures: Lupron, fluoroquinolones, oral contraceptives (two studies), the human papillomavirus (HPV) vaccines, and hysterectomy outcomes.

It is through her work on medication adverse events that Drs. Marrs and Lonsdale began to collaborate and uncover evidence of thiamine deficiency in patients suffering from medication or vaccine adverse reactions.

This book represents a culmination of what we both have learned. A major part concerns the clinical and biochemical research covered between 1962 and 1982 while Dr. Lonsdale was at Cleveland Clinic. This research was published originally in 1987. The finished books were stored in a warehouse that caught fire and only a handful of them were saved. Dr. Lonsdale took early retirement from the Cleveland Clinic as Associate Emeritus and entered a private practice specializing in nutritional therapy. This type of medicine is now known as alternative complementary medicine, and he was able to continue adding to his rapidly increasing awareness concerning the role of vitamins in treating common diseases. He discovered the extraordinary role of thiamine and magnesium deficiency in causing conditions where the standard laboratory studies were negative or deemed to be because of other causes. The changes in brain function were so diverse that Dr. Lonsdale came to be aware that this kind of deficiency was the great imitator of different conditions, each of which was considered to be a separate disease in its own right. This was particularly obvious in children and in 1962 a symposium was published to commemorate the synthesis of thiamine. From that symposium, Zbinden stated that 696 published papers had reported attempted thiamine therapy in 230 different diseases with varying degrees of success.[6]

Dr. Lonsdale found that high-calorie malnutrition was so common that he felt it necessary to republish the 1987 material, but also update it with new insights gleaned between 1982 and his retirement in 2013 and subsequently with his collaboration with Dr. Marrs. Over the last few years we have begun working together to untangle the nutrient deficiencies and mitochondrial damage associated with medication and vaccine adverse reactions, specifically those capable of triggering dysautonomia.

Dysautonomic symptoms have been reported following HPV vaccination.[7] We have also found that this vaccination that we have encountered in many cases unmasks latent thiamine deficiency or dependency disorders along with other nutrient issues. With subsequent research, Dr. Marrs has been able to map many of the mechanisms involved in these reactions. We will be detailing those mechanisms throughout the book.

## THIAMINE AND THE MITOCHONDRIA IN HEALTH AND DISEASE

This book is about thiamine and how its deficiency affects the functions of the brain stem and autonomic nervous system by way of metabolic changes at the level of the mitochondria. Thiamine deficiency derails mitochondrial oxidative metabolism and gives rise to the classic disease of beriberi that, in its early stages, can be considered the prototype for a set of disorders that we now recognize as dysautonomia. We will provide evidence that thiamine deficiency underlies some of the dysautonomic syndromes and make the provocative suggestion that disordered oxidative metabolism may represent a common part of the etiology in both the genetic and acquired forms of dysautonomia.

## BERIBERI AS A PROTOTYPE FOR DYSAUTONOMIA

It is well established that beriberi evolves from thiamine deficiency. A review of clinical and laboratory findings of the dysautonomias demonstrates tremendous similarities with beriberi. Like beriberi, dysautonomia is not one syndrome, but rather denotes a constellation of disorders that are characterized by autonomic dysfunction or sympathetic/parasympathetic imbalance. Inasmuch as the autonomic system regulates organism-wide homeostasis, dysautonomias are marked by a variety of seemingly disparate and often erratic symptoms. From heart rate irregularities to cerebellar ataxia, sleep–wakefulness disturbances to salt and mineral dysregulation, and everything in between, the system-wide autonomic disturbances make diagnosis of these conditions difficult for all but the most astute clinician. This is in large part caused by the underlying contributing etiology—mitochondrial dysfunction where disordered oxidative metabolism is key and thiamine and other nutrient cofactors are critical. Over the subsequent chapters we will review the research and provide clinical studies to support this.

Today there is increasing interest in the role of mitochondria in health and disease. Mitochondria sit at the nexus of health and disease and, in many ways, moderate the complex interactions between the organism and its environment. As will be discussed later in the book, we have obtained information on how trauma, infection, and poor nutrition can interact together in damaging mitochondrial function. They deplete critical cofactors, compromising mitochondrial function and evoking disease processes that extend beyond our current medical conceptualizations of anatomically discrete etiologies. Nutrients, especially thiamine, matter to mitochondrial functioning.

## THE ROLE OF HIGH-CALORIE MALNUTRITION AND ENVIRONMENTAL STRESSORS IN PRECIPITATING DISEASE

In 2015, Dr. Lonsdale hypothesized that thiamine and magnesium deficiencies were keys to disease.[1] In that publication he reported three girls and a boy, all of whom had developed postural orthostatic tachycardia syndrome (POTS) following vaccination with Gardasil. These cases, as well as many others involving vaccine or medication reactions, were also published on HormonesMatter.com,[8] Dr. Marrs' online journal. Each of them was shown to have an abnormal erythrocyte transketolase that proved thiamine deficiency or abnormal homeostasis. These young people were later found to express single nucleotide polymorphisms in thiamine transporter genes. All of them were top-class students and athletes before they became crippled by POTS. We concluded that the effects of marginally high-calorie malnutrition, particularly in the brightest and the best "energy-requiring" brains, coupled with genetic risk and the nonspecific stress of vaccination, precipitated POTS, one of the dysautonomic syndromes that is rapidly becoming more common.

The combination of malnutrition, genetic risk, and vaccination appeared to be necessary to precipitate POTS, masking as beriberi. We know from history[9] that a group of Japanese workers would develop the first symptoms of beriberi together when suddenly exposed to sunlight. This observation had misled the early investigators who were trying to elucidate the cause of this ancient scourge that had affected people for thousands of years. Because several individuals succumbed to the first symptoms of the disease concurrently, they concluded that the cause was a mysterious infection. Since we now know that the disease is caused by thiamine deficiency, we have to conclude that exposure to the ultraviolet light acted as a stress factor and precipitated the disease in marginally malnourished individuals.

That a stressor can initiate disease is an important precept. Actions always mediate reactions and in physiology those reactions are biochemical in nature. No matter the form that the stressor takes, it will require an adaptive response. So a stressor can be defined as any environmental factor that requires an adaptive response to the effects of living in a hostile environment. The biochemical mechanisms that they evoke would not only initiate symptoms of a latent biochemical or genetic risk, but also might be capable of inducing new disease processes. Case histories, appearing later in this book, bear this out. The evidence suggests that the answers lie with the mitochondria and more specifically in disordered oxidative metabolism, the process by which food is converted to cellular fuel.

Dietary vitamins and essential minerals are critical cofactors for the enzymatic reactions participating in mitochondrial respiration and energetics. Mitochondrial functioning therefore can be compromised significantly by nutrient deficiency. When the mitochondria are damaged or inefficient their decline in function leads to diminished cellular efficiency. This leads to pathologic changes in tissues where cellular energy demands are highest, the central nervous system and the heart being the most important.

## MITOCHONDRIA: WHERE GENETICS AND ENVIRONMENT MEET

When mitochondrial illness is contemplated as a diagnosis it is usually based almost solely upon mitochondrial genetics. We will show evidence that while there are undeniable genetic components to the expression of a dysautonomic syndrome, in all but the most severe cases of mitochondrial disease genetic aberrations are neither necessary nor sufficient to evoke it. Secondarily, environmental triggers may be required to initiate the disease process. Indeed, acquired or functional alterations from dietary, pharmaceutical, and other lifestyle variables may account for a larger percentage of dysautonomic illnesses than currently recognized. The notion that environment affects health and disease is not a new one. Hans Selye contemplated the role of stressors in the initiation of disease some 70 years ago, but it is difficult to accept within our current medical model. It suggests that lifestyle choices and medical practices have a heavy influence on the expression of disease. For the clinician, however, understanding the interactions between environment and health, particularly where mitochondrial functioning is concerned, opens many new avenues for treatment for a myriad of previously treatment refractory symptoms.

This book underscores the extraordinary importance of nutritional elements, not only in preventing disease but opening up a new world of potential treatment. Although all noncaloric nutrients work together in a complex team, thiamine and magnesium stand out for a number of reasons. They are essential cofactors in enzymes that preside over energy metabolism. For many years we have known that these two nutrients involve the oxidation of glucose, alpha ketoglutarate, and the branched-chain amino acids. They are cofactors for transketolase that occurs twice in the pentose pathway. Since this pathway is responsible for reducing equivalents, thiamine and magnesium also participate in antioxidation. Recent research, to be discussed later in the book, has recognized that thiamine pyrophosphate is necessary in the peroxisome for alpha-oxidation, has a part to play in the mystery of prion disease, and is involved in the treatment of diabetes. The widespread ingestion of sugar in all its different forms is precipitating dysautonomia that is not being recognized as early beriberi.

Vitamin deficiency diseases are ignored, perceived as being relegated to history because of the artificial vitamin enrichment used by the food industry. We have recognized the importance of the work on stress by Hans Selye and the work of his student Skelton, who was able to initiate the general adaptation syndrome by making the animal thiamine deficient. By reviewing this work in the book we are emphasizing the role of stress in the causation of human disease. For example, we have known for years that diabetes may make its first appearance after some form of stress, suggesting that it triggers an undeniable genetically determined metabolic disease involving glucose metabolism. By recognizing that autonomic dysregulation is really indicative of mitochondrial dysfunction, we will show from multiple case reports that thiamine deficiency plays a huge part in producing symptoms that are being diagnosed falsely as psychosomatic. It is very unfortunate that our present model for disease treats only the symptoms under the oversimplified impression that relieving the symptom will put the disease into remission. The book stresses the necessity of a search for cause and recognizes that metabolism in the brain is the dominating influence in our ability to adapt to the hostility of our environment.

## DO WE NEED A NEW MODEL FOR MEDICINE?

A model has to express a generally accepted concept about how disease differs from health. It is worth remembering that there was literally no idea what disease was in the Middle Ages. There was in fact no model. The relatively recent discovery of microorganisms became the foundation that can simply be stated as "kill the enemy." For many years scientists were trying to find ways of doing this without killing the patient and the discovery of penicillin became the watchword for its success. This has been the focus of medical research ever since. Not only have we sought to kill the bacteria, much research has been focused on killing the virus and even killing the cancer cell. As an analogy, medical science is much like a traveler seeking the right path. Imagine that it came to a fork in the road with a signpost that pointed in one direction with the instruction "kill the enemy." The signpost on the other fork was blank but should have given the instruction "support the defense." Like all analogies, this is insufficient because we should be traveling down both forks in the road.

This book focuses on the methodology by which we support the natural mechanisms that fall under the general heading of immunity. Assuming that the inherited machinery is intact, all it requires is energy to reach perfection. We know of course that the inherited machinery is not always intact and poses a risk factor, but the new science of epigenetics shows us that we can often manipulate genetic changes by lifestyle and nutrition. We recognize that a symptom is nothing more than a signal to the brain to inform it of some form of hazard. The brain recognizes the origin of the signal and directs our attention to its source when we are forced to interpret its meaning. It is a notification process and to treat the symptom alone can be compared with tearing up an important telegram without reading it first.

Thus this book focuses on the generation of cellular energy that has to be mustered to enable us to adapt to a hostile environment. The greater the stress, the more efficient the energy supply has to be, just like a locomotive climbing a gradient. It reinforces the pioneering work of Hans Selye who came to the conclusion that modern civilization caused what he called "the diseases of adaptation." Thiamine and magnesium stand astride the complex entry of glucose into the citric acid cycle and thiamine deficiency has long been known to be the cause of beriberi, a disease that is an excellent example of loss of energy efficiency in mitochondria. The subsequent decline of mitochondrial function reveals its effects by compromising the autonomic–endocrine axis, netting what is now called dysautonomia. By looking at the mitochondria as the central regulators of organismal adaptation, we present a foundation for the construction of a revised model for health and disease; one that was originally initiated in part by Hippocrates in 400 BC and placed the role of nutrition front and center. We have envisioned the etiology of disease by a combination of three factors: genetics, stress, and nutrition. Using an idea derived from Boolean algebra, they are represented as three interlocking circles. Each etiological component for a given disease can be assessed by the size of each circle and the degree of overlap with the other two circles. Several case reports in later chapters clearly denote the fact that all three components are necessary for the expression of the disease. Although it is true that one of the circles may be so dominant that it clearly points to the etiology on its own, it is probably true that the other two circles always contribute, even though they may be relatively minor influences. For example, there is ample evidence that environmental factors are involved in the etiology of type 1 diabetes,[10] although the nature and the timing of the interactions are poorly understood. Now that thiamine has been found to play a part in protecting diabetics from complications, we are beginning to see the impact of scientific nutrition.[11]

## REFERENCES

1. Lonsdale D. Thiamine and magnesium deficiencies: keys to disease. *Med Hypotheses* 2015;**84**(2):129–34.
2. Bettendorff L, Sluse F, Goessens G, Wins P, Grisar T. Thiamine deficiency-induced partial necrosis and mitochondrial uncoupling in neuroblastoma cells are rapidly reversed by addition of thiamine. *J Neurochem* 1995;**65**(5):2178–84.
3. Giacalone M, Martinelli R, Abramo A, Rubino A, Pavoni V, Iacconi P, Giunta F, Forfori F. Rapid reversal of severe lactic acidosis after thiamine administration in critically ill adults: a report of 3 cases. *Nutr Clin Pract* 2015;**30**(1):104–10.
4. Infante MT, Fancellu R, Murialdo A, Barletta L, Castellan L, Serrati C. Challenges in diagnosis and treatment of Wernicke encephalopathy report of 2 cases. *Nutr Clin Pract* 2016;**31**(2):186–90.
5. Brubacher G, Hornig D, Ritzel G. Food patterns in modern society and their consequences on nutrition. *Bibl Nutr Dieta* 1980;(30):90–9.
6. Zbinden G. Therapeutic use of vitamin B1 in diseases other than beriberi. *Ann NY Acad Sci* 1962;**98**(2):550–61.
7. Blitshteyn S. Postural tachycardia syndrome following human papillomavirus vaccination. *Eur J Neurol* 2014;**21**(1):135–9.
8. Lonsdale D. Post gardasil POTS and thiamine deficiency. *Hormones Matter* 2013. [Online] Available at: http://www.hormonesmatter.com/post-gardasil-pots-thiamine-deficiency/.
9. Inouye K, Katsura E. Etiology and pathology of beriberi. In: Shimazono N, Katsura E, editors. *Thiamine and beriberi*. Tokyo: Igaku Shoin Ltd; 1965. p. 1–28.
10. Stene LC, Gale EAM. The prenatal environment and type 1 diabetes. *Diabetologia* 2013;**56**(9):1888–97.
11. Rabbani N, Thornalley PJ. Emerging role of thiamine therapy for prevention and treatment of early-stage diabetic nephropathy. *Can J Diabetes* 2011;**13**(7):577–83.

CHAPTER 1

# The History of Thiamine and Beriberi

## Contents

| | |
|---|---|
| From Kakke to Beriberi | 1 |
|    Thiamine With Malnutrition: Navy Sailors Connect the Dots | 2 |
|    Polished Rice, Pigeons, and the Catatorulin Effect | 3 |
|    Clinical Features of Beriberi: Early Accounts | 3 |
|    Historical Observations of Beriberi Symptoms | 4 |
|       *Appearance* | 4 |
|       *Cardiovascular and Respiratory Disturbances* | 4 |
|       *Gastrointestinal Dysmotility* | 5 |
|       *Nervous System Disruption* | 5 |
| Beriberi in Children | 6 |
|    Infantile Beriberi | 6 |
|    Juvenile Beriberi | 7 |
| Wet and Dry Beriberi and Wernicke's Encephalopathy | 7 |
| Beriberi: The Great Imitator | 8 |
|    Thiamine Deficiency and Autonomic Chaos | 9 |
|    Toward a Broader Understanding of Stress and Autonomic Regulation | 12 |
| From Beriberi to Dysautonomia | 13 |
| Underlying Mechanisms of Autonomic Dysfunction: Thiamine, the Mitochondria, and Oxidative Metabolism | 15 |
|    Thiamine as a Rate-Limiting Factor in Oxidative Metabolism | 16 |
|    Thiamine and the Nervous System | 16 |
| Therapeutic Nutrition for Autonomic Balance | 17 |
|    Stress and Nutrient Demands | 19 |
|    Energy Production and Consumption | 20 |
|    Oxidative Metabolism | 21 |
|    Nutritional Versus Pharmaceutical Therapies | 22 |
| References | 23 |

## FROM KAKKE TO BERIBERI

Evidence of thiamine deficiency syndromes in Japanese society dates back to as early as 808[1] where it was called "Kakke" or "leg disease" because of the large "proportion of cases of partial paraplegia, cases of edema of the

*Thiamine Deficiency Disease, Dysautonomia, and High Calorie Malnutrition*
ISBN 978-0-12-810387-6
http://dx.doi.org/10.1016/B978-0-12-810387-6.00001-0

© 2017 Elsevier Inc.
All rights reserved.

legs, and cases of general dropsy."[2] In the 18th and 19th centuries the term beriberi was adopted and remains with us today.[2] Much of the research on thiamine emanated from Japan where beriberi was rampant.

Until the 17th century the majority of the population in Japan took unpolished rice as the staple food. Polished rice was associated with relative affluence, since it looked better on the table when served. Epidemics of beriberi have been known to occur in association with increased affluence simply because it was expensive to take the rice to the mill. When white rice was served to friends, it became a signature of their newly acquired affluence. As the ingestion of well-milled white rice became nationwide, the incidence of the disease increased. This is because the B group vitamins were in the discarded husks. The pigs, to whom the rice polishings were thrown, were being fed better than the humans, who were unaware of the reason for this as the cause of their beriberi symptoms.

The first national statistics for the disease appeared in 1899 and showed a death rate of 20 per 100,000, a surprisingly low mortality. This dropped to 0.5 in 1959 after its nutritional association was discovered. Of considerable interest to us today is that the peak incidence of beriberi occurs in August and September every year. Although the reason for this is obscure, it might have been associated with the stress of ultraviolet light. For example, factory workers would take their lunch between factory buildings. If the sun came round so that it shone into the corridor between the buildings, some workers would show the first symptoms of the disease. When the underlying cause became known, it had to be concluded that the sun's rays would stress them sufficiently to initiate the symptoms in individuals who were in a state of hitherto asymptomatic marginal malnutrition. Perhaps before sun exposure their symptoms, if any, were relatively trivial, or perhaps ascribed to other factors. It was therefore hardly surprising that the etiology in the early 1900s, before its nutritional association became common knowledge, was considered to be from infection.

## Thiamine With Malnutrition: Navy Sailors Connect the Dots

The discovery of the relationship between thiamine and malnutrition came in the last decades of the 19th century, but it was many years before scientific knowledge caught up. A Japanese naval surgeon by the name of Takaki studied in England from 1875 to 1880. He noted that beriberi was less common in the British Royal Navy than in navy personnel in Japan where the diet on ships was very different. In 1882 a Japanese naval vessel sailed on a 272-day voyage. On its return, 61% of the crew had succumbed to beriberi. Two years later, Takaki sent another ship that completed the same voyage, but was provided with an ample supply of dried milk and meat, giving a carbon-to-nitrogen ratio of 16:1. Only 14 crew members had developed beriberi. Takaki concluded that the lack of nitrogenous food was the cause of the disease, a notable contribution before vitamins were known. Protein and calorie deficiency is still relevant in beriberi in countries where this disease is still endemic.

## Polished Rice, Pigeons, and the Catatorulin Effect

In 1890, Eijkman found that polished rice given to pigeons caused polyneuritis, and the histopathology was similar to that seen in humans with beriberi. Funk and Cooper isolated an "antiberiberi factor" from rice polishings in 1910 and this was crystallized in 1926 and called Vitamine.[3] It was not until 1936 that thiamine was synthesized,[4] leading to an explosion of basic science and clinical experimentation. The work of Sir Rudolph Peters[5] exposed the vitally important association of thiamine with what was later to become the science of oxidative metabolism. He was the first to discover that respiration in a brain cell from thiamine-deficient pigeons was no different from the respiration in thiamine-sufficient cells until glucose was added to the preparation. The effect of failure of the thiamine-deficient cells to respond like the thiamine-sufficient cells was immediately obvious and he referred this as the catatorulin effect. He even noted that this effect was more prominent in cells from the lower part of the pigeon brain, a fact that later became important in a better understanding of thiamine deficiency in the human brain.

## Clinical Features of Beriberi: Early Accounts

After the discovery of thiamine and its application to the treatment of a scourge that had existed for thousands of years and still occurs, particularly where white rice is a staple food, it was natural that a vast amount of research was initiated. In 1962 a symposium was published to commemorate the synthesis of the vitamin. At that time there were 696 published papers where thiamine therapy had been attempted in more than 230 different diseases with varying degrees of success.[6] It should be noted that although a great many symptoms of beriberi have been described, none of them is considered to be pathognomonic.[1]

At that time, beriberi was classified into "wet" or edematous type and "dry" type, both being chronic in their course. Those categories have since been expanded to include neuritic beriberi (sensorimotor polyneuropathy) and gastrointestinal beriberi (gastrointestinal dysmotility), although the vestiges of the original framework remain. A peracute and extremely lethal form is known in Japan as "Shoshin" where "Sho" means acute damage and "shin" means heart. Shoshin denotes acute cardiac collapse and is believed to develop in approximately 5% of beriberi cases.[7] Shoshin has also been referred to as acute pernicious beriberi.[8]

Despite the original classification of beriberi based on cardiac symptoms, reading through clinical observations made in the 1960s we see a far more expansive pattern of symptoms emerging: symptoms that are difficult to account for unless one looks beyond the specific organ systems involved. What follows are the historical observations of beriberi symptoms as reported in an English translation of a book written in 1965 in Japan.[1]

## Historical Observations of Beriberi Symptoms
### Appearance
The general appearance of an individual affected by thiamine deficiency did not always suggest malnutrition, at least in the early stages. Thiamine deficiency was more common in robust manual laborers. Edema was one of the important signs and was always present in early stages of the disease, sometimes confined only to the pretibial area. Slight edema of the face was also common. When edema was present in the calf muscle, tenderness could be elicited by gripping it with the hand. In advanced cases, fluid could be found in the pleura, abdomen, and pericardium. The transudate from the pleura contained much less protein than serum. Low-grade fever was demonstrated in 45% of 159 cases of beriberi in its early stages.

### Cardiovascular and Respiratory Disturbances
Cardiovascular symptoms are common with beriberi. Both systolic and diastolic heart sounds are intensified at the apex, often with a low-grade murmur. The heart may be enlarged, particularly to the right, and might easily be mistaken for other causes of cardiomyopathy.
1. **Electrocardiogram.** Although the majority of cases of mild to moderate beriberi showed no electrocardiographic changes, those with cardiac symptoms could have high P, QRS, and T waves and prolongation of PQ intervals. Occasional ventricular extrasystoles were recorded.
2. **Pulse.** The pulse rate was usually rapid. However, in some cases it could be slow, but would rapidly increase with slight exertion. The sphygmogram showed a sharp rise and fall and frequently an elastic rebound, which followed immediately as typified by a dicrotic pulse.

3. **Blood pressure.** The diastolic pressure was usually below 60 mm Hg, often falling to zero, and was widely recognized as one of the most characteristic signs. The systolic pressure was mildly elevated in the early stages. Arterial tone over the femoral artery was often audible and in the lumbar area it often became audible to someone standing near the patient. The oxygen concentration in arterial blood was low and high in venous blood, indicating defective transfer of oxygen from hemoglobin to the cell.
4. **Vasomotor function.** Beriberi patients demonstrated labile excitability of the autonomic nervous system (ANS). This could be confirmed by testing the pharmacological responses to adrenaline, atropine, and pilocarpine. An injection of 0.1% adrenaline usually produced tachycardia, increased blood pressure, cardiac palpitations, substernal oppression, nausea, and vomiting. Sometimes, however, this resulted in bradycardia and lowering of blood pressure, perhaps demonstrating different stages of the disease. The Japanese investigators concluded that parasympathetic tone was increased in the early stages of the disease and was followed by increased sympathetic activity in the later stages.[1]
5. **Altered respiratory function.** Vital capacity was reduced. Oxygen and carbon dioxide measurements in the alveolar air and the arterial and venous blood showed decreases of carbon dioxide and oxygen in the alveolar air as well as in blood, indicating that there was extensive change in the gas exchange rate in the alveoli.

### *Gastrointestinal Dysmotility*

A "full" sensation in the epigastrium, heartburn, and constipation were common in beriberi. Marked loss of appetite, thirst, nausea, and vomiting were common in Shoshin. In the stomach, early hypoacidity was followed by hyperacidity during recovery before becoming normoacidic. This was thought to be related to the instability of ANS activity. X-ray studies of the bowel showed that peristaltic movement was diminished, markedly increasing the retention time of radioopaque material. This again reflected sympathetic/parasympathetic imbalance.

### *Nervous System Disruption*

As indicated previously in reference to vasomotor function, the ANS was functionally altered early in the course of the disease. Early beriberi must therefore be considered in the differential diagnosis of dysautonomia.

1. **Peripheral neuropathy.** Polyneuritis and paralysis of peripheral nerves were common as the disease progressed. The pattern of progression was discordant, making diagnosis difficult until the later stages. There were often no clear-cut boundaries that could be mapped out by an examining physician. For example, the index finger and thumb, innervated by the radial nerve, could be affected early and more severely than the other fingers, innervated by the ulnar nerve. Loss of deep tendon reflexes in the lower extremities sometimes appeared before demonstration of sensory damage. Nevertheless, loss of sensation was characteristic in its locality, starting in the fingertips and lower abdomen and around the mouth in the distribution of the trigeminal nerve. In the legs, loss of sensation began in the dorsal aspect of the foot. In the arms, beginning in the fingertips, it gradually ascended on the lateral side, then on the medial side, and later on the flexor side.
2. **Vertigo and ataxia.** Vertigo and ataxia were common and Romberg's sign could sometimes be elicited.
3. **Horizontal nystagmus.** It was occasionally reported.
4. **Reduced visual acuity.** Frequent amblyopia, central scotomas, optic neuritis, and narrowing of the visual field were all recorded, and the pallor occurred in the lateral half of the papilla.

### Case Example 1.1 An Unusual Case of Beriberi
A case is recorded of a 39-year-old housewife who complained of lassitude and visual disturbances following a period of "heavy sewing" 3 years previously. She was ataxic and complained of "dizziness" and "shaking." Both patellar and ankle reflexes were absent and there was mild loss of sensation in the lower extremities. Decreased visual acuity, papillary pallor, decreased auditory acuity, and horizontal nystagmus were demonstrated. Administration of 10 mg of thiamine a day relieved the symptoms within 1 month.[1]

## BERIBERI IN CHILDREN

Although the symptoms described above are mostly found in adults, both infantile and juvenile beriberi were also observed.

## Infantile Beriberi

Beriberi infants were, in general, pale, edematous, and ill-tempered. Loss of appetite, vomiting of milk, diarrhea, and green feces marked the gastrointestinal problems. A hoarse cry and blepharoptosis (ptosis) were common.

Neck tone was poor. On the other hand, breast-fed infants of mild beriberi-suffering mothers looked healthy but would suddenly die at or about 3 months of age. They were often regarded as the healthiest infants in the family. The full-blown symptoms of infantile beriberi were sometimes initiated by a simple infection.

## Juvenile Beriberi

Childhood beriberi was originally thought to be rare by these investigators, but they came to realize that in this age group the disease was different from that affecting adults and infants. The phenomenon most frequently observed was motor disturbances of the lower extremities, making walking difficult, and nasal voice, hoarseness, hearing difficulties, blepharoptosis, strabism, and nystagmus were frequently observed. Tendon reflexes could be hyperactive or hypoactive, depending on the state of the disease. Children with beriberi complained of pain or tenderness in the calf or thigh muscles. Occasionally, rigidity of the neck and Kernig's sign (severe stiffness of the hamstring) made the diagnosis difficult.

## WET AND DRY BERIBERI AND WERNICKE'S ENCEPHALOPATHY

The early investigators of beriberi made it very clear that the three cardinal signs of the disease included edema and neurologic and cardio circulatory symptoms, varying in intensity with one of them predominating. They classified it into wet (with edema), dry (without edema), paralytic, dry (atrophic), and the peracute form known as "Shoshin." They knew that there were differences in the clinical course, depending on age, sex, and environment, including nutrition, and that none of the symptoms were pathognomonic. The infantile and childhood forms were completely different from those in the adult and demanded separate descriptions. Unless there were complications, the general nutritional state of the individual was not reduced. The mental state was not affected in the early stages.

Although neurochemistry has advanced tremendously in the past few decades, research in thiamine deficiency has been almost completely confined to alcoholism.[9,10] A realization that a severe form of abnormal thiamine metabolism could produce intermittent, self-contained episodes of cerebellar ataxia,[11] later found to be thiamine dependency,[12] helped to give rise to the genetic aspects of thiamine deficiency in association with dietary deficiency.[13] Naturally occurring inhibitors of thiamine have been known for years[14] and two types of thiaminase have been described, enzymes that attack the methylene bridge of the thiamine molecule.[15]

A new frontier in clinical medicine where thiamine has an expanded role beyond its well-known cofactor function may be opening. For example, its nonenzymatic role in cholinergic neurotransmission has long been suggested. Using the metabolic antagonist oxythiamine, the data indicated synaptic transmission of acetylcholine, supporting its possible neuromodulatory role.[16] Thiamine deficiency frequently occurs in patients with advanced cancer and thiamine supplementation is used for nutritional support. It was therefore considered important to determine whether the benefits of thiamine supplementation outweighed the risks of tumor proliferation. In a study in mice with Ehrlich's ascites tumor, it was found that thiamine supplementation at a dose of 25 times the recommended dietary allowance (RDA) accelerated the tumor growth. At approximately 2500 times the RDA it resulted in 10% inhibition of tumor growth. The mechanism of this inhibitory effect of high-dose thiamine is unexplained.[17]

## BERIBERI: THE GREAT IMITATOR

From the historical nomenclature and the subsequent designation into wet and dry beriberi, we see a clear focus on cardiac function, and with "wet" beriberi, the associated edema. More recently, the taxonomy of beriberi nomenclature has been expanded to include gastrointestinal, neuropathic, respiratory, and dysautonomic symptoms, and although Wernicke's encephalopathy is still primarily associated with chronic alcoholism, there is an increasing awareness of it across nonalcoholic populations where the intake or absorption of thiamine becomes compromised. Table 1.1 illustrates the newer classifications of beriberi and the thiamine deficiency syndromes.

Upon review of the expanded taxonomy of beriberi-like disease, the astute clinician should begin to wonder how such seemingly disparate sets of symptoms would be related to one disease process and the deficiency of one nutrient. The symptoms of beriberi, even by early accounts, are quite diverse, affecting what are typically considered disconnected systems: cardiac function and gastrointestinal motility, for example. By what mechanisms could two such seemingly unrelated sets of symptoms be connected? In other words, how could thiamine deficiency, the recognized cause of beriberi, evoke a predominantly cardiac set of symptoms in one patient and a predominantly gastrointestinal set of symptoms in another? An even more salient

Table 1.1 Beriberi and the Thiamine Deficiency Syndromes and Symptoms

| Thiamine Deficiency Syndromes | Key Symptoms |
|---|---|
| Wernicke's encephalopathy | • Ataxia<br>• Changes in mental status<br>• Optic neuritis<br>• Ocular nerve abnormalities<br>• Diminished visual acuity |
| Wet beriberi | • High-output cardiac failure *with edema*<br>• High pulse pressure |
| Dry beriberi | • High-output cardiac failure *without edema*<br>• High pulse pressure |
| Neuritic beriberi | • Polyneuropathy (sensorimotor) |
| Gastrointestinal beriberi | • Enteritis<br>• Esophagitis<br>• Gastroparesis<br>• Nausea and vomiting<br>• Constipation<br>• Hyper- or hypostomach acidity |
| Dysautonomia | • Sympathetic/parasympathetic imbalance<br>• Postural orthostatic tachycardia syndrome<br>• Cerebral salt wasting syndrome<br>• Vasomotor dysfunction |
| Respiratory distress | • Reduced vital capacity<br>• Low arterial $O_2$, high venous $O_2$ |

question is how would thiamine deficiency evoke the full scope of symptoms listed, cardiac, neuropathic, neurological, and gastrointestinal, in the same patient? Are these each separate disease processes, deserving of a delineated nomenclature and separate treatment plans, or is there some root process involved that is hinted at by the very diversity of the symptoms? If thiamine deficiency is responsible for the conditions known as beriberi, by what mechanisms is this nutrient affects such a broad swath of physiology?

## Thiamine Deficiency and Autonomic Chaos

As evidenced by the historical and more recent expansion of symptomology and confronted with a patient with a host of bizarre and seemingly disparate symptoms and clinical signs, a modern physician might begin to suspect that autonomic function is altered. Beriberi and dysautonomia might then be included in the differential diagnosis, reflecting a sensitivity of the limbic system and brainstem to thiamine deficiency, in a manner similar to that produced by hypoxia. Indeed, thiamine deficiency is sometimes referred to as pseudohypoxia.[18] In contrast to the hypoxic state induced by an injury or obstruction that causes a deficiency in oxygen, the pseudohypoxic state is mediated molecularly by a lack of oxidation. Oxidation is the process by which mitochondria consumes molecular $O_2$ to convert glucose into ATP. Thus pseudohypoxia is a functional disturbance in which thiamine is intimately involved. The early researchers of beriberi recognized the role of thiamine in oxygenation, observing that arterial oxygen concentration was often low while it was higher than normal in venous blood.[22] However, Japanese researchers have learned that thiamine plays an important role in the ability of hemoglobin to pick up oxygen in the lung, deliver it to tissues, and cause its consumption in the process of oxidation.[19] Perhaps one of the more striking examples of thiamine's role in blood oxygenation comes from Dr. Lonsdale's case files,[20] described briefly in Case Example 1.2, more fully in Chapter 5, and on Dr. Marrs' website, Hormones Matter (www.hormonesmatter.com).

### Case Example 1.2 Thiamine and Blood Oxygenation in a Comatose Child

An 18-month-old female infant was admitted to hospital in a coma caused by a Reye's-like syndrome, which had begun 48 h previously with repeated vomiting. The initial treatment, given by neurologists, using exchange blood transfusion, failed. The coma deepened rapidly. Pupils became fixed and dilated and she was judged to be in a terminal state. The respirator that had been used on the assumption that it kept her alive was withdrawn.

One week after her admission there was no change in her condition. She was deeply comatose and all treatment other than normal life support was withdrawn. After receiving consent for the experimental use of thiamine tetrahydrofurfuryl disulfide (TTFD), 100 mg of TTFD by nasogastric tube was administered every 4 h and 150 mg by intravenous injection, a total of 750 mg in 24 h. This was repeated daily.

The lip vermilion quickly became bright red, whereas it had previously been dusky, the color of deoxygenated blood. Healthy flushing of the cheeks returned. At 2 days, spontaneous movement of the limbs returned, her pupils responded to light, and she developed a cough reflex. At 1 week the daily dose of intravenous TTFD was discontinued and the oral dose was decreased to 300 mg a day. After 9 days from the beginning of this treatment, TTFD was decreased to 150 mg a day.

On the 15th day, eye contact could be established and she responded to sounds but was still unconscious, a state known as coma vigilum. Subsequently, she began to take Jell-O from a spoon and began to show primitive crying responses. By the 21st day she was able to chew and could support her own weight with help. She began to walk with her hand held and self-feeding began. Speech returned and gradually improved. She was discharged from hospital 1 month after this treatment had been started. This case is described more fully in Chapter 5.

The example of pseudohypoxia described earlier demonstrates the importance of thiamine in oxidation processes. Although this case was emergent, disturbances in oxidation are sometimes of long term and chronic. A functional loss of oxidation will affect an organ or multiple organ systems simultaneously and those most demanding of ATP are compromised first. This should point the practitioner toward the possibility of a thiamine deficiency disorder.

Regardless of the origins of the hypoxic state, however, hypoxia is dangerous to the organism. Survival reflexes are activated and the sympathetic branch of the ANS is called upon to fight. Autonomic activation, particularly when it appears disordered, is another clue. Although they may not have understood thiamine's role in oxygenation, early researchers recognized the dysautonomic state as an indicator of beriberi and noted the signs that we have now come to recognize as defective oxidation. For example, Inouye and Katsura[1] observed changes in vasomotor function as a core symptom of beriberi. Wide pulse pressure was noted with high or normal systolic and low diastolic pressures, so indicative of the chaotic state of the ANS.

Platt,[22] one of the leading early thiamine researchers, noted that beriberi victims could be divided into certain categories by their chemistry, specifically, how well these patients maintained blood sugar concentrations. He reported that many beriberi victims had normoglycemia and were easily treated with thiamine. More severe cases had hyperglycemia and responded to thiamine with greater difficulty, while others had hypoglycemia and did not respond at all to the administered vitamin.[21] Platt reasoned that the differences in response reflected the severity and chronicity of the biochemical changes incurred. Researchers have also found that glucose regulation is very closely tied with thiamine concentrations in both type 1 and type 2 diabetics.[22] Suffice it to say that thiamine deficiency impacts on the most basic survival mechanisms: oxygenation and oxidation. Both oxygenation of the blood and its delivery to the tissues for the process of cellular oxidation are dependent on thiamine. Its deficiency, particularly by its effects on the functions of the limbic system and brainstem, places the ANS front and center. Both endogenous and exogenous signals from the brain to body organs become chaotic, leading to a vast array of symptoms.

The instability and imbalance of ANS signaling is the core issue in beriberi. The symptomology arising from defective function in many organs in the body is extremely complex. Nevertheless, when viewed from the perspective of disordered autonomic function, a picture emerges pointing us toward a more functional approach: one that considers treatment from the perspective of addressing etiological origins rather than simple symptom amelioration. Before we dig deeper into the mechanisms at play, we invite the reader to reintroduce himself/herself to the work of Hans Selye and his concept of stress.

## Toward a Broader Understanding of Stress and Autonomic Regulation

In his work on stress and physiological adaptation, Selye recognized that the hypothalamic, autonomic, endocrine axis guides our ability to adapt to all the physical and mental phenomena encountered on a daily basis. He recognized that a stressor, no matter its origins, evoked a set of physiological responses that allowed the organism to respond. Grief or a telegram giving bad news provides mental input that is just as stressful to the body as a physical injury, running a race, or receiving an inoculation. Any stress input, whether it be mental or physical, activates the sympathetic branch of the ANS. This action is accompanied by automatic withdrawal of the parasympathetic signal. After the adaptive response is completed, the sympathetic action is automatically withdrawn and the parasympathetic branch takes over. The sympathetic can be regarded as the action system and the parasympathetic as the "rest and be thankful" system.

When there is a mild degree of hypoxia or pseudohypoxia as in thiamine deficiency, this automatic control system becomes chaotic. The automatic mechanisms, infinitely complex and about which we know surprisingly little, become distorted. In beriberi, the ANS is abnormally activated with either sympathetic or parasympathetic dominance[1] at different stages of the disease as it progresses. For example, in the world of today the phenomenon that is diagnosed as a "panic attack" represents a fragmented fight-or-flight reflex and it matters little whether it is called beriberi or panic attack as long as we understand the mechanism. A slow pulse might be called bradycardia or parasympathetic dominance from early beriberi. A rapid pulse may be referred to as tachycardia or seen as a sympathetic signal to the heart. These are functional phenomena and will not be accompanied by abnormal traditional modern laboratory studies. These nervous mechanisms consume a vast amount of energy and are designed for short-term use. Having killed or escaped from the enemy with a fight-or-flight sympathetic reflex, a survivor can retire to a place of safety. As the cortex gets into the act, sympathetic activity may be prolonged, giving rise to an inordinate consumption of energy that results in the sensation of abnormal fatigue or other "functional" symptoms.

That is why the symptoms of beriberi are quite diverse and seem to have no rhyme or reason in their presentation unless they are regarded as abnormal brain body signals. Since body organs are under the control of the ANS, its dysregulation reflects itself in an expression of symptoms that are often mistakenly diagnosed as psychosomatic or "functional," as though the patient is imagining them. Thus beriberi is the great imitator of many conditions that commonly haunt the offices of physicians. It can be viewed as a prototype for dysautonomias: a set of disorders, both genetic and acquired, marked by defective autonomic regulation. The question remains, by what mechanism or mechanisms would something as simple as thiamine impart such a diversity of symptoms? Enter the mitochondria.

## FROM BERIBERI TO DYSAUTONOMIA

Many case reports of autonomic dysfunction have been reported in the literature over the last several decades. In isolation, these cases add little to our knowledge of etiology while obfuscating the prevalence of these conditions. When reviewed in totality, however, case reports reveal common threads and innumerable etiological clues. Dysautonomia indicates a disruption in autonomic function and represents a class of conditions with different genotypes and phenotypes. The dysautonomias are considered primarily genetic, emanating from mutations in both nuclear DNA[23] and mitochondrial DNA.[24]

However, there has been an emerging body of evidence showing that functional dysautonomic syndromes can be initiated by environmental stressors including dietary constraints and pharmaceuticals[25] by mitochondrial damage. As such, both primary and secondary dysautonomias can present at birth but may, in some cases, be triggered later in childhood and even into adulthood. It is the syndromes that develop later in life that seem to perplex practitioners the most, leading to many an unwarranted diagnosis of psychosomatic illness. This is understandable given the complexity of the autonomic system. The sheer variety of different syndromes that could arise from selective malfunction is daunting. Nevertheless, even a cursory understanding of the autonomic system and sympathetic and parasympathetic balance, when combined with a bit of deductive reasoning should quickly point the clinician toward dysautonomia. Consider the symptoms listed previously in Table 1.1 and those that follow within the framework of a disordered autonomic system. Recognize that these symptoms were identified by mid-20th century researchers long before key genetic and mitochondrial discoveries:

Symptoms of dysautonomia recognized by early investigators include:
1. Lack of tears
2. Temperature dysregulation, excessive sweating
3. Inappropriate emotional responsiveness and lability

4. Abnormal cardiovascular reflexes
5. Vomiting, gastroparesis, and/or bowel dysmotility
6. Anorexia and/or hyperphagia
7. Impaired temperature, olfactory, or taste sensations
8. Insulinopenia
9. Balance, motor control, and/or muscular weakness
10. Absent deep tendon reflexes
11. Breath holding

Once dysautonomia is considered as a diagnosis, the similarities with beriberi should point the clinician toward thiamine. Indeed, reports of thiamine deficiency, along with the constellation of symptoms indicative of autonomic dysfunction, have emerged across multiple, seemingly disparate, populations.

Conditions associated with thiamine deficiency include:
- Alcoholism[26]
- AIDS[27]
- Malignancy[28]
- Hyperemesis gravidarum[29]
- Prolonged total parenteral nutrition[30]
- Gastric bypass[31]
- Diabetes[32]
- Postvaccine reactions[33]
- Postmedication reactions[34]
- Psychiatric populations[35]
- Elderly[36] and the young[37]

Clinically, when high-dose thiamine therapy is administered, in many cases dysautonomic symptoms resolve.

### Case Example 1.3 Pharmaceutically Triggered Dysautonomia
The mother of an 18-year-old girl contacted us. Her daughter had received Gardasil vaccine 4 years previously and had succumbed to postural orthostatic tachycardia syndrome (POTS) immediately after the three injections. The mother had done some of her own research and came to the conclusion that her daughter had beriberi. An erythrocyte transketolase study proved thiamine deficiency, thus indicating that the POTS was early beriberi. She was later shown to have single-nucleotide polymorphisms in the SLC19 thiamine transporters, thus suggesting a combination of nutritional deficiency, genetic risk, and nonspecific stress from the vaccination.[56]

## UNDERLYING MECHANISMS OF AUTONOMIC DYSFUNCTION: THIAMINE, THE MITOCHONDRIA, AND OXIDATIVE METABOLISM

It is now well known that dietary thiamine is essential for health and critical for brain function. What the early researchers did not understand, and what many modern physicians yet fail to recognize, is how and why. We now know that thiamine performs critical enzymatic and nonenzymatic functions.[38] Thiamine is the rate-limiting cofactor in a set of mitochondrial enzymes that are central to oxidative metabolism. This is in addition to its roles in nerve myelination,[39,40] neurotransmission,[41–43] immune function,[38,44] central sodium ($Na^+$), and potassium ($K^+$) homeostasis,[41] and a veritable array of other important physiological roles.[45]

By way of its role in oxidative metabolism specifically, thiamine dictates mitochondrial energetics. That is, thiamine availability determines whether and how much ATP is produced. Mitochondria are the power plants of the cell. They provide 90% of the ATP, the cellular fuel required to maintain cellular function and viability via the interconnected processes of the Krebs/tricarboxylic acid (TCA) cycle and the electron transport chain.[46] The production of cellular fuel depends entirely upon the efficient transformation of dietary energy, derived from carbohydrates, fats, and proteins, into cellular energy, or ATP.[47]

The machinery of oxidative metabolism requires nutrients, at least 17,[48] also derived from dietary sources. Vitamins and minerals provide structural components for enzymes and mitochondrial cytochromes,[49] act as electron and proton carriers in ATP[50]– generating the electron transport chain, and scavenge for free radicals,[51] the by-product of ATP production and key initiator of mitochondrial damage.[52] Mitochondrial functioning therefore can be compromised significantly by nutrient deficiency.[53]

Thiamine, along with a cadre of other nutrients, serves as a catalyst and cofactor to all of the enzymatic reactions that participate in oxidative metabolism yielding ATP. Thiamine, however, along with magnesium, sits atop this process as a critical cofactor in the metabolism of carbohydrates, fatty acids, in the hexose monophosphate shunt pathway and the decarboxylating component of alpha-ketoglutarate dehydrogenase, and the branched chain amino acid dehydrogenase.

Organ systems requiring the most ATP are especially susceptible to slight permutations in mitochondrial efficiencies, e.g., the brain, heart, muscles, and gastrointestinal system, where symptoms of beriberi and dysautonomia emerge.

## Thiamine as a Rate-Limiting Factor in Oxidative Metabolism

Among the nutrients involved in oxidative metabolism, evidence shows that thiamine and magnesium are the most critical.[34] As the rate-limiting cofactor in pyruvic dehydrogenase, thiamine pyrophosphate (TPP) takes a central role in the mechanisms involving oxidation of glucose. Since there is no known storage for it in the body, it must be supplied continuously in the diet. TPP is a cofactor for HACL1,[54] oxidation of the branched chain amino acids, leucine, isoleucine, and valine, and occurs twice in the hexose monophosphate shunt. Because this pathway is responsible for producing reducing equivalents, TPP that is invariably dependent on the presence of magnesium can be regarded also as an antioxidant. Even mild deficiency would impact downstream mitochondrial energetics and functional dynamics.

## Thiamine and the Nervous System

Considerable experimental support exists for the involvement of thiamine compounds in the central nervous system.[55] Although thiamine triphosphate (TTP) appears to play a vital role, independent of the cofactor function of TPP, deficiency of TPP alone is sufficient to evoke significant dysfunction. Formation of TTP from TPP is catalyzed by TPP–ATP phosphoryltransferase in the presence of magnesium. Its exact place in cellular metabolism remains somewhat of a mystery, but evidence is in favor of its action being related to excitable membrane.[56]

The first indication that thiamine had an effect on nervous excitation was demonstrated by Minz[57] and was further explored by von Muralt.[58] Cooper and associates investigated the role of the vitamin in nervous tissue, and Cooper and Pincus reviewed the subject. About 80% of thiamine in nervous tissue is TPP. About 5%–15% is in the form of TTP, and the remainder is free thiamine and thiamine monophosphate.[39] Thiamine triphosphatase, diphosphatase, and monophosphatase catalyze the respective hydrolysis reactions from TTP to free thiamine. All require magnesium.[59]

The original observations of Minz[41] concerning the release of thiamine into the medium after electrical stimulation of a nerve have been confirmed by other investigators.[60,61] This release coincides with a shift of the thiamine phosphate esters to a more dephosphorylated form.[39] A similar release occurs after the use of a variety of neuroactive agents,[62,63] so it appears that any condition that results in a change in ion movements dephosphorylates the vitamin and permits its efflux. However, the clinical interpretation and effect of this phenomenon are not presently possible.

Of obvious importance, experimental evidence points to the presence of a saturable thiamine transport system, which may be located in the choroid plexus.[64] Entry of thiamine into the brain via this system would presumably be compromised if prolonged thiamine deficiency had resulted in deterioration of energy metabolism in this mechanism and might lead to a vicious cycle and increasing neurological effect.

However, since the early work demonstrated the cofactor importance of TPP, repeated efforts have failed to show any deterioration of pyruvate dehydrogenase, alpha-ketoglutarate dehydrogenase, or transketolase in nervous tissue of thiamine-deficient animals,[65–68] suggesting alternative mechanisms might be involved.

## THERAPEUTIC NUTRITION FOR AUTONOMIC BALANCE

It should be evident that the influence of thiamine on basic biochemistry is vast. The clinical implications of widespread mitochondrial dysfunction are staggering. If we add this direct damage to nerve conduction and neurotransmission, it is not difficult to imagine the devastation thiamine deficiency would cause. Early researchers knew this. Indeed, much of the research cited throughout the chapter was conducted decades ago. Somewhere along the line, however, we forgot the most basic tenets of organismal biology, that noncaloric nutrients matter as much as those that provide calories and that their absence wreaks havoc on the most essential components of cellular functioning. Consider Case Example 1.4,[69] where the removal of simple carbohydrates from diet improved symptoms, thiamine utilization, and all standard lab measures of health.

### Case Example 1.4 Diet-Driven Thiamine Deficiency in an Older Man

An 84-year-old man began to experience severe insomnia for the first time in his life. He also had painful tenosynovitis (also known as "trigger finger") in the index finger of the left hand. He had edited a journal for some 14 years and for several years had been a member of a bell choir in which he played a heavy base bell in each hand, involving repetitive trauma to the index fingers. He did not crave sugar, his ingestion of simple carbohydrates being minimal to moderate. The only treatment offered was complete withdrawal from all forms of simple carbohydrates, which he did. His weight decreased from 182 to 170 lb without any other change in diet. Insomnia and tenosynovitis gradually improved. Serial laboratory studies over a 6-month period revealed a gradual improvement when simple carbohydrates were avoided. His triglycerides dropped from 206 to 124. Fibrinogen and HsCRP, markers of inflammation, declined. Importantly, prior to the dietary changes, his labs showed thiamine deficiency indicated by elevated thiamine pyrophosphate effect (TTPE) percentages (35%). Elevated TTPE, which will be discussed in Chapter 4, is a marker of thiamine deficiency. With simple dietary changes alone, this gentleman's TPPE returned to normal at 0%, showing increased utilization of thiamine. After 6 months of improvement, however, the gentleman ingested a minimal amount of a simple carbohydrate and symptoms returned. Laboratory values began to increase again, as did symptom expression.

Diet affects biochemistry at the most fundamental levels. Hippocrates recommended dietary therapy almost exclusively, and his fame must have been derived from his success as a physician. It is therefore hardly new to discuss diet in relation to disease. Biochemistry has made spectacular advances in the 21st century and enabled a more scientific approach to nutrition. If such an approach really works, then it has the fundamental quality of safety, which was one of the principles of therapy most emphasized by Hippocrates. Consider the recent history of medicine. It is only a few hundred years since circulation of the blood was discovered. Bleeding the patient was as irrational in the light of present knowledge as was trephining the skull to let out evil spirits. Both of them must have worked, or appeared to work, or the practice would have been rapidly discontinued. Polycythemia and hypertension might have responded to the first procedure and raised intracranial pressure from any source to the second. Until the discovery of penicillin there was no specific therapy, and its value depends on the fact that it is destructive to bacterial life processes with a large margin of safety to the patient. But even penicillin is occasionally lethal, and many of the antibiotics that have since evolved possess numerous toxic qualities. Bacterial resistance is also becoming a serious problem.

The powerful drugs that are used today have one thing in common. They are essentially physiologic inhibitors or stimulants and much of the discussion about any one of them in a manual emphasizes the side effects, or unwanted actions, of which the physician must be aware and attempt to avoid by a proper dose. The principle must assume therefore that the disease is brought about by abnormally active function, which has to be suppressed, or underactive function requiring stimulation. A typical example of the use of this principle was the use of propranolol to block adrenergic receptors in hypertension, and it is not without interest that the same drug has been used in an attempt to treat psychoses,[70,71] although the two conditions are generally thought of as entirely different disease entities. The conclusion is that in both cases the symptoms arise from, or are connected with, an unbalanced and excessive activity of the adrenergic component of autonomic and endocrine function. It is well known that autonomic response is normally balanced in terms of the entire system and a proper mixture of adrenergic and cholinergic drive gives rise to the control of function. Presumably, the excessive and persistent adrenergic drive in the two disease states is based on one of two possibilities: excessive adrenergic and normal cholinergic component or normal adrenergic and ablated or subnormal cholinergic component.

The nutritional approach to therapy is an attempt to restore balance in the system and makes use of biochemical knowledge. It is readily apparent that if this hypothesis is true, the nature of the imbalance would be crucial. But if one component of the total system is subnormal, then a suppression of activity of the normal opposing component would lead to two subnormal members and might result in deterioration rather than improvement of the patient. The aim of nutritional therapy is directed at the weaker side of the imbalance.

## Stress and Nutrient Demands

This hypothesis also involves an understanding of the concept that was studied for many years by Selye[72] and followed up by others[73–75] but has since fallen by the wayside. Selye was struck by the similarity of appearance in all sick patients, irrespective of the cause. It dawned upon him that this appearance represented something to do with the individual being overwhelmed by the nature of the attack, whether it was from infection, trauma, or the environment. He called the attacking force "stress," just the same as an engineer refers to the press or weight that he or she applies to a metal bar to test its tensile strength. If there is a genetically built-in defect in an individual such as an enzyme deficiency, the "machine" is partially crippled and the attacking force—or stress factor—would be expected to worsen the situation in terms of the response of the total organism by exposing or exacerbating the symptoms related to the defective enzyme. A rather typical example of this is intermittent maple syrup urine disease (branched chain ketoaciduria). When the patient has an infection such as a simple cold, branched chain amino acids increase in concentration and keto acids derived from the abnormal metabolism are found in urine.[69] This might be referred to as the host response resistance. The enzyme defect is analogically equivalent to a molecular fault in the tested metal, which would quickly develop stress lines and thus be detectable by the engineer from X-ray studies or other technical means. Selye's concept goes further than that. His reasoning would suggest the idea that the steel bar might be built as well as the tensile strength of the metal would allow, but still be unable to resist the applied force. Using this analogy would suggest that a genetic defect might show up as "stress lines" in an organism, but might just as easily appear if the organism was intact and the attacking agent or force great enough to overwhelm the "normal tensile strength." Since all organisms, including humans, are under stress, as indeed is the metal in the analogy, it is not really surprising that the idea of stress as a cause of disease has not been readily accepted.

If the argument is accepted thus far, the next question to be asked is how the total organism meets stress and how its total commitment to survival is organized. Selye repeatedly emphasized that this was a normal response and was concerned by its breakdown as the cause of disease. He emphasized, too, that the mechanism could be improved with practice and might be the key to adaptation, hence the concept that he called "the diseases of adaptation." The physiology of stress response is the well-known fight-or-flight reflex, primarily adrenergic and capable of extraordinary "superhuman" power: the secret of success in rescue work, battle engagements, or other emergency events that raise the average human being to be above average. What happens if this reflex is chronically sustained in a poorly adapted individual? We can assume that the total commitment to survival calls up every ounce of usable energy and, even in the event that bioenergy regeneration proceeds during the crisis, there may come a time when the use of energy stores exceeds the ability to supply it. Could this perhaps be what we call "shock"?

## Energy Production and Consumption

The third aspect that must therefore be considered in the hypothesis is the process of energy production. What is known about bioenergy and how can it be fitted into the various disease patterns? Essentially, it is necessary to think in Einsteinian terms of the interchangeability of matter and energy. The cell, as a single live unit of the whole organism adapted to its highly specialized role within the species, has to take in fuel and burn it just the same as any internal combustion engine. It does it by unlocking the energy of glucose and building up an ionic gradient that synthesizes ATP by the process of oxidative phosphorylation. The ATP formed can then be used to perform work. If a state of alarm existed for long enough and without respite, it does not seem to be illogical to contemplate that it might result in a deficit of available ATP. The location of the deficit might be related to the organ or system that is called upon most heavily and is likely to originate sensory signals or symptoms that attempt to notify the brain of the crisis that is developing. This could be a protective mechanism that results in the whole organism seeking rest, or a local effect such as the sensations created in a limb after exercise. If this be true, then functional disease patterns could well be the forerunner of organ or system structural disease and would represent the clearest indication that more trouble might be ahead if the signals are ignored. We know that physical rest is not necessarily the answer, for the activated brain of insomnia could be seen as part of the energy using the fight-or-flight mechanism, and the deficit continues to build up in the brain itself. It is here where nutritional therapy might be most valuable by providing the raw materials that the cell cannot synthesize but that may be squandered in carrying out the multitude of reactions that represent the cellular response to stress as defined earlier.

## Oxidative Metabolism

Perhaps one of the factors that has been insufficiently studied is the relation between calories offered and the potential for completely oxidizing them. Like a choked internal combustion engine, hydrocarbons representing incomplete oxidation products could form and circulate in the blood before elimination in urine. Such calories are sometimes referred to as "empty" or "naked," the best example perhaps being alcohol, where its association with thiamine deficiency as a cause of Wernicke's encephalopathy has long been known.

In the chapters that follow, an attempt has been made to look at the mechanisms involved and to try to understand how knowledge of them might be used to our advantage. Nutrition is primarily a preventive approach and there is no doubt that medicine is swinging toward a realization that prevention is indeed better than cure. We may have to accept that cataracts, for example, are incurable except by surgical means, but are in many instances preventable, as Heffley and Williams showed in animal studies.[76] They showed that they could produce cataracts in the eyes of rats by giving them galactose. By adding noncaloric nutrients they were able to prevent the cataracts from forming but were unable to reverse them with nutrients once the cataracts had formed. The equivalent of this in humans is the inborn error known as galactosemia, a cause of cataracts in affected individuals.[77]

The old adage that surgery is an admission of medical failure may well be invoked if the physician is unable to perceive the warning signals that herald the biochemical changes leading to organic damage. If preventive measures are advised and are successful, it is virtually impossible to prove. How could a physician claim that the patient would have developed cataracts without such a measure being taken? It is only in the long run, by making cataract surgery a thing of the past or a relative rarity, that medicine would be able to claim that the measures represent a useful change in the ability of humans to maintain a healthier existence.

Studies of nutritional therapy have, for the most part, been on the basis of pure clinical observation, which is likely to be subjectively biased. Efforts are being made to obtain more objective biochemical measurements that, hopefully, will support the observations and bring credibility to a field that continues, quite rightly, to be under skeptical observation.

## Nutritional Versus Pharmaceutical Therapies

One of the most alarming factors that will have to be considered when nutritional therapy begins is the effect of what we have termed "paradox." The patient's symptoms, particularly if they have been long-standing, are apt to become considerably worse for an unpredictable period, varying from a few days to a few weeks. Although this does not happen too much with the administration of nutrients taken by mouth, it is an extremely common phenomenon when the nutrients are given intravenously. Biochemical changes may appear to reflect this. For example, we have found that creatine may increase drastically before diminishing. Oligoaminoaciduria may become hyperaminoaciduria before becoming normal. This is not new. Paradox was very visible in the treatment of beriberi patients and we have the modern counterpart of unpredictability from dextroamphetamine and barbiturates, particularly in children. This makes double-blind studies of nutrients very difficult since the period of authentic administration has to be long enough, and it appears to "overlap" the placebo period if the authentic compound has been used first in the random selection.

Another difficulty we have recognized is that nutritional therapy is not often successful from the use of a single agent. In some instances we have obtained remission only by the addition of other vitamins or nutrients, and hormone replacement may be required. Since hormones are produced by endocrine glands and their release is automated through the ANS, it is possible that energy deficiency is responsible for the lack of synthesis.

Our experience strongly suggests that nutrient deficiencies are the root of many modern disease processes, including those that involve autonomic system dysregulation. Thiamine in particular, because of its role in the pyruvate dehydrogenase enzymes that sit between glycolysis and the mitochondrial TCA cycle, functions as a critical gatekeeper to the oxidative metabolism of glucose. In the central nervous system where glucose is critical, thiamine deficiency becomes detrimental. The metabolic changes initiated by thiamine deficiency impact brainstem and ANS function giving rise to the classic disease of beriberi that, in its early stages, can be considered the prototype for a set of disorders that we now recognize as dysautonomia. Before we begin the work on dysautonomia in earnest, it is important to review the physiology and chemistry of normal autonomic functioning and the role that thiamine plays throughout. Chapter 2 reviews the autonomic system while Chapter 3 tackles mitochondrial functioning and thiamine chemistry. From then on, the book seeks to show that interpretation of autonomic function, by understanding the "balanced" relation between cholinergic and adrenergic activities, may be used to "decode" the true meaning of the signals (symptoms) experienced by the patient and observed by the physician (signs).

## REFERENCES

1. Inouye K, Katsura E. Etiology and pathology of beriberi. In: Shimazono N, Katsura E, editors. *Thiamine and beriberi*. Tokyo: Igaku Shoin Ltd; 1965. p. 1–28.
2. Arnold D. British India and the "beriberi problem", 1798–1942. *Med Hist* 2010;**54**(3):295–314.
3. Jansen BCP, Donath WF. The isolation of anti-beriberi vitamin. *Geneeskundig Tijdschrift Voor Nederlandsche-indie* 1926;**66**(4):573–4.
4. Williams R. Chemistry of thiamine (vitamin B1). *JAMA* 1938;**110**(10):727–31.
5. Peters R. The biochemical lesion in vitamin B1 deficiency: application of modern biochemical analysis in its diagnosis. *Lancet* 1936;**227**(5882):1161–5.
6. Sauberlich HE. Biochemical alterations in thiamine deficiency—their interpretation. *Am J Clin Nutr* 1967;**20**(6):528–42.
7. Wolf PL, Levin MB. Shōshin beriberi. *N Engl J Med* 1960;**262**(26):1302–6.
8. Engbers JG, Molhoek GP, Arntzenius AC. Shoshin beriberi: a rare diagnostic problem. *Br Heart J* 1984;**51**(5):581–2.
9. Butterworth RF. Cerebral dysfunction in chronic alcoholism: role of alcoholic liver disease. *Alcohol Alcohol Suppl* 1993;**2**:259–65.
10. Latt N, Dore G. Thiamine in the treatment of Wernicke encephalopathy in patients with alcohol use disorders. *Intern Med J* 2014;**44**(9):911–5.
11. Lonsdale D, Faulkner WR, Price JW, Smeby RR. Intermittent cerebellar ataxia associated with hyperpyruvic acidemia, hyperalaninemia, and hyperalaninuria. *Pediatrics* 1969;**43**(6):1025–34.
12. Blass JP, Lonsdale D, Uhlendorf BW, Hom E. Intermittent ataxia with pyruvate-decarboxylase deficiency. *Lancet* 1971;**297**(7712):1302.
13. Brown G. Defects of thiamine transport and metabolism. *J Inherit Metab Dis* 2014;**37**(4):577–85.
14. Vimokesant SL, Hilker DM, Nakornchai S, Rungruangsak K, Dhanamitta S. Effects of betel nut and fermented fish on the thiamin status of northeastern Thais. *Am J Clin Nutr* 1975;**28**(12):1458–63.

15. Evans WC. Thiaminases and their effects on animals. *Vitam Horm* 1975;**33**:467.
16. Hirsch JA, Parrott J. New considerations on the neuromodulatory role of thiamine. *Pharmacology* 2012;**89**(1–2):111–6.
17. Comín-Anduix B, Boren J, Martinez S, Moro C, Centelles JJ, Trebukhina R, Petushok N, Lee WNP, Boros LG, Cascante M. The effect of thiamine supplementation on tumour proliferation. *Eur J Biochem* 2001;**268**(15):4177–82.
18. Sweet RL, Zastre JA. HIF1-α-mediated gene expression induced by vitamin B. *Int J Vitam Nutr Res* 2013;**83**(3):188–97.
19. Ishimaru T, Yata T, Hatanaka-Ikeno S. Hemodynamic response of the frontal cortex elicited by intravenous thiamine propyldisulphide administration. *Chem Senses* 2004;**29**(3):247–51.
20. Lonsdale D. Recovery from Reye's syndrome: a case report. *Hormon Matter* 2016. [Online]. Available at: https://www.hormonesmatter.com/recovery-reyes-syndrome-case-report/.
21. Platt BS. Thiamine deficiency in human beriberi and in Wernicke's encephalopathy. In: Wolstenholme GEW, O'Connor M, editors. *Thiamine deficiency*. Boston: Little Brown and Company; 1967. p. 135–43.
22. Thornalley PJ, Babaei-Jadidi R, Al Ali H, Rabbani N, Antonysunil A, Larkin J, Ahmed A, Rayman G, Bodmer CW. High prevalence of low plasma thiamine concentration in diabetes linked to a marker of vascular disease. *Diabetologia* 2007;**50**(10):2164–70.
23. Shin JW, Jung KH, Lee ST, Moon J, Seong MW, Park SS, Lee SK, Chu K. Novel mutation in the ATL1 with autosomal dominant hereditary spastic paraplegia presented as dysautonomia. *Auton Neurosci* 2014;**185**:141–3.
24. Schwartz F, Baldwin CD, Baima J, Gavras H. Mitochondrial DNA mutations in patients with orthostatic hypotension. *Am J Med Genet* 1999;**86**(2):145–50.
25. Cohen BH. Neuromuscular and systemic presentations in adults: diagnoses beyond MERRF and MELAS. *Neurotherapeutics* 2013;**10**(2):227–42.
26. Vedder LC, Hall JM, Jabrouin KR, Savage LM. Interactions between chronic ethanol consumption and thiamine deficiency on neural plasticity, spatial memory, and cognitive flexibility. *Alcohol Clin Exp Res* 2015;**39**(11):2143–53.
27. Larsen TR, Dragu D, Williams M. Wernicke's encephalopathy: an unusual consequence of the acquired immune deficiency syndrome—case report and literature review. *Case Rep Med* 2013;**2013**.
28. Lu'o'ng KVQ, Nguyễn LTH. The role of thiamine in cancer: possible genetic and cellular signaling mechanisms. *Cancer Genomics Proteomics* 2013;**10**(4):169–85.
29. Di Gangi S, Gizzo S, Patrelli TS, Saccardi C, D'Antona D, Nardelli GB. Wernicke's encephalopathy complicating hyperemesis gravidarum: from the background to the present. *J Matern Fetal Neonatal Med* 2012;**25**(8):1499–504.
30. Ramsi M, Mowbray C, Hartman G, Pageler N. Severe lactic acidosis and multiorgan failure due to thiamine deficiency during total parenteral nutrition. *BMJ Case Rep* 2014;**2014**. pii:bcr2014205264.
31. Walker J, Kepner A. Wernicke's encephalopathy presenting as acute psychosis after gastric bypass. *J Emerg Med* 2012;**43**(5):811–4.
32. vinh quoc Luong K, Nguyen LTH. The impact of thiamine treatment in the diabetes mellitus. *J Clin Med Res* 2012;**4**(3):153–60.
33. Blitshteyn S. Postural tachycardia syndrome following human papillomavirus vaccination. *Eur J Neurol* 2014;**21**(1):135–9.
34. Lonsdale D. Thiamine and magnesium deficiencies: keys to disease. *Med Hypotheses* 2015;**84**(2):129–34.
35. Schwartz RA, Gross M, Lonsdale D, Sham Berger RJ. Transketolase activity in psychiatric patients. *J Clin Psychiatry* 1979;**40**(10):427–9.
36. Gibson GE, Hirsch JA, Fonzetti P, Jordan BD, Cirio RT, Elder J. Vitamin B1 (thiamine) and dementia. *Ann NY Acad Sci* 2016;**1367**(1):21–30.

37. Lallas M, Desai J. Wernicke encephalopathy in children and adolescents. *World J Pediatr* 2014;**10**(4):293–8.
38. Hiffler L, Rakotoambinina B, Lafferty N, Martinez Garcia D. Thiamine deficiency in tropical paediatrics: new insights into a neglected but vital metabolic challenge. *Front Nutr* 2016;**3**:16.
39. Collins GH, Webster HDF, Victor M. The ultrastructure of myelin and axonal alterations in sciatic nerves of thiamine deficient and chronically starved rats. *Acta Neuropathol* 1964;**3**(5):511–21.
40. He X, Sullivan EV, Stankovic RK, Harper CG, Pfefferbaum A. Interaction of thiamine deficiency and voluntary alcohol consumption disrupts rat corpus callosum ultrastructure. *Neuropsychopharmacology* 2007;**32**(10):2207–16.
41. Frank LL. Thiamine in clinical practice. *J Parenter Enteral Nutr* 2015;**39**(5):503–20.
42. Eder L, Hirt L, Dunant Y. Possible involvement of thiamine in acetylcholine release. *Nature* 1976;**264**:186–8.
43. Yamashita H, Zhang YX, Nakamura S. The effects of thiamin and its phosphate esters on dopamine release in the rat striatum. *Neurosci Lett* 1993;**158**(2):229–31.
44. Wertman K, Groh M. The effects of thiamine deficiency on some physiologic factors, phagocytosis and susceptibility to infection. *J Immunol* 1959;**82**(3):241–7.
45. Geng MY, Saito H, Katsuki H. The effects of thiamine and oxythiamine on the survival of cultured brain neurons. *Jpn J Pharmacol* 1995;**68**(3):349–52.
46. Neustadt J, Pieczenik SR. Medication-induced mitochondrial damage and disease. *Mol Nutr Food Res* 2008;**52**(7):780–8.
47. El Bacha T, Luz M, Da Poian A. Dynamic adaptation of nutrient utilization in humans. *Nat Educ* 2010;**3**(9):8.
48. Marrs C. Micronutrient deficiencies and mitochondrial dysfunction. In: Greenblatt JM, Brogan K, editors. *Integrative therapies for depression: redefining models for assessment, treatment and prevention*. CRC Press; 2015. p. 73–95.
49. Huskisson E, Maggini S, Ruf M. The role of vitamins and minerals in energy metabolism and well-being. *J Int Med Res* 2007;**35**(3):277–89.
50. Berg JM, Tymoczko JL, Stryer L. Metabolic pathways contain many recurring motifs. In: Freeman WH, editor. *Biochemistry*. 5th ed. 2002. New York. Available from: http://www.ncbi.nlm.nih.gov/books/NBK22398/.
51. Pieczenik SR, Neustadt J. Mitochondrial dysfunction and molecular pathways of disease. *Exp Mol Pathol* 2007;**83**(1):84–92.
52. Federico A, Cardaioli E, da Pozzo P, Formichi P, Gallus GN, Radi E. Mitochondria, oxidative stress and neurodegeneration. *J Neurol Sci* 2012;**322**(1–2):254–62.
53. Depeint F, Bruce WR, Shangari N, Mehta R, O'Brien PJ. Mitochondrial function and toxicity: role of the B vitamin family on mitochondrial energy metabolism. *Chem Biol Interact* 2006;**163**(1):94–112.
54. Casteels M, Sniekers M, Fraccascia P, Mannaerts GP, Van Veldhoven PP. The role of 2-hydroxyacyl-CoA lyase, a thiamin pyrophosphate-dependent enzyme, in the peroxisomal metabolism of 3-methyl-branched fatty acids and 2-hydroxy straight-chain fatty acids. *Biochem Soc Trans* 2007;**35**(5):876–80.
55. Cooper JR, Pincus JH. The role of thiamine in nervous tissue. *Neurochem Res* 1979;**4**(2):223–39.
56. Barchi RL. Thiamine triphosphates in the brain. In: Gubler CJ, Fujiwara M, Dreyfus PM, editors. *Thiamine*. New York: John Wiley & Sons; 1976. p. 195–212.
57. Minz B. Sur la liberation de la vitamine B1 par le trone isole de nerf pneumogastrique soumis a l'exitation electrique. *CR Soc Biol* 1938;**127**:1251–3.
58. Von Muralt A. The role of thiamine (vitamin B1) in nervous excitation. *Exp Cell Res* 1958;**14**(Suppl. 5):72.
59. Bettendorff L. Thiamine in excitable tissues: reflections on a non-cofactor role. *Metab Brain Dis* 1994;**9**(3):183–209.

60. Gunner HP. Aneurin und nervenerregung versuche mit 35S - markiertem aneurin und areurinantimetabolisen. *Helv Physiol Pharmacol Acta* 1957;(Suppl. 11).
61. Cooper JR, Roth RH, Kini MM. Biochemical and physiological function of thiamine in nervous tissue. *Nature* 1963;**199**:609–10.
62. Itokawa Y, Cooper JR. Ion movements and thiamine in nervous tissue—I Intact nerve preparations. *Biochem Pharmacol* 1970;**19**:985–92.
63. Itokawa Y, Cooper JR. Thiamine release from nerve membranes by tetrodotoxin. *Science* 1969;**166**(3906):759–60.
64. Spector R. Thiamine transport in the central nervous system. *Am J Phys* 1976;**230**(4):1101–7.
65. Gubler CJ. Studies on the physiological functions of thiamine. 1. The effects of thiamine deficiency and thiamine antagonists on the oxidation of α-keto acids by rat tissues. *J Biol Chem* 1961;**236**:3112–20.
66. Koeppe RE, O'Neal RM, Hahn CH. Pyruvate decarboxylation in thiamine deficient brain. *J Neurochem* 1964;**11**(9):695–9.
67. Dreyfus PM, Hauser G. The effect of thiamine deficiency on the pyruvate decarboxylase system of the central nervous system. *Biochim Biophys Acta Gen Subj* 1965;**104**(1):78–84.
68. Brin M. Effects of thiamine deficiency and of oxythiamine on rat tissue transketolase. *J Nutr* 1962;**78**:179–83.
69. Lonsdale D. How dietary mayhem causes disease: the choked engine syndrome. *Hormon Matter* 2014. [Online]. Available at: https://www.hormonesmatter.com/dietary-mayhem-disease-thiamine-choked-engine-syndrome/.
70. Atsmon A. The short-term effects of adrenergic-blocking agents in a small group of psychotic patients. *Psychiatr Neurol Neurochir* 1971;**74**:251–8.
71. Steiner M, Latz A, Blum I, Atsmon A, Wijsenbeek H. Propranolol versus chlorpromazine in the treatment of psychoses associated with childbearing. *Psychiatr Neurol Neurochir* 1973;**76**:421–6.
72. Selye H. The general adaptation syndrome and the diseases of adaptation 1. *J Clin Endocrinol Metab* 1946;**6**(2):117–230.
73. Cassens G, Roffman M, Kuruc A, Orsulak PJ, Schildkraut JJ. Alterations in brain norepinephrine metabolism induced by environmental stimuli previously paired with inescapable shock. *Science* 1980;**209**(4461):1138–40.
74. Lonsdale D. Stress. *Pediatr Digest* 1977;**19**:11–7.
75. Cryer PE. Physiology and pathophysiology of the human sympathoadrenal neuroendocrine system. *New Engl J Med* 1980;**303**(8):436–44.
76. Heffley JD, Williams RJ. The nutritional teamwork approach: prevention and regression of cataracts in rats. *Proc Natl Acad Sci USA* 1974;**71**(10):4164–8.
77. Varela-Lema L, Paz-Valinas L, Atienza-Merino G, Zubizarreta-Alberdi R, Villares RV, López-García M. Appropriateness of newborn screening for classic galactosaemia: a systematic review. *J Inherit Metab Dis* 2016:1–17.

# CHAPTER 2
# The Autonomic Nervous System and Its Functions

## Contents

| | |
|---|---|
| The Autonomic Nervous System: General Arrangement and Function | 28 |
|    Sympathetic and Parasympathetic Divisions | 29 |
|    Enteric Nervous System | 29 |
| Autonomic Signaling: Layered Control | 29 |
|    Adrenomedullary Tract of the Autonomic Nervous System | 31 |
|       *Nerve Tracts and Reflex Loops: Somatic Versus Autonomic* | *31* |
|       *Somatic Spinal Reflex* | *31* |
|       *Autonomic Reflex* | *31* |
|    Adrenocortical Tract of Autonomic Response | 32 |
|       *Hypothalamus* | *32* |
|       *Brainstem* | *33* |
|       *Other Brain Regions Involved in Autonomic Function* | *34* |
|       *Points of Consideration* | *35* |
| Autonomic Chemistry and Neurotransmission | 35 |
|    Acetylcholine and Its Receptors | 36 |
|    Adrenergic Receptors and Response | 37 |
|    Stress Response of Hormones and Receptors | 38 |
|       *Receptor Crosstalk* | *38* |
|    Autonomic Nervous System Modulators: Immune Cells and Other Influencers | 40 |
|       *Points of Consideration* | *40* |
| The Myths of Linearity and Symmetry | 41 |
|    Nonlinear Dose–Response Actions | 41 |
|    Asymmetrical Autonomic Innervation Patterns | 42 |
|       *Points of Consideration* | *43* |
| Autonomic Dysfunction: Clinical Patterns and Clues to Sympathetic Dominance | 44 |
|    Acute Blepharospasm, Sweating, and Piloerection as Clues to Sympathetic System Dominance | 44 |
|       *Points of Consideration* | *45* |
|    Heart Rate, Rhythm, and Pressure Dysregulation | 46 |
|    Postural Orthostatic Tachycardia | 47 |
|       *Points of Consideration* | *47* |
|    Neuropathy, Muscle Weakness, Skin Disorders, and Balance | 48 |
|    Gastrointestinal Dysmotility Syndromes | 49 |
|    Bladder and Bowel Dysfunction as Signs of Autonomic Disturbance | 49 |

| | |
|---|---|
| Sexual and Reproductive Abnormalities Associated With Autonomic Disturbance | 50 |
| Cognitive and Mental Health Symptoms as Signs of Autonomic Disturbance | 50 |
| Autonomic Imbalance | 52 |
| References | 53 |

The anatomy and physiology of the autonomic nervous system (ANS) are taught in virtually all health-related classes from grade school through medical school. Similarly, the basic tenets of stress and adaptation articulated by Selye as the general adaptation syndrome are common knowledge to the layman and professional alike. Indeed, these concepts are so commonplace that one might wonder why we have included a review of autonomic function in a medical textbook where advanced topics are covered. Perhaps most obviously it is important to review normal autonomic function before one can consider a dysautonomic response. Less obvious, however, we find that missing from most examinations of the anatomy and physiology of ANS are the biochemically mediated functional changes and their ensuing clinical presentations. In the absence of injury or evidence of genetic disposition, and in advance of observable white matter lesions that accrue from long standing thiamine deficiency,[1] it is difficult for the physician to diagnose a dysautonomic syndrome without an appreciation of the functional adaptations of the ANS to "stressors." These stressors, whether mediated by outside sources, such as exposures to chemical or dietary toxicants, illness, and life in general, or by aberrant internal adaptations, produce characteristic patterns of autonomic disorder based upon where the triggering event attacks. Understanding these patterns will help the clinician immensely. No attempt will be made to deal with ANS in full since that information is readily available in any textbook on physiology. We do, however, want to provide an overview and emphasize concepts that will aid in the recognition of disordered autonomic function, particularly as it relates to thiamine deficiency.

## THE AUTONOMIC NERVOUS SYSTEM: GENERAL ARRANGEMENT AND FUNCTION

The central nervous system includes the brain and spinal cord and the peripheral nervous system, within which is the somatic branch responsible for voluntary movements. The ANS activates the involuntary responses of vital organs and organismal homeostasis. It is therefore responsible for maintaining life. The ANS operates largely at the border between central and peripheral nervous system functions. The lower brain organizes adaptation to internal and external stimuli while it relies on the cortical brain to interpret and guide further accommodations. It is important to emphasize that if either aspect of communication is impaired, autonomic regulation will be impacted. The autonomic system can be divided into three branches: sympathetic, parasympathetic, and enteric.

## Sympathetic and Parasympathetic Divisions

Also known as the vegetative, visceral, or involuntary nervous system, the ANS controls the activities of heart rate, respiration, digestion, blood flow, glands, and all smooth muscles. Structurally and functionally, it is divided into two tracts that control activation and deactivation of automatic and reflexive functions in a complementary fashion. The sympathetic tract, which is largely responsible for action coordination, innervates viscera through the splanchnic nerves, exiting the spinal cord from the thoracic and lumbar areas. The parasympathetic tract, responsible for tamping down the excitatory influence of the sympathetic branch, innervates through the cranial, sacral, and vagus nerves. Central control of these functions originates from the hypothalamus and the brainstem, the nuclei of which integrate information sent from the central and peripheral nervous systems. This adjusts autonomic function accordingly. Fig. 2.1 illustrates the sympathetic and parasympathetic branches of the ANS.

## Enteric Nervous System

In contrast to the sympathetic and parasympathetic branches of the ANS, the enteric nervous system (gut brain) is located entirely in the periphery and provides intrinsic control of gastrointestinal function. The enteric system operates independently of the central nervous system via complex reflex loops to control peristalsis.[3]

## AUTONOMIC SIGNALING: LAYERED CONTROL

The communication tracts within the ANS include the sensory or afferent messaging that takes signals from the environment and the body to the brain, and the efferent messaging that communicates signals from the brain through the spinal cord to the effector organs and the body. As a master integrator of internal and external signals, the ANS manages multiple, interconnected levels of information processing. In the face of

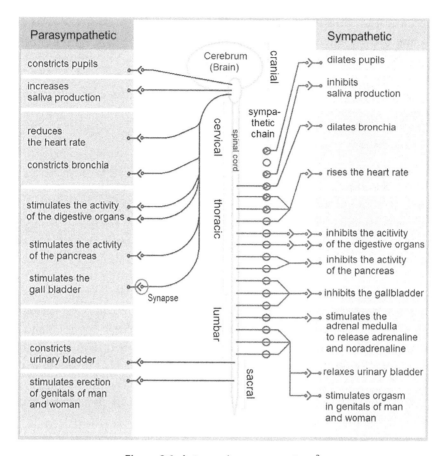

**Figure 2.1** Autonomic nervous system.[2]

a stressor or changes to homeostatic balance, the sympathetic system is activated along parallel descending tracts: one projecting from the hypothalamus through the brainstem and sympathetic ganglia to the medulla region of the adrenal glands (cerebral cortex > hypothalamus > posterior pituitary > brainstem > ganglia > adrenal medulla) and the other from the hypothalamus and the pituitary to the cortical region of the adrenal glands (cerebral cortex > hypothalamus > anterior pituitary > adrenal cortex). The adrenomedullary or sympathetic path is rapid and mediated by the release of acetylcholine (ACh) and the catecholamines epinephrine and norepinephrine, while the adrenocortical tract, or the hypothalamic–pituitary–adrenal (HPA) axis, is slower and mediated by the release of the glucocorticoid (GR) hormones, cortisol being primary among them.

## Adrenomedullary Tract of the Autonomic Nervous System

The adrenomedullary path of the ANS utilizes a two-neuron system, preganglionic and postganglionic, to signal change. The preganglionic neuron has its cell body located in the central nervous system and directs signals down an extended axon to organs in the periphery where it synapses on the postganglionic neuron in the peripheral ganglia. Cell bodies of the postganglionic neurons are located in the periphery. Axons directed toward the adrenal medulla itself receive direct innervation from the preganglionic neurons.[4]

The whole system falls into three outflow tracts anatomically. The sympathetic system has one contiguous outflow tract, flowing from the entire thoracic region of the cord and its first two lumbar segments, while the parasympathetic system is segregated into two outflow tracts: the craniosacral outflow in connection with the nuclei of cranial nerves III, VII, IX, and X and the second, third, and fourth sacral segments of the spinal cord.[4]

A single sympathetic preganglionic fiber may synapse with 20 or more postganglionic neurons inducing more widespread effects. In contrast, the parasympathetic system contains far fewer preganglionic fibers relative to the postganglionic fibers (1:3), indicating a more graded response and localized effect. Additionally, the postganglionic fibers of the sympathetic system are long, whereas those of the parasympathetic system are short.[3] These anatomical differences influence the speed of autonomic activation and deactivation.

### Nerve Tracts and Reflex Loops: Somatic Versus Autonomic

Functions of ANS ganglia are coordinated with those of the somatic nervous system, controlling motor movements. The integration of the somatic and autonomic systems is brought about by reflex pathways at various levels. The two systems may be compared to simplify concepts.

### Somatic Spinal Reflex

In a somatic spinal reflex, three neurons are involved. The afferent has its cell body in the dorsal root ganglion and transmits impulses to the ventral horn through the connector neuron whose cell lies in the dorsal horn of gray matter. Efferent impulses are then relayed to the ventral horn cell and its axon, which leaves via the ventral root. This gives rise to the automatic control of reflex function.

### Autonomic Reflex

Similarly, there are three neurons in the autonomic system. There is an afferent, proceeding from an internal organ, and the nucleus of the cell lies in the dorsal root ganglion or its cranial equivalent. A central process is sent into the gray matter adjacent to the dorsal horn and its axon passes out ventrally to the excitor cell, which is situated peripherally outside the central nervous system. Excitor cells form masses or ganglia, and from them the postganglionic fibers pass to the innervated tissue either to excite or to inhibit the action.

## Adrenocortical Tract of Autonomic Response

In parallel to the adrenomedullary tract of the ANS is the adrenocortical tract, more commonly recognized as the HPA axis responsible for the stress response. Upon initiation of the sympathetic nervous system, corticotropin releasing hormone (CRH) is released from the hypophysiotropic neurons within the paraventricular nucleus of the hypothalamus. CRH binds to receptors in the anterior pituitary and affects the release of adrenocorticotropin releasing hormone (ACTH) into the bloodstream. ACTH binds to receptors in the adrenal cortex, releasing the stress hormone cortisol, which then binds to GR and mineralocorticoid (MR) receptors throughout the body and brain.

### *Hypothalamus*

The hypothalamus sits at the center of the autonomic system and is responsible for integrating signals from both the central nervous system and the viscera to regulate the bodily functions that ensure survival. Together with the brainstem and the pituitary and adrenal glands, the hypothalamus maintains dynamic homeostatic balance between the sympathetic and parasympathetic pathways. From a functional point of view, the hypothalamus can be divided into an anterior portion, which when stimulated electrically gives rise mostly to parasympathetic responses, and a posterior portion, which initiates mostly to sympathetic responses.[5] Anatomically, the hypothalamus is divided more laterally with the major ascending and descending autonomic projections through the hypothalamus coalescing in the paraventricular nucleus.[4]

The physiology of the hypothalamus is easy to understand when it is recognized as a neuroendocrine organ, representing the bridge between the reception of afferent nervous impulses and the "executive command," which is mediated through a combination of efferent autonomic and somatic impulses and the endocrine system. The bodily changes produced by emotional stimuli are initiated in the stress response. The limbic system represents the primary area of control of autonomic function in the forebrain,

and the hypothalamus is considered to be part of this system. The impact of emotional input and expressions of anger, pleasure, fear, and so forth are initiated in this part of the brain. Similarly:
- Stimulation of posterior hypothalamic nuclei causes hypertension, tachycardia, vasoconstriction, shivering, and pupillary dilatation. Somatic responses involve struggling in the anesthetized animal.
- Ablation removes this response and the body temperature responds passively to its surroundings, the animal being unable to protect itself against rising environmental temperature.
- Electrical stimulation of the anterior nuclei causes panting, sweating, and vasodilatation, all the mechanisms that play a part in heat loss and are parasympathetic in action.
- Destruction of this area abolishes these somatic and autonomic reactions when the animal is exposed to a raised environmental temperature.
- The descending pathways from this rostrally placed heat-responsive center pass caudally through the lateral hypothalamic areas and may be interrupted by lesions of the caudal hypothalamus.
- Damage to this automatic mechanism presumably results in failure to adjust to overproduction of heat energy by the animal itself and could be looked at seriously as a cause of fever in certain seizure disorders in humans, fever of unknown cause, or even the concept of so-called psychosomatic fever.
- Bilateral lesions in the ventromedial nuclei cause hyperphagia resulting in obesity; lateral hypothalamic lesions produce anorexia.
- Destruction of the posterior hypothalamus in a cat abolishes the behavioral patterns of estrus, and transection of the brainstem immediately rostral to the thalamus causes the remarkable reaction known as "sham rage." Trivial stimuli cause this vicious reaction in the experimentally treated animal and can be evoked in the conscious animal by electrical stimulation of the posterolateral hypothalamus. It is considered that the neocortex may lower the threshold of rage reactions and that the amygdala and limbic cortex exert inhibitory effects on the hypothalamic rage reaction, but the associations vary in different species and are not clearly defined. Hypothalamic lesions in humans can cause sham rage syndrome.[6]

## *Brainstem*

Autonomic control of basic survival is mediated via the brainstem, which can be functionally divided into three regions: the medulla, the pons, and the midbrain. The medulla controls cardiac, vasomotor, respiratory, and vomiting response while the pons, via cranial nerves V, VI, VII, and VIII, influences hearing, equilibrium, facial sensation, motor movement, salivation, and tears. Finally, the midbrain structures house cranial nerves III and IV, together with the nuclei that govern norepinephrine, dopamine, and gamma-aminobutyric acid synthesis.[8] The dense projections to and from the cerebrum and cerebellum and the periphery through the brainstem are central to homeostasis.

The vasomotor center, situated in the medulla and located in the floor of the fourth ventricle, maintains arteriolar and venous tone by means of vasoconstrictor fibers relayed in the sympathetic system. Asphyxia increases the frequency of the tonic impulses and there is variation with the phases of respiration. The respiratory centers are directly connected with the vasomotor center and are related functionally. Stimulation of an inspiratory center in the medial region of the medullary reticular formation causes an inspiratory movement that is sustained during the stimulus. Stimulation of a more dorsolaterally placed expiratory center causes expiration. An apneustic center in the lower and mid pons and a pneumotaxic center in the rostral pons constitute the higher centers for autonomic respiratory control.

### Other Brain Regions Involved in Autonomic Function

It is well accepted that thoughts and emotions influence and even initiate autonomic responsiveness. Entire books are written on the subject.[3] With that recognition, much work has been done delineating the various innervation paths from nuclei within the brain through the hypothalamus and back. Consider the innervation paths from the prefrontal cortex (PFC), the amygdala, and hippocampus to the hypothalamus and on through to the brainstem and adrenal glands along with reciprocal paths back through the hypothalamus to the hippocampus, amygdala, or PFC. The layers of connectivity are vast.

What is less well recognized is that the reverse is also true: that autonomic dysfunction can precipitate symptoms of psychological distress without the factors traditionally categorized as psychological stressors. That mood lability, anxiety, depression, psychosis, or other disordered cognitive function can be symptoms associated with dysautonomia is not readily appreciated. Indeed, such symptoms are, more often than not, relegated to the realm of the "psychological" and assumed as somehow being separate from "real" or organic diseases. The dense interconnectivity of the autonomic system shows that this is simply not logical, as we will see when we explore changes in biochemistry in the remaining chapters, where symptoms are precipitated by disordered oxidative metabolism. Not only are there mood and cognitive symptoms present, but they are often key to the early identification of autonomic dysfunction, particularly when in conjunction with symptoms acceptable by all as those of dysautonomia.

*Points of Consideration*

At the most basic level, the sympathetic and parasympathetic nerves produce antagonistic effects on the organs that they both supply, and under natural conditions they act synergistically to produce a balanced action. Thus increased rate of the heart is produced mainly by decreased vagal tone, but also by increased sympathetic tone. However, even from a purely anatomical perspective, the relationship between activation and deactivation is far more complex than a simple on/off system of homeostatic balance would imply. Inputs that determine response are received from numerous regions of the brain and the body; each is assessed and assimilated before the response is produced. Understanding the anatomical components of the ANS will aid the clinician in recognizing the array of seemingly disparate symptoms as belonging to autonomic function. Beyond that, however, the anatomy provides little information about how these symptoms emerge and/or what to do about them. For that perspective, we must understand the chemical components of ANS signal transduction. The gradations of ANS response are mediated at the chemical level, dependent upon a combination of neurotransmitters, hormones, immune cells, and at the most basic level, nutrients that drive the availability of the cellular energy.

## AUTONOMIC CHEMISTRY AND NEUROTRANSMISSION

Traversing the structural highways of nerves that make up the ANS are multiple levels of chemical transactions that sense, signal, and effectively control the adaptive interactions between the organism and the environment. Mediating those transactions and the communication within neurons and between the synapses are the neurotransmitters and their cognate receptors. Modifying the strength and duration of ANS activation is a complement of hormones, immune cells, and other chemical signaling agents.[7]

At its foundation, ANS activation is controlled by the release of two chemicals: ACh and norepinephrine or noradrenaline. To that end, the preganglionic nerve fibers of both the parasympathetic and the sympathetic systems are cholinergic and located within the central nervous system. They synapse in the peripheral nervous system to postganglionic neurons and then again at the target organ. Postganglionic fibers in the parasympathetic system are cholinergic, whereas those in the sympathetic system are adrenergic and release norepinephrine.

## Acetylcholine and Its Receptors

ACh chemistry will be discussed more thoroughly in Chapter 3, but briefly, it is generally an excitatory neurotransmitter that initiates its actions via two classes of receptors: the nicotinic and the muscarinic type. The nicotinic ACh receptors (nAChRs) are fast-acting (micro-to submillisecond), ligand-gated, ion-gated channels while the muscarinic receptors (mAChR) are the slower-acting (millisecond to second), metabotropic, or G-protein coupled receptors.[8] Both are located in neuronal and nonneuronal tissue.

The nicotinic receptors in the musculature are composed of five functional subunits that change conformation when bound to the neurotransmitter.[9] Those in the nervous system, though also comprised of five subunits, have differing degrees of complexity. Some appear as homodimers (where a single subunit repeats) and some as heterodimers (multiple subunit repeats). The subtype or conformation of the nAChR determines their role in regulating myriad physiological processes that range from metabolic rate to inflammation, in addition to the general inhibitory/excitatory balance of the ANS.[10] Binding to the nicotinic receptors confers a fast-acting signal. Type 1 nicotinic receptors are located at the neuromuscular junctions, while type 2 are distributed throughout the autonomic ganglia, central nervous system, and adrenal medulla.[11]

Animal studies indicate that thiamine binds to the presynaptic nicotinic receptors exhibiting anticholinesterase activity and increasing ACh release in the central nervous system. This is an effect that is resistant to the blockade of the nAChRs by the pharmacological agent scopolamine.[12]

In contrast to the fast-acting nicotinic receptors, whose actions are mediated by conformational changes among the subunits of the receptor, the slower-acting muscarinic receptors are composed of five different subtypes of receptors (M1–M5), each tasked with different sets of functions and differentially distributed throughout the brain and body.

Differences in receptor conformation (nAChR)[13] or receptor expression and activity (mAChR)[14] are important to our purposes, inasmuch as those changes can be induced by pharmaceutical[15,16] and environmental[17] agents, as well as nutritional factors such as thiamine deficiency.[18] This may help to explain interindividual differences in autonomic response. Changes in receptor conformation or binding propensity determine the degree and direction of influence that ACh can exert at any given time. For example, ACh binding to M2- or M4-type receptors in the heart, central nervous system, or smooth muscle tempers ACh release, whereas ACh that binds to the M1, M3, or M5 increases ACh release.[19] This then influences the general balance of autonomic activation/deactivation, sometimes more subtly than one might expect and certainly more subtly than from a direct injury.

In the case of the muscarinic receptors, allosteric binding sites that cooperatively enhance or limit the actions of the primary ligand are common. A thiamine derivative, thiochrome, allosterically binds to M1- to M4-type muscarinic receptors, increasing ACh affinity to the M4 receptors by three- to fivefold.[20] Since the M4 autoreceptor is inhibitory, slowing ACh release, the impact of thiamine deficiency would result in altered ACh feedback mechanisms at the receptor level. This would potentially activate a more dominant sympathetic response, particularly in the tissues where the M4 receptors in the heart, central nervous system, and musculature predominate.

## Adrenergic Receptors and Response

The adrenal gland serves as the peripheral endocrine component of the ANS. It is divided into the cortex (adrenocortical path), where cortisol and other steroid hormones are synthesized, and the adrenal medulla (adrenomedullary path). Upon receiving cholinergic input from the sympathetic system via the splanchnic nerves, the chromaffin cells from the adrenal medulla release stored epinephrine and norepinephrine.[21] The catecholamines then bind to adrenergic receptors and further activate the sympathetic response.

The adrenergic receptors come in two classes of receptor: alpha (1, 2) and beta (1, 2), each with two principal subtypes. Both classes of adrenergic receptors are G-protein coupled and the ligand–receptor complex ultimately determines the signal transduction pathway and consequent activation or deactivation of the cell.

Epinephrine and norepinephrine bind to and activate both alpha receptors with different affinities and potencies. In the peripheral nervous system, alpha 1 receptors are located postsynaptically and mediate excitatory effects while the alpha 2 receptors are presynaptic autoreceptors that temper norepinephrine release. This is in contrast to the alpha adrenergic receptors within the central nervous system. There, both the alpha 1 and alpha 2 receptors are located postsynaptically. Additionally, although norepinephrine will activate both subtypes of beta receptors, epinephrine will activate only the beta 1 receptors. Both classes of adrenergic receptors are expressed in most tissues. However, receptor expression is uneven.[22] For example, the beta 1 receptors dominate in the heart while the beta 2 receptors dominate in vascular and nonvascular smooth muscle. As a result, activation of beta 1 receptors in the heart leads to an increase in heart rate and contractile force, whereas activation of the beta 2 receptor leads to vascular and nonvascular smooth muscle relaxation[23] and a complementary decrease in heart rate.

Like the other receptors, the adrenergic receptors can be modified allosterically by pharmacological agents and physiologically relevant endogenous factors.[24] Although the research is in its preliminary stages, thus far it is known that the alpha receptors are modifiable by the presence of cholesterol, sodium, and the cytokine immunoglobulin G (IgG), while the beta-type receptors are sensitive to zinc,[25] magnesium, manganese, and IgG.[25]

## Stress Response of Hormones and Receptors

Laying astride the sympathetic pathway to the adrenal medulla and other organs is the adrenocortical path, more commonly referred to as the stress pathway or the HPA axis. The hypothalamic release of CRH with arginine vasopressin or antidiuretic hormone, followed by pituitary ACTH (and the analgesic beta endorphin), initiates the release of cortisol into general circulation. Cortisol then binds to GR and MR receptors throughout the body and brain. Cortisol, together with epinephrine, reaches virtually all tissues and organs and actively alters the background environment of the organism, and thus is considered a key regulator of autonomic responsiveness.

On the HPA side, cortisol is essential for the redistribution of energy and resources needed to face a threat via its role in glucose control, immune system regulation, and inflammation. Cortisol's effects on individual tissues and organs and its role in the HPA stress response are well known, and so will not be covered here. However, we would like to point out some of the less well-appreciated aspects of this system that impact and are impacted by autonomic function. These involve the hormone–receptor crosstalk that mediates cortisol's effects both centrally and peripherally, and the diversity of communication pathways beyond the traditionally considered autonomic and HPA systems.

### *Receptor Crosstalk*

As with the actions of ACh and epinephrine, the direction, duration, and scope of response is mediated at the receptor level. In contrast, however, steroid-to-receptor binding is, for all intents and purposes, promiscuous.

That is, steroid hormones bind not just to their cognate receptors but to other hormone receptors as well. For example, cortisol binds readily to both the MR and GR receptors with the receptors sharing 56% sequence homology.[26] Under basal conditions, circulating cortisol concentrations are approximately 1000-fold higher than aldosterone concentrations, the cognate receptor for the MR receptors.[27] Cortisol binds with MRs with a high affinity resulting in considerable MR occupation even when cortisol concentrations are at their lowest diurnally.

In contrast, lower-affinity GRs become increasingly activated only with greater concentrations of cortisol, when MRs are already largely occupied. To some extent, the cortisol–MR binding is reduced by a prereceptor enzymatic reaction mediated by two isoforms of 11beta-hydroxysteroid dehydrogenase enzyme (11beta-HSD 1, 2).[28] However, a number of conditions, mostly those with underlying hypoxia or pseudohypoxia from thiamine deficiency,[29] are key components, downregulating these enzymes, limiting aldosterone to MR binding, and promoting increased sodium retention and hypertension.[29] In contrast, the enzymes are upregulated in adipose tissue, which reduces circulating cortisol that then increases central obesity and further metabolic dysregulation.[30]

Steroid hormone promiscuity does not end with cortisol's coregulation of the MR receptors. Progesterone and many of its metabolites also bind strongly both to GR and MR receptors. In fact, progesterone and its metabolites bind to the GRs and MRs slightly more strongly than either cortisol or aldosterone.[26] When bound to the GRs, progesterone induces a number of GR-like effects.[31] When bound to the MRs, however, its actions are largely antagonistic.[30] There are exceptions, however.

MR receptors are susceptible to modification both genetically and epigenetically. Researchers have noted gain-of-function MR mutations[32] where MRs are constitutively activated by progesterone, effectively negating its antialdosterone effects. In addition, there is emerging evidence suggesting that steroid hormone receptors are susceptible to epigenetic modification that changes receptor function and sensitivity to steroid ligands.[33] Functional changes in the MR become especially problematic for women during the luteal phase of menstruation, during pregnancy, and with the use of progestins in oral contraceptives and hormone replacement therapies, because the elevated progesterone concentrations would increase salt reabsorption and elevate blood pressure.

Fourth-generation contraceptive pills with drospirenone, a 17a-spirolactone analog that binds 500 times more tightly to the MR than progesterone,[34] are particularly dangerous for women with genetic or epigenetic gain-of-function alterations in these receptors. It is not yet clear how common MR gain-of-function alterations are, but even without these receptor disturbances it should be evident that naturally or synthetically manipulated fluctuations in progesterone across the menstrual cycle or pregnancy would impact autonomic responsiveness, particularly as it relates to cardiovascular function.

## Autonomic Nervous System Modulators: Immune Cells and Other Influencers

Adding additional layers of complexity, numerous endogenous and exogenous compounds influence the adrenal response to sympathetic activation. Over the last decade, researchers have identified direct immune-to-adrenal activation pathways. These are local immune-adrenal circuits that operate independently of sympathetic system input, which are sensitive to circulating pathogens or inflammatory markers[35] and initiate the release of cortisol that then signals the need for a sympathetic response.

Conversely, common pharmaceuticals can alter this response. Serotonin (5-hydroxytryptamine; 5-HT) is synthesized in perivascular mast cells of the adrenal cortex and released with sympathetic activation.[28] Once released, 5-HT binds with local 5-HT$_4$ receptors stimulating the release of both cortisol and aldosterone. Excess 5-HT is catabolized by local monoamine oxidase A enzymes.[28] Although there is little research on the topic, the use of serotonin reuptake inhibitors (SSRIs) is likely to alter the adrenal–serotonergic pathway and autonomic function. Chronically high concentrations of serotonin, mediated by long-term SSRIs, have been found to blunt cortisol response and immune function[36] possibly via desensitized 5-HT receptors.[37]

### Points of Consideration

Admittedly, considering receptor binding adds a level of complexity for the diagnostician interested in understanding dysautonomic function. However, it is important to recognize the complexity of possible alterations. Beyond discrete anatomical tracts of the sympathetic and parasympathetic nervous systems, and even beyond the hormonal stress response mediated by the HPA axis, are a myriad of intervening variables that adjust dynamically to modify autonomic response. As a result, we should expect a diversity of symptoms to fall under the umbrella of dysautonomia. Some symptoms may follow the sympathetic/parasympathetic tracts closely, whereas others may not and may reflect compensatory reactions at the molecular level that are ultimately somewhat unique to the individual. Moreover, some symptoms may be attributable to or exacerbated by lesser known medication side effects.

## THE MYTHS OF LINEARITY AND SYMMETRY
### Nonlinear Dose–Response Actions

As should be evident from the preceding sections, autonomic signaling, and indeed most chemical signaling within an organism, is not a linear one-to-one process. As a result, our expectations for linear dose–response curves, where a given response is directly proportional to the dose, may be misguided. More often than not, small doses or, if we are speaking in terms of the circulating concentrations of a chemical, lower concentrations will confer one response, moderate doses or concentrations another, and high doses or concentrations yet another. The nonmonotonic and curvilinear nature of dose–response curves is not commonly recognized, but it does exist[38,39] across the entirety of organism physiology, but particularly in regard to autonomic function.

For example, if ACh is injected into a cat in doses less than 0.01 µg, it lowers the blood pressure by its peripheral effect on blood vessels.[40] This dilator action is abolished by atropine. Larger doses produce slowing and decreased contraction of the heart, which results in considerable fall in blood pressure caused by a vagus effect. After injections of atropine, however, large doses of ACh produce a marked rise in blood pressure and cardiac acceleration caused by stimulation of the sympathetic ganglia, and adrenaline is discharged. This action is enhanced after destruction of the medulla and spinal cord. It slows, weakens, or arrests the isolated perfused heart.

If ACh is injected into human skin there is total vasodilatation, sweating, and stimulation of pain receptors. That is, the actions of ACh on the central nervous system are excitatory or inhibitory according to the experimental conditions. Similarly, the experimental actions of ACh are rapidly hydrolyzed in alkaline solution at room temperature to form choline, and this instability partly explains the transient nature of its action. Cholinesterase accelerates its destruction and can be influenced by drugs that inhibit the action of this enzyme.

Adrenaline, formed biochemically from tyrosine, affects all sympathetically innervated structures and has an action similar to that produced by sympathetic stimulation. Noradrenaline, its immediate precursor, acts similarly but is more potent in elevating blood pressure and less potent in relaxing smooth muscle. There are other differences between noradrenaline and its methylated derivative, adrenaline, but it may be said broadly that they are essentially the neurotransmitters that together are responsible for the mediation of sympathetic response.

## Asymmetrical Autonomic Innervation Patterns

Like the nonmonotonic dose–response actions, another long-held belief is that innervation patterns are always symmetrical. With the ANS in particular, this is not always the case. For example, researchers investigating autonomic response to cold pressor and facial cooling tests[41] found striking asymmetry with right hemisphere sympathetic dominance. Similarly, Dr. Lonsdale identified significant differences in right/left blood pressure when measured simultaneously in patients with diagnosed dysautonomia. These observations were never published but are included here as an example of asymmetrical innervation with dysautonomia.

Briefly, repeated simultaneous bilateral pulse pressures were taken in 17 Caucasian patients diagnosed with dysautonomia and 13 healthy controls. The patient group included 9 females and 8 males, ages 14–76 years (average 44.6 years), while the control group included 12 females and 1 male, ages 24–66 years (average of 51.8 years). Erythrocyte transketolase activity and thiamine pyrophosphate effect were performed in all 17 patients.[42]

Some of the patients had multiple measurements. Of the 17 patients, 16 had asymmetrically different blood pressures measured simultaneously in both arms. The thiamine pyrophosphate effect (TPPE) was positive in 10, showing thiamine deficiency, and negative in 7. Table 2.1 illustrates these observations.

Based purely on observation, the higher pulse pressures are noted in the left arm of the patients compared to controls. Similarly, pulse pressures appear higher in the positive TPPE patients compared to the negative TPPE

**Table 2.1** Asymmetrical Pulse Pressure and Thiamine Deficiency

| Subjects | Number | Mean Pulse Pressures | | | |
|---|---|---|---|---|---|
| | | Right | Left | Right | Left |
| Total | 17 | 48.7 | 57.3 | 8 | 16 |
| +TPPE | 10 | 56.4 | 66.3 | 3 | 11 |
| −TPPE | 7 | 32.8 | 47.7 | 1 | 6 |
| Controls | 13 | 44.6 | 47.1 | 7 | 6 |

TPPE, Thiamine pyrophosphate effect.

patients. Finally, across all patients there appears to be little difference in the right arm pulse pressure compared with the controls, whereas the left arm pulse pressure is distinctly greater than that in the controls.

*Points of Consideration*

Many of the patients had a lifelong history of polysymptomatic illness, one having begun at the age of 7 years after falling from a second floor window. The range of symptoms experienced by this patient cohort was broad and illustrates the diversity of symptoms that can be experienced when ANS function is disturbed. The symptoms in this patient cohort included the following:

- Thirteen had either undiagnosed daily headaches or migraine.
- Thirteen experienced constant and/or recurrent alternating unilateral recumbent nasal congestion, indicating asymmetric exaggeration of the normal ANS controlled nasal cycle.[43]
- Two had received a proven diagnosis of sleep apnea, two had Lyme disease, one of whom had proven deficient esophageal peristalsis, and two had had mononucleosis.
- Four patients, one of whom had been found elsewhere to be homozygous for the MTHFR C677T mutation, had elevated blood homocysteine and one of whom had melanin pigmentation on both arms suggesting vitamin B12 deficiency.[44] This individual, in whom the TPPE was repeatedly in the thiamine deficiency range, was addicted to sugar in any form, experiencing a severe reaction after consumption of blackstrap molasses taken as a "health food."
- One patient with a lifelong history of daily headaches had a previous diagnosis of membranous glomerulonephritis, myelodysplasia, and esophageal ulceration. Echocardiography revealed mild tricuspid insufficiency.
- A male patient had a 20-year history of alternating urgency diarrhea and constipation, panic attacks, and bipolar symptomology.
- A female patient had experienced 12 Pap smears, each of which had been positive for human papillomavirus (HPV) infection.
- Another female patient had a hysterectomy at age 38 years for endometriosis.
- Echocardiograms had shown mitral valve prolapse in one patient and mitral regurgitation without prolapse in another.
- A 38-year-old man had mild aortic and tricuspid regurgitation and a 14-year-old boy had an "insignificant patent foramen ovale."
- Another 38-year-old man had migraine headaches and had passed six renal calculi.

- A man, also 38 years of age, presented with an 18-month history of chest pain, extreme fatigue, and tinnitus (he reported that studies elsewhere had shown that he had complex IV deficiency marked by repeatedly low blood levels of thiamine, even after the administration elsewhere of 600 mg of a water-soluble thiamine salt daily for an extended period).
- One patient had been reported to have elevations of anti-DNA and antistreptolysin O titers.
- Another man reported that he had been found elsewhere to be infected with *Blastocystis hominis* and three of the women had suffered recurrent yeast infections of the vagina.

Sweet and/or salt craving was admitted in 14 of these patients and appeared to be an important etiologic component. Of the 14 addicted to sugar, 9 had abnormal erythrocyte transketolase changes, indicating loss of thiamine homeostasis.

Beriberi is the prototype for functional dysautonomia in its early stages. It was hypothesized that excessive ingestion of simple carbohydrates resulted in defective oxidative metabolism in ANS control mechanisms, resulting in exaggeration of normal asymmetric reflex action, an effect similar to that induced by mild, chronic hypoxia. Abnormal thiamine homeostasis has been reported in a number of degenerative brain diseases.[45] Of these 17 patients, aside from having symptoms directly related to ANS dysfunction, several experienced infections that demonstrated poor immunity. Several had conventional diagnoses in association with their dysautonomia. This begs the question: does the conventional diagnosis have an etiology separate from that of dysautonomia or are both of them, as well as the poor immunity, the result of long-term oxidative dysfunction?

## AUTONOMIC DYSFUNCTION: CLINICAL PATTERNS AND CLUES TO SYMPATHETIC DOMINANCE

Now that we have outlined the basic anatomy and physiology of the autonomic system, let us look at the clinical symptoms when components of this system become dysregulated.

### Acute Blepharospasm, Sweating, and Piloerection as Clues to Sympathetic System Dominance

Structures of the eye supplied by the sympathetic system are as follows:
- Dilator pupillae muscles.
- Smooth muscle fibers in the upper and lower lids, called respectively the superior and inferior tarsal muscles, which retract the upper and lower lids.

- Smooth muscle fibers of the retroocular muscle of Müller, which lies in the orbital fascia and pushes the globe forward. This is important in considering exophthalmos as a sign of adrenergic overdrive and enophthalmos as a sign of its interruption.

Stimulation of the cervical sympathetic tract causes dilatation of the pupil and retraction of the lids resulting in a "staring" gaze. The effect on the globe in humans is variable, although it can move the dog's globe forward by as much as 5 mm. The blood vessels are constricted. Sectioning of the cervical sympathetic nerves causes Horner syndrome; this consists of a constricted pupil, narrowed palpebral fissure, ptosis of the upper lid, and slight elevation of the lower lid, together with diminished sweating of the face on the same side. The blood vessels are dilated.[46]

There is a center in the superior colliculi for the control of sympathetic fibers to the eye. The path from midbrain to the connector cells in the thoracic cord is the tectospinal tract, so that a disturbance in brainstem, cervical, or upper thoracic cord, upper chest, neck, or interior of the skull can lead to changes in sympathetic innervation of the eye and the eccrine glands.

Fibers to the eccrine sweat glands are anatomically sympathetic but functionally cholinergic. The apocrine sweat glands are probably activated by circulating adrenaline. The erector pili muscles are smooth muscle fibers that erect skin hairs, producing the appearance of "goose skin" in humans when stimulated. The appearance of "goose bumps" and unusual sweating may be the only clinical signs of sympathetic domination.

## Points of Consideration

How might eyelid constriction, sweating, and goose bumps be connected functionally? Let us unpack a few cases. Open angle glaucoma is associated with dysautonomia, and specifically, parasympathetic neuropathy.[47] Parasympathetic inhibition induces a state of sympathetic dominance, which can then be associated with blepharospasm, the involuntary constriction of the eyelids and the pupils. A common treatment for the symptoms of blepharospasm includes a series of botulinum toxin or Botox injections. Botulinum toxin inhibits ACh release. Together with its role at the adrenal medulla, ACh is the neurotransmitter at all the parasympathetic innervated organs, at the sweat glands, and for the piloerector muscle of the sympathetic ANS. Blocking ACh thus can be said to induce a functionally equivalent state of parasympathetic neuropathy or sympathetic dominance. Since parasympathetic neuropathy leads to certain types of glaucoma, it is not surprising that blocking ACh via Botox would induce it. Neither should it be surprising that sympathetic dominance would produce a host of symptoms that include not only the eyes and the sweat glands, but also the heart and metabolic function.

The brief case reported below, describing a patient with acute blepharospasm, was but the tip of a proverbial symptom iceberg. The eyes offer an excellent opportunity to observe autonomic function but the clinical presentation can be bizarre as the Case Example 2.1 illustrates.[48-50] This case is described in more detail in Chapter 5.

### Case Example 2.1 Blepharospasm and Piloerection as Evidence of Disordered Autonomic Function and Thiamine Deficiency

The case of an 8-year-old girl with acute blepharospasm[5] is described by Dr. Lonsdale (unpublished). She developed suppurative parotitis at the age of 18 months, which was then followed by recurrent photophobia, clouding of the cornea, and persistent piloerection of the skin (the clue to sympathetic activity). Photophobia gradually became permanent and was accompanied by nasal congestion. Acetone was frequently detected in her breath. Polydipsia, tachycardia, periorbital edema, and fever occurred through the years intermittently. She had a grossly abnormal glucose tolerance and after insulin treatment was started, piloerection disappeared. She was treated with thiamine tetrahydrofurfuryl disulfide (TTFD) 300 mg a day with consequent clinical improvement.

## Heart Rate, Rhythm, and Pressure Dysregulation

Dysfunction of the ANS is seldom considered in the treatment of patients in a state of heart failure. Sympathetic/parasympathetic imbalance has been reviewed to summarize the current knowledge concerning mechanisms for disturbed parasympathetic and sympathetic circulatory control and heart failure with reduced ejection fraction and its clinical and prognostic implications.[51] The brain and heart are the organs that have a fast rate of oxidative metabolism and are affected early by any mechanism that induces oxidative deficiency. Beriberi is a prototype for dysautonomia in its early stages and it may be a combination of autonomic and myocardial failure that produces the typical beriberi heart.[52]

From an anatomical standpoint, this makes sense. Connector fibers in animals go to the stellate ganglion, and in humans to all three ganglia of the cervical sympathetic chain. Postganglionic fibers go to the heart and increase the force of contraction, rate, conductivity, and excitability. The bronchi are dilated by inhibition of smooth muscle action in their walls and pulmonary arteries are constricted. The coronary arteries are normally dilated, perhaps a major clue to autonomic dysfunction when catheterization fails to find arterial obstruction.

Ganglion cells for regulating functional control of the heart lie in the sinoatrial and atrioventricular nodes. The postganglionic fibers supply the nodes, the bundle of His and its ramification, the musculature of the atrium, and the base of the ventricles. The apex of the ventricles does not receive parasympathetic innervation. Constrictor fibers are distributed to the coronary arteries. This innervation carries a tonic stream of inhibitory impulses to the heart, slowing its rate, shortening the period of systole, and reducing contractility.

Cardiac innervation is important to our understanding of the prolonged QT syndrome, which causes sudden death in humans, and which can be treated by surgical removal of the left stellate ganglion or by the use of a beta blocker.[53] Other causes of sudden death have been described, believed to be related to autonomic action on the heart in at least some cases.[54]

## Postural Orthostatic Tachycardia

ANS dysregulation of the heart muscle can be seen clearly in the recently recognized dysautonomia called postural orthostatic tachycardia syndrome (POTS). The primary manifestation of the syndrome is orthostatic intolerance with an excessive tachycardic response (>30 bpm increase from baseline) upon standing. Secondarily, however, the syndrome is marked by a wide variety of additional autonomic disturbances. As one might expect, the full scope of symptoms comorbid with POTS is quite diverse (Dysautonomia Information Network).[54a] Briefly however, comorbid symptoms of POTS include[55] the following:
- Lightheadedness, fainting, and general weakness.
- Gastrointestinal dysmotility including gastroparesis and/or excessive vomiting.
- Heart palpitations, shortness of breath, and tremulousness.
- Loss of sweating or excessive sweating, and heat and/or cold intolerance.
- Light and/or noise sensitivity.
- Mood lability.

### Points of Consideration

As with our discussion of blepharospasm, the diversity of symptoms recognized with POTS is indicative of widespread autonomic disturbance and should point the clinician accordingly. In Dr. Lonsdale's experience, the etiology of POTS, like that of other autonomic disturbances, resides within the chemistry, specifically, mitochondrial chemistry and oxidative capacity. When oxidative capacity is impaired, autonomic dysfunction emerges.

By way of example, brief Case Example 2.2 illustrates both the breadth of symptoms associated with this syndrome and the underlying chemical disturbance.

### Case Example 2.2 POTS and Thiamine Deficiency Post-Gardasil Vaccine

An 18-year-old girl received three injections of the HPV vaccine, Gardasil. With each injection she had suffered nondescript symptoms attributed to mere coincidence. After the third injection, however, she experienced POTS. After 4 years, during which she was crippled, her mother had come to the conclusion that her daughter had beriberi. Erythrocyte transketolase test showed an accelerated thiamine pyrophosphate effect, proving thiamine deficiency. She subsequently had clinical improvement by ingestion of nutrient supplements that included TTFD. Two other girls and a boy with post-Gardasil POTS all had erythrocyte transketolase-proven thiamine deficiency and responded to nutrient supplementation.

## Neuropathy, Muscle Weakness, Skin Disorders, and Balance

Sympathetic postganglionic fibers reach the limbs via the appropriate spinal nerves and are distributed to large arteries, skin, and skeletal muscle vessels. Some preganglionic fibers in the lower limb end in ganglia outside the sympathetic chain, which might account for some failures of sympathectomy.[56] Disturbances of sympathetic/parasympathetic innervation to the limbs, when absent injury or illness and comorbid with other ANS symptoms, should point us to an autonomic neuropathy of metabolic origin. For example, unexplained altered sensory perceptions such as pins and needles, burning feet, itching, hyperalgesia, muscle weakness, and ataxia suggest autonomic neuropathy affecting the small fiber myelinated and unmyelinated nerves[57] as illustrated in Case Example 2.3.[58]

### Case Example 2.3 Peripheral Neuropathy, Paresthesia, and Weakness

A boy suffering from anorexia nervosa was reported with upper and lower extremity glove-and-stocking paresthesias, weakness, vertigo, high-pitched voice, inattention, ataxia, and binocular diplopia after a voluntary 59-kg weight loss. He was studied by brain magnetic resonance imaging and nerve conduction and the findings were diagnostic of peripheral neuropathy and Wernicke encephalopathy secondary to thiamine deficiency.[59]

## Gastrointestinal Dysmotility Syndromes

Preganglionic fibers to abdominal structures pass through the ganglia of the sympathetic chain without relaying and continue as the splanchnic nerves, which are therefore still preganglionic. They relay in the celiac, superior mesenteric, renal, spermatic, and ovarian ganglia, and in the hypogastric ganglia on the lateral walls of the rectum. Postganglionic fibers pass to the various organs via the large arteries that supply them. The system is distributed to the small and large intestine and related sphincters. It supplies the pyloric sphincter, pyloric region of the stomach, and cardiac sphincter. Electrical stimulation of splanchnic nerves causes inhibition of peristaltic movements and diminution of tone throughout the intestine, together with stimulation of the sphincters, which become tightly closed. This distribution of functional response is emphasized since it is theoretically possible to produce pathophysiologic or functional changes by a chronically unbalanced autonomic stimulation of one system relative to the other.

Dr. Lonsdale reported a 14-year-old boy with eosinophilic esophagitis (EoE) who was addicted to sugar. Thiamine deficiency was demonstrated from an abnormal thiamine pyrophosphate effect of erythrocyte transketolase. He responded clinically and biochemically to treatment with TTFD.[59] The case was also posted online[60] and one of the comments was from the mother of a patient with EoE and gastroparesis. The vagus has no sympathetic nerve supply and innervates the esophagus and the entire alimentary tract and suppresses inflammation via the spleen.[61] It was therefore hypothesized that thiamine deficiency resulted in failure of cholinergic neurotransmission affecting esophageal motility, suppression of eosinophilic inflammation, and gastroparesis as a central biochemical lesion.

## Bladder and Bowel Dysfunction as Signs of Autonomic Disturbance

Sympathetic stimulation throughout the splanchnic area causes arteriolar constriction and forms an important part of "peripheral resistance" where shifts in blood volume take place. The detrusor muscle of the bladder is inhibited, whereas the sphincter and trigonal area are contracted. Connector cells for the sacral outflow of the parasympathetic systems lie in the second and third segments of the sacral cord, the preganglionic fibers passing out in their corresponding ventral roots to form a single pelvic nerve on each side. The cell ganglia are found in the vicinity of the substance of the innervated organs. Relays in the hypogastric ganglia on the lateral walls of the rectum supply the bladder, prostate, most of the large intestine, and the blood vessels of the penis. Functionally, the system stimulates the detrusor muscle of the bladder and inhibits the sphincter. The colon and rectum contract and the anal sphincters are relaxed. Imbalance between sympathetic and parasympathetic function may be the explanation for poor bladder control in the elderly as oxidative metabolism gradually becomes less efficient.

### Sexual and Reproductive Abnormalities Associated With Autonomic Disturbance

The muscle coat of the epididymis, ejaculatory ducts, seminal vesicles, and prostate are stimulated with the result that ejaculation of semen occurs. The ureters, uterus, Fallopian tubes, and vas deferens receive both motor and inhibitory fibers without supply from the parasympathetic system. Understanding the physiological effects within the organs of reproduction is necessary to appreciate the common abnormalities and distortions of sexual relationships such as impotence, failure to ejaculate, or unusual emotional states during coitus. It is worth drawing attention to the fact that erection of the penis is under parasympathetic control, but ejaculation appears to be governed by sympathetic activity caused by stimulation of this system. Therefore the completion of successful coitus in humans is highly dependent upon a balanced relation between adrenergic and cholinergic stimulus. Sympathetic secretory fibers are supplied to the adrenal medulla and cause discharge of adrenaline and noradrenaline. Thus all forms of both physical and psychic stimulus, which may be viewed generally as stressful, will produce a compound adrenergic response involving both the autonomic and endocrine systems.

### Cognitive and Mental Health Symptoms as Signs of Autonomic Disturbance

Cognitive disturbances,[62,63] particularly mild ones, together with psychiatric symptoms[64] have long been considered somehow separate from the more organic or physical disease processes allowing many a physician to misdiagnose or, worse yet, ignore important clues to underlying autonomic dysfunction entirely. This disconnect is all the more perplexing considering how frequently associations between stress, autonomic function, and mental illness[65] have been elucidated over the decades since the work of Selye, and how densely connected the limbic system is to the central regulators of autonomic function, the hypothalamus[66] and the brainstem.[67] Except for the tacit acknowledgment of connectivity, Descartes' mind/body dualism holds strong in modern medicine and unfortunately in dysautonomia research, where the vast preponderance involves cardiac function.

As difficult as it has been to recognize fully psychiatric and cognitive disturbances as signs of possible ANS dysfunction, it has been almost impossible to acknowledge that changes in biochemistry, particularly those emanating from disordered oxidative metabolism, may also provoke dysautonomic responses, of which psychiatric and cognition are key components. This makes little sense when one considers the totality of the ANS anatomy and physiology and its role in environmental adaptation. Whether the environmental adaptations are precipitated internally or externally does not matter. Indeed, the reactions are reciprocal. The brain, as the largest consumer of metabolic energy per unit mass than any other organ,[68] is acutely sensitive to permutations in oxidative metabolism—internal stressors that will ultimately necessitate autonomic adjustment. As such, one should expect a relationship between metabolic control and neuropsychiatric morbidity.

At the extreme end of this spectrum, a growing body of evidence links the cognitive dysfunction in aging[69] and Alzheimer's[70] to disordered oxidative metabolism. Similarly, many of the errant genes involving psychosis are linked largely to those affecting oxidative metabolism[71] and impaired neurodevelopment in infants is also linked to disordered oxidative metabolism.[72] Oxidative metabolism affects autonomic stability. To the extent that it becomes disrupted, autonomic maladaptations accrue,[73] affecting everything from cardiac function[74] to wakefulness,[75] gastrointestinal motility,[76] sodium and potassium balance,[77] insulin,[78] mood stability,[79] and cognitive function. A metaanalysis of autonomic disturbances across psychiatric populations found an increased rate of autonomic dysfunction in otherwise healthy patients, irrespective of psychotropic used, with the greatest disturbances found in patients with psychotic disorders.[80]

Indeed, one might argue that as the largest consumer of molecular energy, symptoms involving nervous system function, such as mood and cognition, might emerge first before other more global adaptations are noticeable. Some evidence suggests this may be the case. By way of example, the molecular mechanisms involved in the expression of panic, e.g., sympathetic activation, involve a form of hypoxia linked to thiamine-induced disordered oxidative metabolism.[29,81,82] Studies in the pathogenesis of panic disorder (PD) have shown signs of cerebral hypoxia as the underlying cause. In fact, PD patients remain clinically unwell between attacks and have shown electroencephalogram abnormalities in the nonpanic state.

Provocative studies using carbon dioxide mixtures can induce an attack and suggest that they have hypersensitive $CO_2$ chemoreceptors and that PD represents fragmented fight-or-flight reflexes.[83]

## AUTONOMIC IMBALANCE

It is obvious that the opposing force of the sympathetic and parasympathetic systems is the key to maintaining a balance of function throughout the entire organism. If the sympathetic system is removed in the cat or dog under experimental conditions, apparent "good health" surprisingly remains. Reproduction in the female occurs, the blood pressure shows only a temporary fall, and the blood vessels maintain a sufficient degree of tone for peripheral resistance. The heart rate and size of the pupil quickly return to normal. With emotional stimulus, however, there is no change in blood sugar, no increase in red blood cell count, and no rise of blood pressure as would be normally seen. The animals are sensitive to cold and lose heat more rapidly than intact animals. They are apparently able to maintain a placid existence, but do not respond to stress as well—although even this is not always in evidence, for some of the animals are able to run or fight as vigorously as intact animals. It is possible that alternative "backup" mechanisms of adaptation may be mediated through the endocrine system alone, as was shown by the detailed writings of Selye and others. Balance between the two systems in an intact animal must be maintained by a constant supply of afferent or "input" signals, and the response is dependent upon the result of data processing, which is carried out in the central control within the brain. The brainstem, hypothalamus, and cerebral cortex all play a part in the control.

Humans are far more complex than cats, however. When interpreting autonomic symptoms we must remember that autonomic disorder, particularly when emanating from metabolic disturbances, will present with an array of symptoms that are not necessarily consistent with an organ-based compartmentalized approach to diagnoses. Moreover, since the limbic system is such a huge component of autonomic response, symptoms traditionally considered psychosomatic in nature may in fact be indicative of disturbed metabolism. For example, a middle-aged woman consulted Dr. Lonsdale, presenting with pain in the right shoulder, which was correctly interpreted as referred pain and led to cholecystectomy. It has long been taught in medical school that cholecystitis is related to what is known as the three F's (fair, fat, and forty), strongly suggesting that dietary indiscretion and perhaps menopause both have a role in etiology.

Unfortunately, removing the gallbladder did not relieve the shoulder pain. For the next 10 years, the patient complained that the pain in the right shoulder persisted and radiated across her body to the left hip. It was thus written off as being "psychological." On questioning, she admitted that its sporadic appearance was associated with any form of mental or physical stress. It was explained to her in simple terms that the initial trauma had registered a "file in her brain" and that the pain persisted because of dysfunctional brain oxidative metabolism. Her diet was corrected by proper instruction, the removal of sugar, and she was supplied with a few nutritional supplements. The pain had vanished in 1 or 2 months.

The modern explanation would be an obvious one: that this was indeed psychosomatic and that suggestion or the placebo effect was responsible for removing the pain. We would agree, except that we believe we are explaining the mechanism. We have given consideration to the fact that all pain is a function of the brain, irrespective of whether it is associated with an inflamed and swollen joint, trauma, or other manifestation of bodily disease. The brain receives a signal from the site of the causative factor and it is the brain that initiates the sensory pattern of resultant pain. In the pages that follow we will continue to explore the hypothesis that all sensory and motor phenomena initiated by the brain, sometimes even without an endogenous stimulus, are exaggerated and distorted in the presence of mild hypoxia or pseudohypoxia. Thus psychosomatic disease becomes a reality that requires solution by finding the biochemical lesion. It provides an explanation of why the boy described earlier in this chapter with thiamine deficiency–related eosinophilic esophagitis, hyperalgesia, and many other functional symptoms had been misdiagnosed with psychosomatic disease for years.

## REFERENCES

1. Robertson DM, Wasan SM, Skinner DB. Ultrastructural features of early brain stem lesions of thiamine-deficient rats. *Am J Pathol* 1968;**52**(5):1081.
2. By Geo-Science-International – Own work, CC0. https://commons.wikimedia.org/w/index.php?curid=47377075.
3. Lovallo WR. *Stress and health: biological and psychological interactions*. Sage publications; 2015.
4. Martin JH. *Neuroanatomy text and atlas*. Stamford, CT: Appleton & Lange; 1996.
5. Chatfield PO. Fundamentals of clinical neurophysiology. *Psychosom Med* 1958;**20**(4):340.
6. Savard G, Bhanji NH, Dubeau F, Andermann F, Sadikot A. Psychiatric aspects of patients with hypothalamic hamartoma and epilepsy. *Epileptic Disord* 2003;**5**(4):229–34.
7. O'connor TM, O'halloran DJ, Shanahan F. The stress response and the hypothalamic-pituitary-adrenal axis: from molecule to melancholia. *Qjm* 2000;**93**(6):323–33.
8. Purves D, Augustine GJ, Fitzpatrick D, Katz LC, LaMantia AS, McNamara JO, Williams SM. *Two families of postsynaptic receptors*. 2001.

9. Karlin A, Akabas MH. Toward a structural basis for the function of nicotinic acetylcholine receptors and their cousins. *Neuron* 1995;**15**(6):1231–44.
10. Albuquerque EX, Pereira EF, Alkondon M, Rogers SW. Mammalian nicotinic acetylcholine receptors: from structure to function. *Physiol Rev* 2009;**89**(1):73–120.
11. Kirstein SL, Insel PA. Autonomic nervous system pharmacogenomics: a progress report. *Pharmacol Rev* 2004;**56**(1):31–52.
12. Meador KJ, Nichols ME, Franke P, Durkin MW, Oberzan RL, Moore EE, Loring DW. Evidence for a central cholinergic effect of high-dose thiamine. *Ann Neurol* 1993;**34**(5):724–6.
13. Papke RL. Merging old and new perspectives on nicotinic acetylcholine receptors. *Biochem Pharmacol* 2014;**89**(1):1–11.
14. Gehlert DR, Morey WA, Wamsley JK. Alterations in muscarinic cholinergic receptor densities induced by thiamine deficiency: autoradiographic detection of changes in high-and low-affinity agonist binding. *J Neurosci Res* 1985;**13**(3):443–52.
15. Gill-Thind JK, Dhankher P, D'Oyley JM, Sheppard TD, Millar NS. Structurally similar allosteric modulators of α7 nicotinic acetylcholine receptors exhibit five distinct pharmacological effects. *J Biol Chem* 2015;**290**(6):3552–62.
16. Tuček S, Proška J. Allosteric modulation of muscarinic acetylcholine receptors. *Trends Pharmacol Sci* 1995;**16**(6):205–12.
17. Buccafusco JJ, Beach JW, Terry AV. Desensitization of nicotinic acetylcholine receptors as a strategy for drug development. *J Pharmacol Exp Ther* 2009;**328**(2):364–70.
18. Butterworth RF. Thiamin deficiency and brain disorders. *Nutrition Research Reviews* 2003;**16**(2):277.
19. Eglen RM. Muscarinic receptor subtypes in neuronal and non-neuronal cholinergic function. *Auton Autacoid Pharmacol* 2006;**26**(3):219–33.
20. Lazareno S, Doležal V, Popham A, Birdsall NJM. Thiochrome enhances acetylcholine affinity at muscarinic M4 receptors: receptor subtype selectivity via cooperativity rather than affinity. *Mol Pharmacol* 2004;**65**(1):257–66.
21. Schinner S, Bornstein SR. Cortical-chromaffin cell interactions in the adrenal gland. *Endocr Pathol* 2005;**16**(2):91–8.
22. Minneman KP, Pittman RN, Molinoff PB. Beta-adrenergic receptor subtypes: properties, distribution, and regulation. *Annu Rev Neurosci* 1981;**4**(1):419–61.
23. Brodde OE, Michel MC. Adrenergic and muscarinic receptors in the human heart. *Pharmacol Rev* 1999;**51**(4):651–90.
24. Gentry PR, Sexton PM, Christopoulos A. Novel allosteric modulators of G protein-coupled receptors. *J Biol Chem* 2015;**290**(32):19478–88.
25. Swaminath G, Steenhuis J, Kobilka B, Lee TW. Allosteric modulation of β2-adrenergic receptor by $Zn^{2+}$. *Mol Pharmacol* 2002;**61**(1):65–72.
26. Quinkler M, Meyer B, Bumke-Vogt C, Grossmann C, Gruber U, Oelkers W, Diederich S, Bahr V. Agonistic and antagonistic properties of progesterone metabolites at the human mineralocorticoid receptor. *Eur J Endocrinol* 2002;**146**(6):789–99.
27. Lefebvre H, Duparc C, Prévost G, Bertherat J, Louiset E. Cell-to-cell communication in bilateral macronodular adrenal hyperplasia causing hypercortisolism. *Front Endocrinol* 2015;**6**.
28. Ferrari P, Lovati E, Frey FJ. The role of the 11β-hydroxysteroid dehydrogenase type 2 in human hypertension. *J Hypertens* 2000;**18**(3):241–8.
29. Sweet RL, Zastre JA. HIF1-α-Mediated gene expression induced by vitamin B. *Int J Vitam Nutr Res* 2013;**83**(3):188–97.
30. Frey FJ, Odermatt A, Frey BM. Glucocorticoid-mediated mineralocorticoid receptor activation and hypertension. *Curr Opin Nephrol Hypertens* 2004;**13**(4):451–8.
31. Leo JC, Guo C, Woon CT, Aw SE, Lin VC. Glucocorticoid and mineralocorticoid crosstalk with progesterone receptor to induce focal adhesion and growth inhibition in breast cancer cells. *Endocrinology* 2004;**145**(3):1314–21.

32. Geller DS, Farhi A, Pinkerton N, Fradley M, Moritz M, Spitzer A, Meinke G, Tsai FT, Sigler PB, Lifton RP. Activating mineralocorticoid receptor mutation in hypertension exacerbated by pregnancy. *Science* 2000;**289**(5476):119–23.
33. Martinez-Arguelles DB, Papadopoulos V. Epigenetic regulation of the expression of genes involved in steroid hormone biosynthesis and action. *Steroids* 2010;**75**(7):467–76.
34. Sitruk-Ware R. Pharmacology of different progestogens: the special case of drospirenone. *Climacteric* 2005;**8**(Suppl. 3):4–12.
35. Deak T. Immune cells and cytokine circuits: toward a working model for understanding direct immune-to-adrenal communication pathways. *Endocrinology* 2008;**149**(4):1433–5.
36. Hernandez ME, Mendieta D, Pérez-Tapia M, Bojalil R, Estrada-Garcia I, Estrada-Parra S, Pavón L. Effect of selective serotonin reuptake inhibitors and immunomodulator on cytokines levels: an alternative therapy for patients with major depressive disorder. *Clin Dev Immunol* 2013;**2013**.
37. Vidal R, Valdizán EM, Mostany R, Pazos A, Castro E. Long-term treatment with fluoxetine induces desensitization of 5-HT4 receptor-dependent signalling and functionality in rat brain. *J Neurochem* 2009;**110**(3):1120–7.
38. Vandenberg LN, Colborn T, Hayes TB, Heindel JJ, Jacobs Jr DR, Lee DH, Shioda T, Soto AM, vom Saal FS, Welshons WV, Zoeller RT. Hormones and endocrine-disrupting chemicals: low-dose effects and nonmonotonic dose responses. *Endocr Rev* 2012;**33**(3):378–455.
39. Conolly RB, Lutz WK. Nonmonotonic dose-response relationships: mechanistic basis, kinetic modeling, and implications for risk assessment. *Toxicol Sci* 2004;**77**(1):151–7.
40. Inouye K, Katsura E. Etiology and pathology of beriberi. In: Shimazono N, Katsura E, editors. *Thiamine and beriberi*. Tokyo: Igaku Shoin Ltd; 1965.
41. McGinley JJ, Friedman BH. Autonomic responses to lateralized cold pressor and facial cooling tasks. *Psychophysiology* 2015;**52**(3):416–24.
42. Massod MF, Mcguire SL, Werner KR. Analysis of blood transketolase activity. *Am J Clin Pathol* 1971;**55**(4):465–70.
43. Eccles R, Eccles KS. Asymmetry in the autonomic nervous system with reference to the nasal cycle, migraine, anisocoria and Meniere's syndrome. *Rhinology* 1981;**19**(3):121–5.
44. Hoffman CF, Palmer DM, Papadopoulos D. Vitamin B12 deficiency: a case report of ongoing cutaneous hyperpigmentation. *Cutis* 2003;**71**(2):127–30.
45. Jhala SS, Hazell AS. Modeling neurodegenerative disease pathophysiology in thiamine deficiency: consequences of impaired oxidative metabolism. *Neurochem Int* 2011;**58**(3):248–60.
46. Kisch B. Horner's syndrome, an American discovery. *Bull Hist Med* 1951;**25**:284.
47. Clark CV, Mapstone R. Systemic autonomic neuropathy in open-angle glaucoma. *Doc Ophthalmol* 1987;**64**(2):179–85.
48. Elsron JS, Marsden CD, Grandas F, Quinn NP. The significance of ophthalmological symptoms in idiopathic blepharospasm. *Eye* 1988;**2**(4):435–9.
49. Corridan P, Nightingale S, Mashoudi N, Williams AC. Acute angle-closure glaucoma following botulinum toxin injection for blepharospasm. *Br J Ophthalmol* 1990;**74**(5):309–10.
50. Pasquale LR. Vascular and autonomic dysregulation in primary open-angle glaucoma. *Curr Opin Ophthalmol* 2016;**27**(2):94–101.
51. Floras JS, Ponikowski P. The sympathetic/parasympathetic imbalance in heart failure with reduced ejection fraction. *Eur Heart J* 2015:ehv087.
52. Lonsdale D. Dysautonomia, a heuristic approach to a revised model for etiology of disease. *Evid Based Complement Alternat Med* 2009;**6**(1):3–10.
53. Schwartz PJ, Periti M, Malliani A. The long QT syndrome. *Am Heart J* 1975;**89**(3):378–90.
54. Engel GL. Sudden and rapid death during psychological stress: folklore or folk wisdom? *Ann Intern Med* 1971;**74**(5):771–83.

54a. http://www.dinet.org/content/information-resources/pots/pots-symptoms-r96/.
55. "Do You Have a Question for Our Medical Advisors?" POTS Symptoms. Dysautonomia Information Network, 2013. http://www.dinet.org/index.php/information-resources/pots-place/pots-symptoms.
56. Street E, Ashrafi M, Greaves N, Gouldsborough I, Baguneid M. Anatomic variation of rami communicantes in the upper thoracic sympathetic chain: a human cadaveric study. *Ann Vasc Surg* 2016;**34**.
57. Hovaguimian A, Gibbons CH. Diagnosis and treatment of pain in small-fiber neuropathy. *Curr Pain Headache Rep* 2011;**15**(3):193–200.
58. Renthal W, Marin-Valencia I, Evans PA. Thiamine deficiency secondary to anorexia nervosa: an uncommon cause of peripheral neuropathy and Wernicke encephalopathy in adolescence. *Pediatr Neurol* 2014;**51**(1):100–3.
59. Lonsdale D. Is eosinophilic esophagitis a sugar sensitive disease. *J Gastric Disord Ther* 2016;**2**(1).
60. Lonsdale D. Eosinophilic esophagitis may be a sugar sensitive disease- hormones matter. *HormonesMatter* February 08, 2016. https://www.hormonesmatter.com/eosinophilic-esophagitis-sugar-thiamine-sensitive/.
61. Rosas-Ballina M, Tracey KJ. The neurology of the immune system: neural reflexes regulate immunity. *Neuron* 2009;**64**(1):28–32.
62. Bassi A, Bozzali M. Potential interactions between the autonomic nervous system and higher level functions in neurological and neuropsychiatric conditions. *Front Neurol* 2015;**6**.
63. Nicolini P, Ciulla MM, Malfatto G, Abbate C, Mari D, Rossi PD, Pettenuzzo E, Magrini F, Consonni D, Lombardi F. Autonomic dysfunction in mild cognitive impairment: evidence from power spectral analysis of heart rate variability in a cross-sectional case-control study. *PLoS One* 2014;**9**(5):e96656.
64. Anderson JW, Lambert EA, Sari CI, Dawood T, Esler MD, Vaddadi G, Lambert GW. Cognitive function, health-related quality of life, and symptoms of depression and anxiety sensitivity are impaired in patients with the postural orthostatic tachycardia syndrome (POTS). *Front Physiol* 2014;**5**:230.
65. Alkadhi K. Brain physiology and pathophysiology in mental stress. *ISRN Physiol* 2013;**2013**.
66. Herman JP, Ostrander MM, Mueller NK, Figueiredo H. Limbic system mechanisms of stress regulation: hypothalamo-pituitary-adrenocortical axis. *Prog Neuropsychopharmacol Biol Psychiatry* 2005;**29**(8):1201–13.
67. Smith SM, Vale WW. The role of the hypothalamic-pituitary-adrenal axis in neuroendocrine responses to stress. *Dialogues Clin Neurosci* 2006;**8**(4):383.
68. Kidd P. Neurodegeneration from mitochondrial insufficiency: nutrients, stem cells, growth factors, and prospects for brain rebuilding using integrative management. *Altern Med Rev* 2005;**10**(4):268–93.
69. Wallace DC. A mitochondrial paradigm of metabolic and degenerative diseases, aging, and cancer: a dawn for evolutionary medicine. *Annu Rev Genet* 2005;**39**:359.
70. Kapogiannis D, Mattson MP. Disrupted energy metabolism and neuronal circuit dysfunction in cognitive impairment and Alzheimer's disease. *Lancet Neurol* 2011;**10**(2):187–98.
71. Prabakaran S, Swatton JE, Ryan MM, Huffaker SJ, Huang JJ, Griffin JL, Wayland M, Freeman T, Dudbridge F, Lilley KS, Karp NA. Mitochondrial dysfunction in schizophrenia: evidence for compromised brain metabolism and oxidative stress. *Mol Psychiatry* 2004;**9**(7):684–97.
72. Roth SC, Baudin J, Cady E, Johal K, Townsend JP, Wyatt JS, Reynolds EO, Stewart AL. Relation of deranged neonatal cerebral oxidative metabolism with neurodevelopmental outcome and head circumference at 4 years. *Dev Med Child Neurol* 1997;**39**(11):718–25.

73. Zelnick N, et al. Mitochondrial encephalomyopathies presenting with features of autonomic and visceral dysfunction. *Pediatr Neurol* 1996;**14**(3):251–4.
74. Kanjwal K, et al. Autonomic dysfunction presenting as orthostatic intolerance in patients suffering from mitochondrial cytopathy. *Clin Cardiol* 2010;**33**(10):626–9.
75. Liu Z-W, Gan G, Suyama S, Gao X-B. Intracellular energy status regulates activity in hypocretin/orexin neurones: a link between energy and behavioural states. *J Physiol* 2011;**589**(Pt 17):4157–66. http://dx.doi.org/10.1113/jphysiol.2011.212514.
76. Tougas G. The autonomic nervous system in functional bowel disorders. *Gut* 2000;**47**(Suppl. 4). iv78–iv80.
77. Lonsdale D. Thiamine and magnesium deficiencies: keys to disease. *Medical Hypotheses* 2015;**84**(2):129–34.
78. Maassen AJ, et al. Mitochondrial diabetes: molecular mechanisms and clinical presentation. *Diabetes* 2004;**53**(Suppl. 1):S103–9. http://dx.doi.org/10.2337/diabetes.53.2007.S103.
79. Tobe EH. Cerebellar dysregulation and heterogeneity of mood disorders. *Neuropsychiatr Dis Treat* 2014;**10**:1381–4.
80. Alvares GA, Quintana DS, Hickie IB, Guastella AJ. Autonomic nervous system dysfunction in psychiatric disorders and the impact of psychotropic medications: a systematic review and meta-analysis. *J Psychiatry Neurosci* 2016;**41**(2):89.
81. Maddock RJ, Buonocore MH, Copeland LE, Richards AL. Elevated brain lactate responses to neural activation in panic disorder: a dynamic 1H-MRS study. *Mol Psychiatry* 2009;**14**(5):537–45.
82. Pappens M, De Peuter S, Vansteenwegen D, Van den Bergh O, Van Diest I. Psychophysiological responses to $CO_2$ inhalation. *Int J Psychophysiol* 2012;**84**(1):45–50.
83. Dratcu L. Panic, hyperventilation and perpetuation of anxiety. *Prog Neuropsychopharmacol Biol Psychiatry* 2000;**24**(7):1069–89.

# CHAPTER 3
# Mitochondria, Thiamine, and Autonomic Dysfunction

## Contents

| | |
|---|---|
| Understanding Mitochondrial Disorders: Moving Beyond Genetics | 60 |
|     Primary and Secondary Mitochondrial Disorders | 61 |
|     The Totality of Mitochondrial Genetics | 62 |
|     Mitochondrial Energetics | 63 |
| Mitochondrial Basics of Macro- and Micronutrients | 64 |
|     Beyond Macronutrients: Cellular Respiration Is Vitamin Dependent | 65 |
| From Diet to ATP: The Essential Nutrients in Mitochondrial Functioning | 67 |
|     Acetyl-CoA Synthesis | 68 |
|     Alpha Oxidation | 68 |
|     Beta Oxidation | 68 |
|     Lactate | 68 |
|     Electron Carriers | 69 |
|     Electron Transport Chain | 69 |
|     Redox Homeostasis: Antioxidants | 69 |
| Thiamine Chemistry and Mitochondrial Function | 70 |
|     Thiamine | 70 |
|     *Thiamine Monophosphate* | 72 |
|     *Thiamine Pyrophosphate* | 72 |
|     *A Deeper Perspective of TPP and the Pyruvate Dehydrogenase Complex* | 73 |
|     *TPP Allosterically Regulates TCA and ETC Proteins* | 74 |
|     *Thiamine in Nerve Function* | 75 |
|     *Thiamine in the Brain* | 77 |
| From Diet to Mitochondria: Understanding Thiamine Transporters | 77 |
|     Thiamine Transporters | 77 |
| Modern Thiamine Deficiency and Mitochondrial Damage | 79 |
|     High Calorie Malnutrition: An Underappreciated Culprit in Disease | 79 |
|     Modern Nutrient Deficiency in Context | 80 |
|     Thiamine Sufficiency Is Fragile | 81 |
|     *Naked Calories and Thiamine Deficiency* | 81 |
|     *Naturally Occurring Thiamine Inhibitors: Thiaminases* | 83 |
|     *From Cattle Research* | 84 |

| | |
|---|---|
| Pharmacologically Induced Thiamine Deficiency and Mitochondrial Damage | 85 |
| Environmental Chemicals Block Thiamine Uptake | 89 |
| Nutrient Deficiency, Mitochondria, and the Autonomic System | 90 |
|   Recognizing Thiamine Deficiency in Clinical Care | 90 |
| Rethinking Nutrition | 93 |
| References | 93 |

Mitochondrial defects contribute to a staggering array of disease processes. Whether the defect is a result of heritable genetic flaws, acquired genetic damage, or the more insidious functional disturbances, mitochondropathies sit at the nexus of many a modern disease. While once considered rare, mutations in mitochondrial DNA (mtDNA) are increasingly recognized in broad swathes of the population. Estimates of prevalence range from 1:4000[1] to as many as 1 in 500[2] when considering functional disturbances in the mitochondria. When we consider that functional disturbances in the mitochondria may be initiated by epigenetic alterations[3] in the nuclear DNA (nDNA) that interact with the mitochondria,[4] in mtDNA themselves,[5] by environmental factors such as toxicant exposure,[6] nutrient deficiency,[7] or some combination thereof, it is conceivable that the prevalence of mitochondrial disorders may be much greater. No matter the origins, when mitochondria are affected, we can be guaranteed two things: the autonomic system will be disrupted in some manner and thiamine will be involved.

In the previous chapter we went from a high-level view of the autonomic system from structure to function and from architecture to chemistry, highlighting regional presentations of dysautonomic symptoms while hinting at the molecular mechanisms. In this chapter we will approach dysautonomia from the bottom up; from the molecular cascades within mitochondria upward through cell signal transduction pathways that govern dysautonomic responses. We will look at thiamine chemistry from diet through metabolism, consider its role in enzymatic and nonenzymatic reactions, and elucidate its consequent impact on autonomic function.

## UNDERSTANDING MITOCHONDRIAL DISORDERS: MOVING BEYOND GENETICS

Although the impression most have of mitochondrial disease is that it is a disorder that presents itself at birth, in reality it can appear at any age. With advances in genetics and molecular biology over the last decade, it has been found that mitochondrial disease is not at all rare. Indeed, mitochondria are implicated in a wide range of seemingly independent disease processes including cardiomyopathy,[8] types 1 and 2 diabetes,[9] obesity,[10] schizophrenia,[11] bipolar disorder,[12] dementia and Alzheimer's disease (AD),[13] Parkinson's disease,[14] epilepsy,[15] cardiovascular disease,[16] chronic fatigue syndrome,[17] retinitis pigmentosa,[18] gastrointestinal dysmotility syndromes,[19] thyroid disorders,[20] neuropathy,[21] and cancer,[22] to name but a few. Most salient to our purposes, mitochondrial distress underlies beriberi and dysautonomic function.[23,24] The sheer diversity of conditions linked to mitochondrial function begs an important question about the origins of disease: how can so many disparate disease processes be connected to mitochondrial damage? Perhaps a better question is: why are we not addressing the mitochondria in all disease processes? And by association, why are we not looking for ways to improve mitochondrial functioning? The answers lie, to some degree, in the limits of the nomenclature used to describe mitochondrial disease. That is, despite decades of evidence to the contrary, we lay the blame of illness at the feet of genetics and with that fail to recognize the tractability of mitochondrial function, a tractability with a time course that extends well before mutations arise.

## Primary and Secondary Mitochondrial Disorders

Traditionally, mitochondrial disorders have been classified as primary or secondary, where primary mitochondrial disorders represent inherited mtDNA mutations and secondary disorders indicate the more functional or acquired disease processes attributable to lifestyle variables. With the increasing recognition of the inherent modifiability of mitochondrial function and subsequent pleiotropic clinical manifestations, the distinction between primary and secondary mitochondrial disease has become blurred but unfortunately has not entirely disappeared. We hold tightly to the notion that genetics equals disease or health. With mitochondria, perhaps even more so than in any other field, genetics, especially mitochondrial genetics, is but one component of a far more complicated picture. For while it is true that inherited mutations in mtDNA can wreak havoc on organismal health, it is also true that there is no one-to-one correspondence between mutation and disease expression.[25] MtDNA mutations explain a mere 15% of mitochondrial disease.[26] Moreover, in families with clear genotypic patterns caused by mtDNA mutation, the phenotypic expression of disease is often quite disparate.[27] In some cases, individuals within the same family, expressing the same constellation of mtDNA mutations, exhibit widely different health and disease profiles. Not only are the symptoms expressed differently, but at what age they are expressed varies as well. Some individuals are ill from birth or early childhood, while others do not become ill until adulthood, if at all.[28] This suggests that more is at play than simple heritable genetics. The evidence is clear, with the mitochondria, there appears to be a requisite threshold of stressors, a mutational load that has to be reached before pathogenesis becomes manifest.[29]

The technical term for the diversity of mtDNA-mediated disease expression is heteroplasmy, representing the aggregate ratio of normal mtDNA to mutated mtDNA. As mtDNA defects increase, so too does the propensity for disease. The mechanisms by which heteroplasmy propagate, however, emerge from environmental interactions: from stressors, either external or internal. This means that while it is true that mtDNA mutations are heritable, they are also inducible, and if they are inducible, they are responsive to environmental variables: variables that can be modified and manipulated for good or for ill. This is an important point that is often forgotten in our rush to identify genetic culprits.

## The Totality of Mitochondrial Genetics

It is well known that mtDNA is inherited from the mother. Mitochondria from the sperm enter the ovum but do not contribute genetic information to the embryo. Paternal mitochondria are marked with ubiquitin to select them for later destruction inside the embryo.[30] Thus a defect in cellular transmission of mitochondria gives rise to a form of maternal inheritance. What are less well appreciated are the tightly coordinated interactions between nDNA and mtDNA that maintain mitochondrial function. Indeed, the majority of ~1500 mitochondrial proteins required for proper mitochondrial functioning are transcribed from nuclear genes and translated in the cell cytosol before being transported into the mitochondria,[31] suggesting a paternal contribution to this otherwise maternal inheritance pattern. Moreover, just as nDNA is susceptible to epigenetic alterations, environmental interactions that effectively modify the activity of a gene, so too is mtDNA,[26] perhaps even more so because of the lack of protective histones. Conversely, mitochondria are capable of initiating epigenetic changes in nDNA, a reciprocity that has only recently begun to be untangled.[3] The final common products of these interactions may be an accumulation of what are designated as *de novo* mtDNA mutations: mutations that arise at any time across the lifespan, from the oocyte through old age[32] through a myriad environmental insults. So, far from being hardwired, mitochondrial functioning adapts across the lifespan, with some of those adaptations resulting in mutation.

Despite the recognition that life engenders secondary or *de novo* mutations, and that once these mutations reach a certain threshold disease emerges, we are still trapped by a nomenclature that attributes disease to genetics. Whether inherited or acquired, the concept of mitochondrial heteroplasmy is a concept based upon genetic alterations. It fails to recognize the functional derangements that must precede the induction of a mutation. That is, before epigenetic changes are recognized and *de novo* mutations reach detectable heteroplasmic proportions, there are functional changes in mitochondrial activity; modifications in operating capacity to ensure cell survival that either will be managed effectively or not, and, if not, provoke damage.

What determines whether and when mitochondrial stressors result in mutation, and whether or when these mutations result in pathology, may have as much to do with the type of stressor as with the individual's capacity to adapt and withstand the insult. This, we believe, is the missing piece in the mitochondrial puzzle. This is where oxidative metabolism comes into play; where $Ca^{2+}$ sequestration, metal homeostasis, steroidogenesis, and inflammasome signaling come into play; where mitochondrial morphology, fission and fusion capacity, and mitochondrial death cascades are important; and where mitochondrial functioning, at the most fundamental levels, determines how and where disease processes emerge. Permutations in these functions, whether resulting from, or in advance of, mtDNA mutations, are central to modern disease and are, more often than not, ignored in favor of genetic answers.

## Mitochondrial Energetics

Mitochondrial energetics is at the foundation of cellular function. This is so fundamental to life that its lack of consideration in modern medicine until recently has been truly amazing. Mitochondria are the "engines" of each cell, where food is converted into energy. To the extent that the mitochondria are inefficient or incapable of meeting the demands of a changing environment, not only do the mitochondria begin to fail but the cells in which they reside fail as well, initiating tissue and organ injury. These functional changes in the mitochondria can not only induce disease independent of mtDNA damage, but also, when they are severe or chronic enough, induce mtDNA damage. Thus, mitochondrial efficiency and flexibility are key components of organismal health and in many ways determine whether an environmental stressor can be prevented or managed effectively. Just as the autonomic system maintains organismal homeostasis and survival in the face of an ever-changing environment, the mitochondria must respond to the molecular cues precipitated by those same stressors to maintain cellular homeostasis and survival. In that regard, the mitochondria are akin to a mini autonomic nervous system, sensing danger, signaling the appropriate response, and adapting accordingly. How well the mitochondria respond and adapt is determined not just by genetics but by the available resources, for example, the nutrient cofactors that power mitochondrial functions.

## MITOCHONDRIAL BASICS OF MACRO- AND MICRONUTRIENTS

The most recognized role of mitochondria is to convert dietary fuel into cellular energy or ATP. That is, through a series of enzymatic reactions, carbon molecules from dietary macronutrients (fats, amino acids, and carbohydrates) are extracted or catabolized by the process of oxidative phosphorylation or oxidative metabolism. The electrons gained are then shuttled along to power other enzymatic reactions with the net result being the production of ATP molecules. ATP then escapes the mitochondrial matrix through an exchanger in the inner mitochondrial membrane and is available to power all energy-requiring mitochondrial and cellular functions. This is the traditional view of mitochondria: dietary fuel in, energy out.

Consistent with this perspective, when considering the nutrients required for mitochondrial functioning, a vast majority of the research speaks of macronutrients, the fats, proteins, and carbohydrates that are ultimately converted to ATP. Some of the latest research suggests a reduction in these macronutrients leads to increased mitochondrial performance and reduction in aging and age-related degenerative diseases.[33] The presumption is that all nutrients are created equally, e.g., that calories are calories and no matter the origins of those calories, the end result will be ATP. Indeed, from the mitochondrial perspective, each fuel, no matter its origins, will be broken down into its carbon skeleton, and through series of reactions the final output will be ATP—cellular energy. In that sense, the fuel source makes little difference: the net result will always be ATP. However, and this is a big however, what this perspective fails to recognize is that to get from fats, proteins, or carbohydrates to ATP, there is an entire factory of enzymatic reactions that absolutely require noncaloric micronutrients—vitamins and minerals—to function properly. Mitochondria cannot process the dietary fuel into cellular fuel without the accompanying micronutrients. Simply reducing the macronutrients, while it may reduce the ultimate processing demand on mitochondria, thereby eliciting favorable compensatory reactions and allowing the enzymes to "catch up," does nothing to address what is likely the core problem–that the enzyme machinery within the mitochondria are starving, and because they are starving, not only are they incapable of meeting the processing demands to maintain homeostasis, but also they are initiating a number of compensatory reactions that induce damage and many of the disease processes we see in modern medicine.

## Beyond Macronutrients: Cellular Respiration Is Vitamin Dependent

To illustrate the importance of dietary micronutrients, let us briefly consider the most basic of operations, cellular aerobic respiration. For efficient aerobic respiration and the conversion of carbohydrates, the most abundantly consumed foodstuffs in the Western diet, into ATP, we need a ready supply of oxygen plus 22 essential micronutrients. Absent either oxygen and/or micronutrients, aerobic respiration falters. To compensate, energy is generated anaerobically, a far less efficient process. The production of ATP from glucose, through mitochondrial pathways, has an approximately 13 times higher yield during aerobic respiration compared with fermentation. Although anaerobic metabolism is an effective adaptive mechanism in the short term, it is ultimately disastrous to cellular function in the long term.

Lack of oxygen availability causes the shift from aerobic to anaerobic respiration. On the surface, the transport of oxygen appears to be straightforward. In the absence of injury, blockage, respiratory illness, or excessive exercise demands, oxygen availability is ever-present and automatically used in oxidation. However, research over the last few decades shows that oxygenation requires vitamins and minerals. That is, whether or how effectively blood oxygenation and cellular respiration occur is dependent on dietary vitamins and minerals.[34] Early beriberi researchers knew this decades ago. One of the cardinal signs of beriberi was disparate oxygenation in arterial versus venous blood, with arterial blood showing consistently reduced oxygenation.[35] However, it has been shown by Japanese investigators that intravenous administration of the thiamine derivative, thiamine propyl disulfide, causes an increase in oxyhemoglobin levels without any change in deoxyhemoglobin.[36] Similarly, cocarboxylase (also known as thiamine pyrophosphate, TPP), administered to dogs subjected to endotoxic shock, inhibited deterioration in metabolic function and improved maintenance of normal oxygen consumption. Significant improvements in mean arterial pressure and cardiac index were also observed.[37]

Molecular oxygen deficiency, called pseudohypoxia, develops in response to limited nutrient cofactors, specifically thiamine. Just like an ischemic hypoxia, the thiamine-deficient hypoxia forces the switch to the less efficient anaerobic metabolism. In the short term, this switch is a life-saving, compensatory reaction. In the long term, however, the net reduction in ATP becomes problematic, initiating additional reactions that ultimately prove devastating to the mitochondria and the cells/tissues/organs in which they reside.

Among the compensatory reactions observed in hypoxia is a concomitant increase in hypoxia inducible factor (HIF1α)-mediated gene expression. HIF1α and its counterparts (HIF1β, HIF2α, and HIF3α) are the master regulators of oxygen homeostasis,[38] activated in states of cellular oxygen deprivation.[39] The sole purpose of the HIF proteins is to adapt to the low-oxygen state and facilitate cell survival. HIF activation signals at least 100 other proteins that serve to bring more oxygen and fuel to the cells: proteins involved in angiogenesis, erythropoiesis and iron metabolism, glucose metabolism, growth factors, and, interestingly enough, apoptosis[39] (selective cell death is an important component of survival). HIF proteins also interact with thiamine activated mitochondrial enzymes[40] involved in oxidative metabolism, suggesting potential sensing and signaling mechanisms that connect thiamine deficiency, reduced oxidation, and HIF activation. Notably, overexpression of HIF has been identified in cancer and ischemic diseases, but also in myriad other seemingly diverse disease processes such as endometriosis,[41] a variety of autoimmune diseases,[42] and, of course, in thiamine deficiency disorders.

Micronutrient deficiencies lead to hypoxia, perhaps not as obviously as in emergent cases, such as stroke, heart attack, or other injury, or even as would be expected with strenuous exercise, but it is the equivalent of hypoxia all the same. The implications of this are staggering. Cellular respiration is dependent not only on the inhaled oxygen, but also on the presence of dietary vitamins and minerals. These vitamins and minerals are not supplied equally in all foods and are easily depleted by common pharmaceuticals. Since thiamine deficiency induces HIF-1α-mediated gene expression similar to that observed in hypoxic stress,[34] it is difficult not to wonder if deficiencies in thiamine and/or other micronutrients might represent final common pathways to disease initiation and/or maintenance. As we

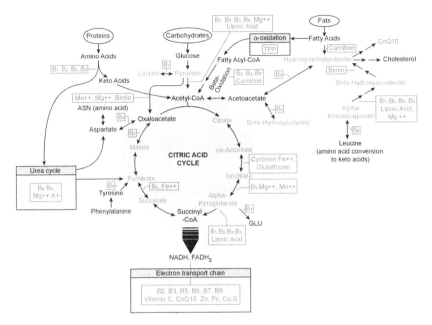

**Figure 3.1** Basic glycolysis. *CoA*, coenzyme A; *GABA*, gamma-aminobutyric acid; *PDHC*, pyruvate dehydrogenase complex; *αKDGH*, alpha-ketoglutarate dehydrogenase.

unpack the nutrient requirements for mitochondrial functioning (Fig. 3.1), it is useful to consider whether current dietary practices provide the required resources to stave off disease.

## FROM DIET TO ATP: THE ESSENTIAL NUTRIENTS IN MITOCHONDRIAL FUNCTIONING

From the most basic function of oxygen hemostasis through the complex chemistry that converts food fuels into cellular fuels, vitamins and minerals are critical. From pyruvate to acetyl coenzyme A (acetyl-CoA), the first steps in cellular bioenergetics where carbohydrate metabolism takes place require no less than 10 nutrients. The enzymes of the pyruvate dehydrogenase complex (PDHC), which sit atop this process and effectively govern the entry of carbohydrates into citric acid cycle, also called the tricarboxylic acid (TCA) cycle, are profoundly dependent upon thiamine (B1). Other nutrients such as riboflavin (B2), niacin (B3), pantothenic (B5) acid, and lipoic acid, in addition to iron, sulfur, cysteine, magnesium, and manganese, are also required as we move down the glycolysis pathway.

## Acetyl-CoA Synthesis

Acetyl-CoA, derived from pyruvate oxidation, or from the beta-oxidation of fatty acids, both being dependent on the presence of thiamine as the rate-limiting factor, is the only fuel to enter into the TCA or citric acid cycle. It is the oxidation of the acetate portion of acetyl-CoA that produces carbon dioxide and water. The energy thus released is then captured in the form of ATP. Mitochondrial matrix calcium levels can reach a marked increase, necessary for the activation of isocitrate dehydrogenase, one of the key regulatory enzymes of the citric acid cycle.

Acetyl-CoA is the substrate for acetylcholine, the primary neurotransmitter of the autonomic system, common to both the sympathetic and parasympathetic branches and myelin, the protective sheath surrounding axons[43] of the nervous system.

## Alpha Oxidation

TPP is now known to be essential as a cofactor for 2-hydroxyacyl CoA lyase (HACL1)[44] in alpha oxidation in the peroxisome. This enzyme is involved in the alpha oxidation of phytanic acid and 2-hydroxy straight-chain fatty acids. Although the HACL1 gene has been mapped to chromosome 3p25, no diseases have been linked to this gene locus so the phenotype is unknown. The authors note that it can be expected that under clinical conditions when dietary thiamine is restricted, alpha oxidation would be impaired, leading to the accumulation of phytanic acid and 2-hydroxy straight-chain fatty acids. Finding these in urine would give us new information in depicting the effects of thiamine deficiency.

## Beta Oxidation

Beta oxidation, a sequel to alpha oxidation, oxidizes fatty acids and requires L-carnitine.[45]

## Lactate

Lactate recycling requires thiamine. In the absence of molecular oxygen, anaerobic metabolism recycles lactic acid and pyruvate acts as the hydrogen acceptor. The enzymes involved in these reactions—the PDHC and lactate dehydrogenase[46]—are both thiamine dependent. In the musculature when lactate builds up, whether by exercise-induced exertion and the accompanying demand for oxygen or by thiamine deficiency, muscle fatigue ensues. In critical care, thiamine deficiency appears common. Case Example 3.1 illustrates the role of thiamine in effective lactate utilization.[47]

### Case Example 3.1 Thiamine-Deficient Lactic Acidosis

Three hospitalized patients were reported who had received parenteral nutrition without vitamin supplementation. All of them had severe lactic acidosis and unstable circulatory state, a severe form of impaired near-coma consciousness, and Wernicke's encephalopathy. Intravenous administration of thiamine and magnesium resulted in a rapid and marked restoration of acid-base balance, hemodynamic stability, and the disappearance of neurological disturbances.

## Electron Carriers

Each of these pathways is energy dependent, using the energy released from these processes to reduce the electron carriers nicotinamide adenine dinucleotide ($NAD^+$), yielding NADH, and flavin adenine dinucleotide (FAD), yielding FADH2. NAD and FAD require niacin and riboflavin, respectively.[48]

## Electron Transport Chain

From there, energy from the electrons is used to pump hydrogen ions (protons) into the mitochondrial intermembrane space. The five complexes of the electron transport chain (ETC) require additional nutrients including ubiquinone, riboflavin, iron, sulfur, and copper.[49] Ubiquinone or coenzyme Q (CoQ) carries electrons from complexes I and II to complex III.[50] Vitamins B2, B6, B12, folate, pantothenic acid, niacin, and vitamin C are required for CoQ synthesis. Heme synthesis, a prerequisite for complex IV, requires seven nutrients: pyridoxine (B6), pantothenic acid (B5), zinc, riboflavin, iron, copper, and biotin (B7).[7] Biotin deficiency leads to loss of complex IV functionality directly via a reduction in heme synthesis.[51] Nutrient deficits affecting complex IV lead to oxidant leakage and DNA damage, resulting in mitochondrial deterioration and cellular aging.[7] Finally, ATP synthesis occurs in complex V. Impediments to ATP production imperil cell function and viability, eventually leading to cell death.

## Redox Homeostasis: Antioxidants

As a byproduct of ATP production during both physiological and abnormal electron transport, the mitochondria release reactive oxygen species (ROS). During normal activities, 1%–5% of all oxygen consumed by the cell is converted to ROS. Excess ROS are cytotoxic. However, at low concentrations,

ROS act as critical signaling molecules that are absolutely requisite for signal transduction and gene expression in a variety of processes involved in injury response.[52] Redox homeostasis, an equilibrium of sorts[53] between pro- and antioxidants, is maintained by a number of factors, nutrients among them. CoQ,[54] lipoic acid,[55] and vitamins C,[56] E,[57] niacin,[58] folate,[59] and vitamin D[60] are the nutrient-free radical scavengers or antioxidants. These nutrients, along with glutathione,[61] known as the master antioxidant (which is dependent upon vitamin C and thiamine[62] and other dietary precursors),[63] are all critical for ROS equilibrium via multiple mechanisms. Lipoic acid, for example, is involved in approximately 200 antioxidant and protective enzymatic reactions.[48]

Damaged or nutrient-deficient mitochondria increase ROS production, as does macronutrient overload, while simultaneously impairing redox capacity.[64] Without the proper balance of micronutrients to maintain mitochondrial efficiencies and buffer ROS production, the feedforward cascade of oxidative damage, cellular aging, and disease ensues.

## THIAMINE CHEMISTRY AND MITOCHONDRIAL FUNCTION

It should be evident that nutrients are critical for mitochondrial function. Thiamine, specifically, fulfills a special role as a gatekeeper of sorts, governing each of the energy pathways. In addition to its role in energy metabolism, thiamine is critical for other aspects of mitochondrial functioning. Culture of neuroblastoma cells in the presence of thiamine deficiency leads to signs of necrosis. Mitochondria are uncoupled and their cristae become disorganized. Glutamate from glutamine is no longer oxidized and accumulates. When thiamine is added to the cells, oxygen consumption increases, respiratory control is restored, and normal mitochondrial morphology is recovered within 1 h.[23] The remainder of this chapter covers the role of thiamine in mitochondrial function (Fig. 3.2).

### Thiamine

Thiamine, one of the earliest vitamins to be discovered and synthesized, is found in lean pork and other meats, wheat germ, liver and other organ meats, poultry, eggs, fish, beans, peas, nuts, and whole grains. Dairy products, fruit, and vegetables are not good sources. The recommended daily allowance is 0.5 mg per 1000 kcal. Although this may be adequate for a normal individual consuming a healthy diet, it may only be a marginal consumption. Considerable losses occur during cooking or other heat

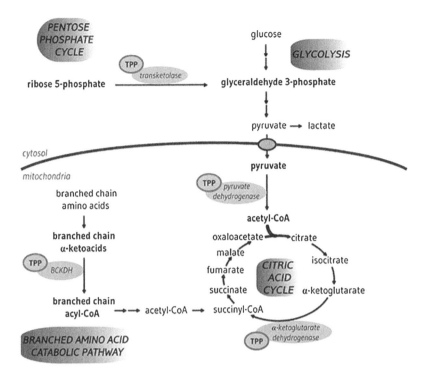

BCKDH, branched chain α-ketoacid dehydrogenase complex; CoA, coenzyme A; TPP, thiamin pyrophosphate.

**Figure 3.2** The role of thiamine pyrophosphate in mitochondrial function. *BCKDH*, Branched-chain α-ketoacid dehydrogenase complex; *CoA*, coenzyme A; *TPP*, thiamine pyrophosphate.

processing of food. Polyphenolic compounds in coffee and tea can inactivate thiamine, so heavy use of these beverages could compromise thiamine nutrition.[65]

Although TPP is the best-known thiamine compound, at least three other thiamine phosphates occur naturally in most cells. Thiamine triphosphate (TTP) and the recently discovered adenosine TTP illustrate the complexity of thiamine biochemistry.[66]

Thiamine consists of a pyrimidine ring (2,5-dimethyl-6-aminopyrimidine) and a thiazolium ring (4-methyl-5-hydroxyethyl-thiazole) joined by a methylene bridge and occurs in mammalian systems in at least four forms: free thiamine and three phosphorylated compounds. Some evidence exists for a methylated thiamine.[67] The presence in mammalian cells of free thiamine and thiamine monophosphate (TMP), respectively, the precursor and the dephosphorylation product of active coenzyme, can be understood in relation to the well-known activity of TPP.

### Thiamine Monophosphate

TMP is an intermediate in the hydrolysis of TPP to thiamine, not in its synthesis. TPP is directly formed by thiamine pyrophosphorylation from ATP. Excess thiamine may be stored to a limited extent in liver and erythrocytes in the form of TPP. When circulating thiamine levels decrease, the stored TPP can be hydrolyzed to TMP, which is then hydrolyzed to thiamine and released into the circulation. No specific thiamine pyrophosphatases or thiamine monophosphatases have been described and no biological role of TMP is known. By the action of alkaline phosphatase, TMP can also be formed in the intestine from TPP present in the ingested food.[68]

### Thiamine Pyrophosphate

Also known as thiamine diphosphate or cocarboxylase, TPP fulfills multiple biochemical roles in energy metabolism.

1. TPP is a cofactor for enzymatic reactions that cleave alpha-keto acids. It has long been known that it activates decarboxylation of pyruvate in the PDHC and is the rate-limiting factor. The complex is a group of enzymes and cofactors that form acetyl-CoA. This condenses with oxaloacetate to form citrate, the first component of the citric acid cycle. Since pyruvate is derived from glucose via the Embden–Meyerhof pathway, it should be emphasized that the energy drive from oxidation of glucose is dependent upon TPP. A mutation in the decarboxylating component of pyruvate dehydrogenase was responsible for intermittent episodes of clinical thiamine-responsive cerebellar ataxia.[69]
2. TPP has the same role in the decarboxylating component of alpha-ketoglutarate dehydrogenase, a link in the sequential metabolism of pyruvate through the citric acid cycle. A mutation has been described in three siblings resulting in death at 30 months of age.[70]
3. TPP is active in branched-chain amino acid (leucine, isoleucine, and valine) dehydrogenase that is similar in structure to pyruvate dehydrogenase. Thiamine and magnesium are the cofactors for the decarboxylating component of the enzyme complex. Thiamine-responsive maple syrup urine disease has been reported.[71]
4. Although glyoxalase and methylglyoxal were reported in thiamine-deficient rats[72] and diabetes was the first disease state where evidence emerged for increased formation of methylglyoxal, further clinical

studies are required. The development of high-dose thiamine therapy for early-stage diabetic nephropathy suggests that the glyoxalase system is likely to be a continuing future focus.[73] Accumulation of triosephosphates and the increased formation of methylglyoxal in intracellular hyperglycemia are implicated in diabetic complications. To assess the effect of thiamine supplementation on the accumulation of triosephosphates and methylglyoxal formation in cellular hyperglycemia, an in vitro experiment with human red cells in hyperglycemic conditions showed that thiamine supplementation increased the activity of transketolase, decreasing the concentration of triosephosphates and the formation of methylglyoxal.[74]

From a clinical standpoint, enzymatic failure and thiamine dependency have been described in each of these enzyme complexes.[75]

*A Deeper Perspective of TPP and the Pyruvate Dehydrogenase Complex*
The process of oxidative dehydrogenation is a complicated reaction. For oxidation of pyruvate, three enzymes and five coenzymes are necessary, the whole complex being known as the PDHC. Its integrated activity is regulated by ATP concentration. First, a hydroxyethyl derivative of the thiazole ring of TPP is formed. Then the hydroxyethyl group is transferred to one of the sulfur atoms of the cyclic disulfide group in lipoic acid. This is covalently bound to dihydrolipoyl transacetylase, the second enzyme in the complex. Lipoic acid is reduced to its dithiol form; the acetyl group is enzymatically transferred to the thiol group of CoA, forming acetyl-CoA that leaves the complex in its free form. Dihydrolipoyl dehydrogenase, which contains the reducible coenzyme FAD, reoxidizes dihydrolipyl transacetylase to its disulfide form, and FAD acts as a hydrogen receptor. The reduced FAD (FADH2) is reoxidized by $NAD^+$, regenerating FAD and forming NADH. NADH carries the electrons to the ETC.

TPP also serves as coenzyme in many enzyme systems involving conversion of alpha-keto acids to acytoins, aldehydes, carboxylic acids, and acyl phosphates.[69]

It is a cofactor in the transketolase enzyme that occurs twice in the hexose monophosphate shunt (HMPS).[76] The HMPS, also called the pentose phosphate cycle, is an alternative glucose oxidation pathway that provides pentose phosphate for nucleotide synthesis and supplies reduced nicotinamide adenine dinucleotide phosphate for synthetic pathways that include steroid hydroxylation and fatty acid synthesis. The proportion of glucose metabolized by this route is high in lactating mammary gland, adrenal cortex, leukocytes, and erythrocytes and TPP must thereby play a critical role in these metabolic processes. Since this pathway is present in erythrocytes, measurement of transketolase activity in these cells is a useful laboratory test for TPP deficiency.

## TPP Allosterically Regulates TCA and ETC Proteins

Beyond its coenzyme role, TPP also regulates the expression and activity of a plethora of additional mitochondrial proteins throughout the TCA and ETC including succinate thiokinase, succinate dehydrogenase, malate dehydrogenase, glutamate dehydrogenase, and pyridoxal kinase.[77] For example, in thiamine-deficient mice, succinate thiokinase and succinate dehydrogenase, enzymes not typically associated with thiamine deficiency, are decreased as much as or more than the pyruvate dehydrogenase enzymes (Fig. 3.2). Succinate thiokinase (also called succinyl-CoA synthetase) forms a multienzyme complex with the alpha-ketoglutarate dehydrogenase enzymes[78] and catalyzes the succinyl-CoA to succinate. Succinate dehydrogenase is present in the TCA cycle, where it oxidizes succinate to fumarate[79] and uses electrons generated from that reaction to catalyze the reduction of ubiquinone to ubiquinol for complex II of the ETC. In that way, succinate dehydrogenase couples the TCA to the ETC. There is some indication that the enzyme acts as a ubiquinone (CoQ10) sensor and regulator of sorts.[80] Recall that CoQ10 is critical to electron transport, suggesting that a diminished thiamine risks not only TCA impairment but also ETC impairment. As an example, deficiencies in succinate dehydrogenase are linked to a range of disparate disease processes, including encephalopathies.[81] Similarly, CoQ10 deficiencies are emerging as a critical component of mitochondrial disease.[82] Thiamine deficiency is linked to both.

As might be expected, when succinate dehydrogenase activity diminishes, compensatory reactions ensue. One of those compensatory reactions, designed to maintain ATP flux and help with the removal of excess alpha-ketoglutarate, succinyl-CoA, and succinate, involves the upregulation of the malate shunt.[83] Malate dehydrogenase, part of the malate shunt responsible for the interconversion of malate to oxaloacetate and the subsequent removal of oxaloacetate from the mitochondria, is also modulated by thiamine. In culture, malate dehydrogenase activity is allosterically modulated by thiamine, showing twofold upregulation in the presence of TPP.[84] Similarly, thiamine deficiency reduces malate dehydrogenase by almost

20%.[77] The end result is an estimated reduction of ATP from 38 to 13 relative units.[77]

Similarly, both glutamate dehydrogenase and pyridoxal kinase are also influenced by thiamine. Glutamate dehydrogenase, a key enzyme involved in glutamate degradation, accounts for as much as 10% of the total protein content in the mitochondrial matrix of astrocytes. The enzyme complex links amino acid metabolism with the TCA in the brain.[85] Thiamine deficiency reduces glutamate dehydrogenase activity, effectively increasing extracellular concentrations of glutamate and the propensity of glutamatergic lesions in vulnerable regions of the brain.[86]

Finally, pyridoxal kinase and pyridoxine 5'-phosphate oxidase are two enzymes responsible for converting dietary vitamin B6 into the active cofactor form pyridoxal 5'-phosphate (PLP). PLP is active in over 140 enzymatic reactions throughout the body, including within the ETC of the mitochondria.[87] Pyridoxal kinase is downregulated with thiamine deficiency[84] contributing to reduced ETC efficiency and diminished ATP. Additionally, because of its role in tryptophan degradation, diminished PLP produces several metabolites that are neurotoxic, including quinolinic acid.[88]

### Thiamine in Nerve Function

In 1938 Minz[89] first suggested a relationship between thiamine and nervous excitation when he observed that thiamine was released into the bathing medium when the pneumogastric nerve from an ox was stimulated. In 1979 Cooper and Pincus[90] reviewed the evidence that there was a possibility that thiamine has a function in the nervous system distinct from its activity as a cofactor to enzymes. Like Minz, they found that nerve stimulation in experimental animal systems resulted in the decline of the level of TPP and TTP from the stimulated nerve. The released metabolites were in the form of TMP and free thiamine, making it difficult to interpret the function of the vitamin in nerve conduction. They found that thiamine appeared to be uniformly distributed in nervous tissue and was highly localized in membrane structures. After intracerebroventricular injection of radioactive thiamine into rats, the distribution of the esters was found to be thiamine 8%–12%, TMP 12%–14%, TPP 72%–74%, and TTP 2%–3%.[91]

In 1969 Cooper and associates published their finding of TTP deficiency in Leigh's disease, also known as subacute necrotizing encephalomyelopathy (SNE).[92] The pathophysiology of this disease is similar, but not identical, to that of Wernicke's disease. Their diagnosis depended upon finding a substance in urine that reportedly inhibited the formation of TTP.[93] The substance was never identified and this important research was eventually discontinued for lack of funding. Urine from several patients suspected of thiamine deficiency symptoms that was sent to Cooper's laboratory was reported positive for this test and responded to thiamine supplementation. None of these patients could be considered to be examples of Leigh's disease (D. Lonsdale, Unpublished observations). It was the only laboratory study ever reported to indicate TTP deficiency and there is presently no known clinically available method of depicting this vitally important link in our knowledge of thiamine metabolism in the brain. Although SNE is now considered the most common pediatric presentation of mitochondrial disease,[94] thiamine pyrophosphokinase, the enzyme that synthesizes TPP, has been implicated as one of the mutations that causes it and it is considered to be a treatable condition.[95] All of this information begs the question whether mitochondrial dysfunction is always genetically determined or whether it can be acquired as a result of prolonged cofactor deficiency, environmental trauma, recreational drugs, or even from prescription drugs.

Bettendorff and associates reported their research on TTP using the electric organ of the eel *Electrophorus electricus*.[96] They found that 87% of the total thiamine content of the electric organ in the eel was in the form of TTP, suggesting the great importance of this ester in nerve physiology since this organ is an adaptation of a nerve–muscle junction to create a condenser. They indicated that the real substrate of TTP phosphatase is probably a 1:1 complex of $Mg^{2+}$ and TTP. Incubation of rat brain homogenates with thiamine and TPP led to synthesis of TTP that appeared to be an activator of chloride channels having a large unit conductance.[97] In mammalian tissues TTP concentrations are regulated by a specific thiamine triphosphatase.[98] It must be stated, however, that the role of TTP is still incompletely understood.

Considerable experimental support exists for the involvement of thiamine compounds in the central nervous system and TTP appears to play a vital role that is independent of the cofactor function of TPP. Its formation from TPP is catalyzed by TPP–ATP phosphoryltransferase in the presence of magnesium. Its exact place in cellular metabolism remains somewhat of a mystery, but evidence is in favor of its action being related to excitable membrane. Thiamine triphosphatase, diphosphatase, and monophosphatase catalyze the respective hydrolysis reactions from TTP to free thiamine. All require magnesium.

## Thiamine in the Brain

TPP is the rate-limiting cofactor in pyruvic dehydrogenase and as such it plays a central role in the mechanisms involving oxidation, particularly glucose. Since there is no known storage for it in the body, it must be supplied continuously in the diet. As glucose is the only fuel that the central nervous system normally uses, lack of thiamine would be expected to interfere with its function, and it does. The response to any form of stress results in acceler-

> **Case Example 3.2 Intermittent Ataxia Precipitated by Thiamine Deficiency**
> The best example of this was reported in a child with intermittent episodes of cerebellar ataxia caused by thiamine dependency. Attacks of ataxia were initiated invariably by a source of environmental stress. This included a simple infection such as a cold, a mild head injury, and even an inoculation. On one occasion he experienced an attack of asthma and became unconscious when he entered an air-conditioned store from a 90°F environmental temperature, thus exhibiting acute environmental temperature change as a source of stress. He had never experienced asthma before and we believe that this illustrates that the pathophysiology was mediated through autonomic dysfunction.

ated activity in the central control of adaptive mechanisms and the need for thiamine rises in proportion to the rate of glucose utilization. Case Example 3.2 illustrates how stress increases the demand for thiamine.[69]

## FROM DIET TO MITOCHONDRIA: UNDERSTANDING THIAMINE TRANSPORTERS

## Thiamine Transporters

As an essential micronutrient, thiamine is derived entirely from diet. Absorption of thiamine takes place in the lower intestine (explaining why gastric bypass patients are susceptible to thiamine deficiency[99]), mediated by a group of membrane transporter proteins, classified as solute carriers (SLCs). The SLC group of membrane transporter proteins includes 395 members organized into 52 families.[100] The SLC gene family of SLCs for thiamine is a family of three transporter proteins with significant structural similarity, transporting substrates with different structure and ionic charge. SLC19A1 mediates the transport of reduced folate and its analogs and SLC19A2 mediates the transport of thiamine. SLC19A3 is also capable of transporting thiamine.[101] Mutations in the gene(s) encoded for SLC19A2 cause thiamine-responsive megaloblastic anemia (TRMA) and SLC19A3 mutations cause biotin-responsive basal ganglia disease.[102]

Over the years, additional mutations have been observed in these transporters, suggesting the possibility that SLC mutations are not as rare as once thought. For example, a novel transition mutation of the SLC19A2 was identified in a girl with Rogers syndrome, now called TRMA. Her symptoms included megaloblastic anemia, diabetes, and deafness. Although muscle biopsy was negative, biochemical analysis showed severe pyruvate dehydrogenase and complex I deficiencies. Supplementation with high dose thiamine restored complex I activity in the fibroblasts.[103] Thirteen patients from seven families with mutations in SLC19A2 have been studied for a median of 9 years. The anemia and diabetes mellitus responded to oral thiamine hydrochloride, but during puberty thiamine supplements became ineffective. Almost all patients require insulin therapy and regular blood transfusions after puberty.[104] TRMA syndrome can manifest at any time between infancy and adolescence. Not all cardinal findings are present initially. The anemia typically improves with a pharmacological dose of thiamine. Variable improvement in diabetes occurs, but the hearing loss is apparently irreversible. Although a delay in the onset of deafness may be possible, a 2-year-old girl has been reported with diabetes and anemia with a novel mutation in the SLC19A2 gene. The patient with this new mutation did not suffer from hearing loss.[105]

A 3-year-old boy was reported with a novel SLC19A2 gene mutation. He had insulin-dependent diabetes and respiratory illness, both with onset at 11 months, bilateral profound hearing loss with onset at 7 months, refractory anemia at 2 years, and decreased visual acuity and photophobia. His condition improved markedly several days after the initiation of 100 mg/day of thiamine was started. The authors emphasized early diagnosis for potentially effective treatment.[103] A 30-day-old patient has been reported with a mutation in the SLC19A3 gene. An increased level of lactate in the blood and cerebrospinal fluid, a high excretion of alpha-ketoglutarate in urine, and increased concentrations of branched-chain amino acids leucine and isoleucine in plasma were found. After treatment with thiamine and biotin, irritability and opisthotonus disappeared and the patient recovered consciousness. Biochemical disturbances reportedly disappeared within 48 h.[106]

The potential importance of the interrelationship of genetics, stress, and energy was illustrated by hypothesizing that sudden infant death syndrome may require a variable combination of all three components, the third component being abnormal thiamine metabolism.[107] To illustrate the genetic/stress aspect, five adolescents with post-Gardasil postural orthostatic tachycardia syndrome (POTS) were reported to have variable single nucleotide polymorphisms (SNPs) in 19A2, 19A3, and 25A19 thiamine transporters. This concept was again emphasized in 2013 when an 18-year-old girl was brought to Dr. Lonsdale's attention because she developed POTS after receiving human papilloma virus (HPV) vaccination. A subsequent transketolase test revealed thiamine deficiency. As a result of this, two other girls and a boy suffering from post-HPV vaccination POTS all demonstrated thiamine deficiency.[108] Although a small number of cases like these prove nothing, it begs the question: how common are SNPs in formulating a risk of this nature?

## MODERN THIAMINE DEFICIENCY AND MITOCHONDRIAL DAMAGE

### High Calorie Malnutrition: An Underappreciated Culprit in Disease

From the preceding sections it should be clear that dietary micronutrients are indispensable to mitochondrial functioning, with thiamine top among them. Inasmuch as mitochondria govern the most fundamental of all cellular functions, bioenergetics, in addition to regulating inflammatory cascades,[109] steroidogenesis,[110] ion homeostasis,[111] heme synthesis,[7] ROS production and detoxification, and cell life and death,[112] mitochondrial fitness must be considered central to organismal health. Unfortunately, nutrient therapies represent at once both the potential height of mitochondrial medicine[113–120] for those lucky enough to find such practitioners and lack of medical insight for the unfortunate rest of the population.[121]

Which side of the fence one falls on depends entirely on how one views health and disease—hardwired or malleable. We believe in the malleability of mitochondrial function and therefore the diseases originating from mitochondrial dysfunction. Both chemistry and clinical experience support this hypothesis. This begs the question: how is it that, in regions where obesity has reached epidemic proportions, nutrient deficiency is possible? The answer lies in the type of calories consumed. Highly processed carbohydrates, of high macronutrient but low micronutrient content, induce oxidative stress.[122]

High calorie malnutrition, caused mainly by excessive ingestion of simple carbohydrates, is widely encountered in Western countries and does as much to derail mitochondrial functioning as the malnutrition derived of scarcity. As an example, in recent years nutrient deficiencies have been observed across all economic and social strata. Although the estimates of malnutrition vary by study, nutrient, and population sampled, invariably, the data show a high degree of both frank and marginal vitamin and mineral deficits where Western diets predominate.[123] Malnutrition is evident in overweight and sedentary individuals[124] and in apparently fit and highly active individuals[125] including athletes.[126,127] Nutrient deficiencies, including thiamine, are especially common in the chronically[128] and critically ill.[129] And the prevalence of chronic illness has increased multifold over just a few generations.[130,131]

Where there are noncaloric nutrient deficiencies, hypoxia or pseudohypoxia are likely and oxidative metabolism will be necessarily impaired. With disordered oxidative metabolism, illness follows. More specifically, with disordered oxidative metabolism, high-energy organ systems such as the brain and nervous system, cardiovascular system, the gastrointestinal tract, and the musculature will all be affected.

## Modern Nutrient Deficiency in Context

Although poor diet is a leading component of modern nutrient deficiency, it is not the only precipitating factor. A number of variables have coalesced over recent decades that predispose even the most conscientious among us to a risk of micronutrient deficiency and the ensuing multimorbidity,[132] variables that should be recognized by health practitioners but are not. Industrial agricultural practices, for example, have depleted crop nutrients significantly, and thus dietary nutrient availability. Nutrient composition of conventionally grown fruits and vegetables provide up to 38% less vitamin and mineral content than they did just a few generations ago[133] and the difference between conventionally grown versus organically grown produce is even more striking.[134] Today's crops, bred for appearance and pesticide resistance rather than nutrition, carry 95% less genetic variety, produce 200,000 fewer metabolites,[135] are grown in topsoils almost completely depleted of minerals (65%–85% depleted in most Western countries),[136] and are sprayed with microbiome and mitochondrial-damaging chemicals.[137] In other words, conventionally grown fruits and vegetables provide fewer raw nutrients and more toxicant exposures than in previous generations. The toxicant exposures in particular have been deemed carcinogenic by the World Health Organization via multiple mechanisms including provoking oxidative damage in the kidneys and liver.[138]

Moving up the food chain, grain-fed animals, artificially fattened with antibiotics[139] and hormones,[140] produce meats that not only contain significantly fewer essential vitamins, fatty acids, and amino acids compared with organic, grass-fed, pasture-grazed animals,[141,142] but when eaten contribute to additional toxicant exposures.[143,144]

When we look at the food industry, modern farming practices, and the totality of modern lifestyle variables capable of damaging mitochondria, it is not difficult to understand the increasing rates of chronic illness observed in Western cultures.[133] Similarly, given the role nutrients play in mitochondrial functioning and the energy demands of the nervous system, particularly the autonomic nervous system, the necessary treatment becomes clear. Replace what is missing through both supplementation and dietary correction.

## Thiamine Sufficiency Is Fragile

Nutrient sufficiency, it appears, is far more fragile than many recognize. Thiamine is particularly vulnerable to both high calorie malnutrition and the medical and environmental variables that target mitochondrial functioning. With its role in energy metabolism, even subclinical deficiency risks serious sequelae.

### *Naked Calories and Thiamine Deficiency*

The term "naked" or "empty" calories is used to refer to food that has no vitamin or mineral content to recommend it. Since thiamine metabolism is closely tied to oxidation of carbohydrate, it is relevant to consider the wisdom of refined sugar in the modern American diet. Anorexia was an almost universal symptom of beriberi and it cleared quickly after thiamine supplementation. Animals become hypophagic in experimentally induced thiamine deficiency. This suggests that there is a centrally mediated protective reflex that prevents further ingestion of calories. The Japanese experience with high calorie malnutrition, illustrated in Case Example 3.3, demonstrates the vulnerability of thiamine to sugar.

### Case Example 3.3 Naked Calories and Beriberi in Japanese Teens

In 1976 the Japanese newspaper *Nihom Keizai Shimbun* reported a "strange disease" in southern Japan. Patients had complained of edema of the lower extremities, palpitations, and numbness. Polyneuritis, hypotension, and other physical signs were observed. In a series of more than 100 cases, the diagnosis had been made of "unknown virus," mononucleosis, and "unknown disease." The patients were all adolescents living in the suburbs and were all from affluent families. Like adolescents in America and other highly industrialized societies, they were congregating at the soda fountain and consuming large amounts of carbohydrates, which included highly flavored imported carbonated beverages. Their disease was recognized as beriberi, and the newspaper commented that although 23,000 patients died annually from the disease in the first quarter of this century in Japan, it was thought that the condition had disappeared in relationship to improved nutrition.

Indeed, this was illustrated as long ago as 1936 by Peters in his pioneering work that showed the catatorulin effect when glucose was added to the thiamine-deficient cells in pigeon brain.[145] Since thiamine is the rate-limiting factor in energy synthesis, its dietary deficiency or lack of metabolic homeostasis figures high in this type of malnutrition. Whether we call it early beriberi or high-calorie thiamine deficiency matters little since it is the biochemical lesion that represents the diagnostic riddle.

We know from history that beriberi is polysymptomatic, has a very prolonged morbidity, and also has a low mortality. Today, the polysymptomatic conditions so frequently observed in the offices of physicians are often diagnosed as psychosomatic. This is particularly true if modern laboratory tests are all normal. If, however, there are changes in the laboratory studies, secondary to energy deficit, they are frequently ascribed to other "modern" conditions. If malnutrition is not recognized as the cause at this stage and is allowed to continue, there is considerable evidence that cellular damage follows, giving rise to a multitude of diseases, each of which is given a diagnostic name.[146] The tragic effect on millions is that they languish, sometimes for years, with symptoms that are so easily reversible in their early stage of appearance. Carbohydrate in the multitudinous and tempting forms in which it is consumed today is virtually an end in itself. Perhaps it is advisable to pause for a moment and consider whether such dietary indiscretion is a much more frequent cause of morbidity than is generally considered.

Even rudimentary clinical observation cannot miss the clear association of hyperactivity and sugar in many children today. Also considered by some investigators to cause hyperactivity are food-coloring substances, found predominantly in refined carbohydrate foods.

To illustrate this principle, there is a neurologic disease known as Cuban molasses disease, which occurs in cattle that consume high concentrations of molasses in their food. It can be relieved or prevented by merely adding a higher percentage of fiber in the form of grass to the feed lots. This suggests that fiber is a most important nutritional component that has its effect in regulating or modifying carbohydrate absorption, thus making fresh fruit and vegetables the only source of sugar nutrition that should be consumed.

The enormous emphasis on refined carbohydrate foods of the modern world may have behavioral effects that have far-reaching consequences. Since aggressive personality changes are so often induced, it may be that there is a strong connection between high carbohydrate calorie malnutrition and the accelerating incidence of violence. Perhaps the critical knowledge required is the ratio of ingested calories to oxidative capacity of brain cells. A thorough examination of the clinical expressions of thiamine-dependent metabolism in the central nervous system appears to provide extremely important clues to the behavioral characteristics of humans. Advice concerning dietary indiscretion often falls on deaf ears. Most people are willing to take pills, and supplementary thiamine, magnesium, and a well-rounded multivitamin may produce dramatic results in the face of only partial dietary correction.

### *Naturally Occurring Thiamine Inhibitors: Thiaminases*

Naturally occurring thiamine inhibitors are common in many types of foods and regular and excessive consumption of these foods can produce thiamine deficiency in some individuals, particularly those with additional risk factors such as a family or personal history of alcoholism, poor diet, comorbid thiamine-reducing medications, or latent SLC issues.

1. Drinking coffee or tea and chewing tea leaves[147] is known to reduce biologic effectiveness of dietary thiamine by way of the phenolic substances (caffeic acid, chlorogenic acid, and tannic acid).[148]
2. Consumption of red cabbage, blueberries, red currants, red beets, some cereals, beans, chickpeas, and lentils and oilseeds.[149]
3. Chewing betel nut.[149]
4. Consumption of raw fish results in athiaminosis.[149]

Thiamine can be destroyed by activating one of two enzymes: thiaminase I (thiamine: base 2-methyl-4-aminopyrimidine-5-methenyl transferase. EC 2.5.1.2) and thiaminase II (thiamine hydrolase. EC 3.6.99.2). Evidence of food-activated thiamine inhibition was first demonstrated by Japanese researchers in the 1950s. Fujita demonstrated that thiamine could be formed in the presence of thiaminase I if a base-exchanged pyrimidine derivative and the thiazole moiety of thiamine were present.[150] His work suggested that a natural ecologic role of the enzyme is in synthesis of the vitamin in primitive organisms, but the equilibrium of the reaction favors destruction of the intact molecule rather than its synthesis.

Thiaminase I is found in raw fish, including shell fish, and in ferns and other plants, and is produced by a number of bacteria. Fujita studied its possible role in human nutrition and described "thiaminase disease" with an incidence of 3% in an urban Japanese population. Diagnosis was established by screening feces and ascertaining the degree of destruction of thiamine in vitro at pH 5.6 and 37°C in 2 h. Many, but not all, of the subjects found to have fecal thiaminase were experiencing symptoms. Symptoms improved after oral thiamine supplementation. Some subjects whose stools contained thiaminase were placed on a thiamine-deficient diet. They developed symptoms of thiamine deficiency earlier than the control subjects on a similar diet, but without thiaminase in their feces.[151] Both enzymes split thiamine at the methylene bridge, but thiaminase I, by a base exchange reaction, causes the base to become linked to the pyrimidine moiety. This newly formed molecule then becomes a thiamine analog inhibitor, which prevents the host animal from using dietary thiamine.[150]

*Bacillus thiaminolyticus*, an aerobe found in the human colon, and *Clostridium thiaminolyticum*, an aerobe found in the small intestine, produce thiaminase I. Aerobic *Bacillus aneurinolyticus* is found in the colon and produces thiaminase II. All three species of bacteria produce spores. *C. thiaminolyticum* is a subgenus of *Clostridium sporogenes*,[152] the organism that has been associated with bilateral cortical necrosis (polioencephalomalacia) in cattle and sheep.[152] Thiaminase I has been found to be activated by nicotinic acid and its amide, forming an analog identified as $N$-(2′-methyl-4′-aminopyrimidyl-(5′)methyl-3-carboxypyridinium)chloride hydrochloride.[153] A relatively simple assay has been established for the detection of thiaminase in animals that could be adapted to human studies.[154]

## From Cattle Research

Bilateral cortical necrosis may be a model for considering the etiology of some human brain disease, which is presently not identifiable in biochemical terms. For example, the disease has been induced experimentally by exposing a calf to amprolium,[155] a known thiamine analog inhibitor. This substance is used as a coccidiostat in chicken feed,[156] and although its concentration is considered to have no bearing on human nutrition, the chickens are produced for human consumption and might result in disease under unusual circumstances. It is also possible that an overwhelming infection of human bowel with *C. sporogenes* might generate neurologic symptoms if thiaminase was found to be produced by the infecting organism.[157]

### *Pharmacologically Induced Thiamine Deficiency and Mitochondrial Damage*

Concomitantly, most, if not all, pharmaceuticals[158] and all environmental chemicals[159] damage mitochondria via multiple mechanisms, further derailing nutrient absorption[160] and metabolic capabilities. Mitochondrial testing is not required by the Food and Drug Administration and pharmaceutically induced damage is only beginning to be appreciated. An in vivo analysis of some 550 pharmaceuticals found that 34% induced mitochondrial damage by disrupting reactions within the ETC.[161] Given that each drug was investigated independently and in culture, it is not difficult to envisage how real-life applications of polypharmacy, coupled with environmental exposures, poor diet, and heritable dispositions, might increase the damage, at least additively if not synergistically.

For detailed lists on medication-induced nutrient depletion, visit the websites of the Linus Pauling Institute,[162] the University of Maryland,[163] and/or the Natural Medicine's Comprehensive Database: Drug Influences on Nutrient Levels and Depletion.[164] For a more detailed description of the mechanisms by which drugs damage mitochondria, see "Drug-induced mitochondrial neuropathy in children: a conceptual framework for critical windows of development,"[6] from which Figs. 3.3 and 3.4 were taken.

By way of example, however, let us examine more closely the mechanisms of mitochondrial damage associated with one of the most popularly prescribed medications worldwide, metformin.[165] Metformin, prescribed for type 2 diabetes, effectively blocks dietary thiamine uptake by acting as a thiamine transporter inhibitor.[166] This means that while metformin is present, the SLC transporters will preferentially pull metformin into the mitochondria instead of thiamine and all of those processes dependent upon thiamine will be starved. Metformin's actions on the thiamine transporters are in addition to its depletion of vitamin B12,[167] which impairs homocysteine metabolism,[168] the derailment of mitochondrial complex I activity,

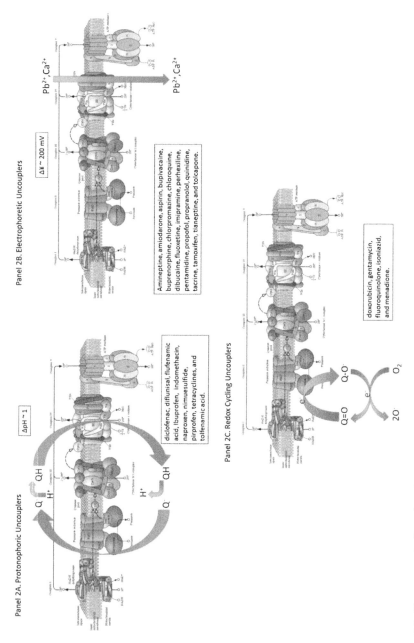

**Figure 3.3** Pharmaceutically induced mitochondrial uncoupling.

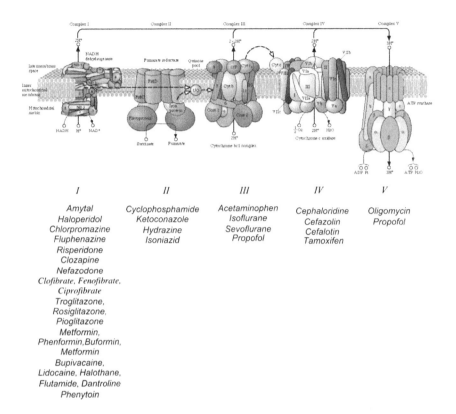

Figure 3.4 Pharmaceutically induced electron transport inhibition.

presumably by depleting the CoQ10 crucial to electron transport, and the depletion of folate.[169] The net effects of metformin are damaged and inefficient mitochondria that produce up to 48% less ATP,[170] leaving those who take the drug with a reduced oxidative capacity[171]; a reduction of exercise-induced insulin sensitivity (by up to 54%[172]); an increase in mitochondrial uncoupling; and at the cell level an increased propensity for Warburg-like reallocation of resources. In other words, the energetic stress caused by metformin leads to compensatory reactions consistent with those in tumorogenesis.[173] Consider the implications of a drug that effectively derails mitochondrial functioning prescribed to at least 49 million Americans annually[174]; individuals that because of diet and sometimes latent genetic factors[175] already bear a degree of mitochondrial damage[176] and thiamine deficiency.[177,178] From that perspective, metformin seems contraindicated, despite its ability to lower circulating glucose. The comorbid conditions that plague many metformin users, physical and mental fatigue, myalgia, neuropathy, cognitive decline, and heart rate irregularities, represent not separate disease processes but manifestations of mitochondrial decline with beriberi and dysautonomic function as the underlying cause.

Metformin is but one medication, however, and is rarely prescribed in isolation. It is often coprescribed with statins that further derail mitochondrial functioning, severely depleting CoQ10.[179] For women, along with metformin, hormonal birth control or replacement therapy is common. Synthetic hormones deplete a whole host of nutrients (thiamine,[180] riboflavin, pyridoxine, folate, vitamin B12, ascorbic acid, and zinc[181]) while damaging mitochondria via multiple mechanisms.[182] Moreover, a quarter of the female population are long-term users of antidepressants and/or anxiolytics.[183] Add to this mix the regular use of nonsteroidal antiinflammatory drugs (which uncouple proton activity across the ETC) to combat menstrual pain, the periodic infection necessitating antibiotics (which uncouple proton activity and redox activity, effectively increasing ROS independently),[6] and we have a recipe for an iatrogenically mediated and sustained state-disordered oxidative metabolism.

Even though polypharmacy among the elderly is common and recognized,[184] it is not often recognized in younger populations, and yet children, teens,[185] and young adults[186] represent the largest growing market for many pharmaceuticals, particularly psychotropic medications. In women, specifically, polypharmacy is becoming an increasingly common problem during pregnancy with the Centers for Disease Control reporting a nearly threefold increase in women using four or more medications during pregnancy.[187] Accordingly, as of 2012, half of all adults were managing at least one chronic condition and a quarter of all adults were managing two or more chronic health conditions.[188] In children, the rate of pharmaceutical-induced mitochondria is climbing.[6]

Pharmaceuticals damage the mitochondria via multiple mechanisms.[159] Many deplete thiamine directly.[189] It is therefore easy to see how symptoms of beriberi and dysautonomia might emerge and be misdiagnosed as discrete disease processes, when in reality they represent manifestations of disordered oxidative metabolism. Mitochondrial dysfunction, although considered rare, may not be. Similarly, thiamine deficiency, a risk all too commonly relegated to chronic alcoholics or patients requiring extended parenteral feeding, is now emerging across multiple populations, bringing with it corresponding symptoms of the long-forgotten beriberi and Wernicke's encephalopathy.[190]

## Environmental Chemicals Block Thiamine Uptake

In much the same way that pharmaceuticals target mitochondria, evidence suggests that environmental chemicals do the same.[159] RoundUp with glyphosate, for example, damages complex I and III of the electron transport cycles, reducing ATP production by some 40%.[191] Early evidence of this was demonstrated over 30 years ago[192] and has been largely ignored by the regulatory agencies, the public, and most presciently health-care providers. Exposures to glyphosate through ingestion of conventionally grown foods or the use of household chemicals are difficult to avoid and often merit cumulative effects. Across research protocols, glyphosate and its adjuvants have been found in up to 99% of populations tested[193] with significantly higher glyphosate concentrations in individuals who eat conventionally grown, genetically modified foods compared with those who eat predominantly organically, and in the chronically ill versus healthy individuals.[194] This is disturbing when one considers that:

1. RoundUp with glyphosate destroys beneficial gut bacteria, which not only impairs nutrient absorption, but when the more pathogenic species of gut bacteria dominate, disposes one to additional gut and systemic disease processes as well.[195]
2. Glyphosate chelates essential dietary metals[196] such as iron, zinc, and manganese, contributing to mineral deficiencies and vitamin deficiencies. Minerals are required for the enzyme activity that regulates vitamin synthesis.
3. Glyphosate disrupts the endocrine system and damages DNA.[197]

Although glyphosate is ubiquitous in the environment with 527 million pounds of product used worldwide in 2011,[198] it is but one of thousands of environmental chemicals capable of disrupting mitochondrial functioning by multiple mechanisms.[199]

Clinically, among the most extreme examples of environmentally induced multisystem mitochondriopathy is Gulf War syndrome. With the widespread exposures to environmental and pharmaceutical toxicants, fully one-third of Gulf War vets developed complex, multisystem illnesses that have been clearly linked to mitochondrial damage[82] and nutrient depletion[200] with corresponding autonomic dysregulation[201] and direct effects on cholinergic transmission.[202] Despite enormous political and economic efforts to obfuscate linkages, a growing body of evidence consistently demonstrates environmentally induced mitochondrial damage at the foundation of this disease process.

## NUTRIENT DEFICIENCY, MITOCHONDRIA, AND THE AUTONOMIC SYSTEM

Yuval Noah Harari writes in *Sapiens: A Brief History of Humankind* that the position of *Homo sapiens* was, until quite recently, solidly in the middle of the food chain.[203] For more than 2 million years, human neural networks kept growing and growing on the unknown whim of evolution. The fact is that what Harari refers to as a "jumbo brain" is hard to fuel. The human brain accounts for about 2%–3% of total body weight but consumes 25% of the body's energy when the body is at rest. The energy requirement during activity must be enormous, particularly when it is mental. By comparison, other apes require only 8% of rest-time energy for the brain. The fact is that we do not sufficiently associate deviations in behavior or health with poor-quality nutrition. In the current climate of high calorie low micronutrient consumption and inescapable toxicant exposure, nutrient sufficiency is remarkably precarious, and when nutrients decline, oxidative metabolism slows. With energetic demands of the brain, even slight permutations in oxidative metabolism are likely to have far-reaching consequences. The autonomic system in particular, tasked with organismal homeostasis, will struggle with basic functions and become increasingly disordered, affecting the basic regulation of everything from breathing and heart rate and rhythm to thermogenesis and gastrointestinal motility. With ATP in short supply, uncharacteristic and unremitting fatigue may be among the most consistently dismissed clues of mitochondrial involvement.[204]

Thiamine deficiency, like other similar nutritional disorders, is considered erroneously to be rare or nonexistent in developed countries. It is still widely prevalent in underdeveloped societies, particularly where rice is staple. It is well established that beriberi is closely associated with ingestion of high-calorie foods, particularly carbohydrates. Early investigators[205] strongly suspected that the sudden death attributed to thiamine-deficient beriberi was a centrally mediated phenomenon, although heart failure was considered to be the dominant cause at that time. It was further recognized that the state of glucose metabolism influenced the response to thiamine therapy. Patients with hypoglycemia did not respond, whereas those with hyperglycemia sometimes responded and those with normoglycemia always responded quickly. This probably represented the decline in the efficiency of metabolism as the disease progressed.

### Recognizing Thiamine Deficiency in Clinical Care

If thiamine deficiency results in inefficient energy metabolism through its effect in the mitochondria, then one should anticipate a chaotic state of

brain/body function where the symptoms are essentially unpredictable. The polysymptomatic presentation of beriberi is a model for mitochondrial disease. In considering thiamine deficiency, it is important to remember:
1. Symptoms involve the cardiovascular and nervous systems, the autonomic system in particular.
2. Symptoms vary with age and method of inducing the deficiency. The disease is especially acute and lethal in infancy.
3. Severe behavioral and learning problems can be signs of thiamine deficiency in children.
4. The clinical spectrum is widely protean in nature.[206]
5. Marginal deficiency can exist for long periods, even years, but an acute crisis can be precipitated by stress, including pregnancy, surgery, injury, or febrile illness.[213] This is particularly important in identifying the disease in well-developed societies where marginal malnutrition exists, often without clinical recognition.

As we have suggested throughout, beriberi is one of the classic nutritional deficiency disorders, and it is possible that it may not be recognized today, even in its complete expression. Two brothers were reported with unknown cardiomyopathy.[207] The symptoms and physical signs were those of cardiac beriberi. Beriberi was not evidently considered in the differential diagnosis. Wolf and associates reported two cases of Shoshin beriberi in 1960, and they suggested that the disease was not uncommon in the United States, although it was rarely diagnosed.[208] Cardiac beriberi was reported in two cases in 1971,[209] both of which could easily have been treated as heart failure of unknown cause. The rooted opinion that the disease has been stamped out in all its forms creates a danger of misdiagnosis.

Adolescents and children in the United States may develop psychologic and somatic symptoms related to diet,[210,211] and dietary correction, together with supplements of water-soluble vitamins, was shown to result in correction of red cell transketolase[215] (a measure of thiamine deficiency). The research suggests that the intake of naked calories might increase vitamin needs drastically, and thiamine and carbohydrate metabolism are related. Refined sugar and many varieties of sweets have become virtually an addictive trend in America. Peters showed that there was no difference in respiratory rate of thiamine-deficient brain cells compared with thiamine-sufficient cells until glucose was added.[147]

Experimental thiamine deficiency in human subjects[212] causes typically nervous system symptoms including depression, parasthesiae, weakness, dizziness, backache, muscle pain, palpitations, precordial distress on exertion (pseudoangina), insomnia, anorexia, nausea, vomiting, weight loss, hypotension, bradycardia at rest, and tachycardia with sinus arrhythmia on exertion. These symptoms develop after severe deprivation for several weeks and are often misdiagnosed as psychosomatic today.

Moderate prolonged thiamine deficiency, without caloric restriction, results in emotional instability, mood changes, and lack of cooperation, fearfulness with agitation, and many somatic symptoms. These were the same symptoms reported in a group of young Americans whose red cell transketolase studies plainly indicated thiamine deficiency.[219] Wernicke's disease has been reported as a complication of intravenous hyperalimentation.[213] In another similar report the patient had developed Wernicke's encephalopathy, in spite of the fact that she had received 24 mg of thiamine a day in the intravenous fluid. This suggested that the vitamin was either still insufficient or was not biologically activated.[214]

Thiamine deficiency produces functional changes, particularly in the autonomic system in its early stages, making it the prototype of dysautonomia.[215] The autonomic neuropathy seen in diabetes[216] is similar to that in beriberi, and insulinopenia, observed in familial dysautonomia,[217] suggests the possibility of a primary central mechanism involved in diabetes. Thiamine deficiency is also indicated in neurodegenerative diseases such as AD where the abnormality of the cholinergic system is part of the pathophysiology.[218,219]

Mastrogiacoma and associates studied thiamine, its phosphate esters, and its metabolizing enzymes in autopsied specimens of brain in AD and controls.[220] In the AD group the mean levels of free thiamine and TMP were normal. Concentrations of TPP were reduced by 18%–21% although the TPP metabolizing enzymes were normal. The authors hypothesized ATP deficiency since that is required for increased phosphorylation in thiamine esters.

Thiamine deficiency in rats caused encephalopathy and DNA synthesis decreased significantly in cortex, brain stem, cerebellum, and subcortical structures. This was reversible by the administration of thiamine.[221] The limbic system, brain stem, and cerebellum are peculiarly sensitive to thiamine deficiency, perhaps because of their high metabolic rate. The variability of the enormous number of symptoms that are generated as a result of its deficiency is because of the effect in the hypothalamic, autonomic, endocrine axis, the metabolic machinery that enables us to adapt to environmental changes. The changes in the brain are similar if not identical to those produced by hypoxia[222] and are the reason why thiamine deficiency is sometimes referred to as pseudohypoxia.

## RETHINKING NUTRITION

The symptoms and multimorbidity expressed so commonly in modern disease should remind us that this is exactly how beriberi was expressed in rice-consuming cultures. The approach should obviously begin with dietary correction. However, we have learned from hard-won experience and indeed from the history of thiamine megadoses required in the treatment of beriberi that simple dietary correction is not sufficient. High calorie malnutrition, is so widespread and so damaging to the enzymes that preside over energy metabolism that noncaloric nutrient supplementation is a necessity. In fact, water-soluble vitamins given by intravenous infusion are often necessary to begin the resuscitation of the cofactor-deprived enzymes.

## REFERENCES

1. Picard M, Wallace DC, Burelle Y. The rise of mitochondria in medicine. *Mitochondrion* 2016;**30**.
2. Vandebona H, et al. Prevalence of mitochondrial 1555A-G mutation in adults of European descent. *N Engl J Med* 2009;**360**:642–4.
3. Minocherhomji S, Tollefsbol TO, Singh KK. Mitochondrial regulation of epigenetics and its role in human disease. *Epigenetics* 2012;**7**:326–34.
4. Zheng LD, Linarelli LE, Liu L, Wall SS, Greenawald MH, Seidel RW, Estabrooks PA, Almeida FA, Cheng Z. Insulin resistance is associated with epigenetic and genetic regulation of mitochondrial DNA in obese humans. *Clin Epigenetics* 2015;**7**(1):1.
5. Chinnery PF, Elliott HR, Hudson G, Samuels DC, Relton CL. Epigenetics, epidemiology and mitochondrial DNA diseases. *Int J Epidemiol* 2012. http://dx.doi.org/10.1093/ije/dyr232.
6. Wallace KB. Drug-induced mitochondrial neuropathy in children: a conceptual framework for critical windows of development. *J Child Neurol* 2014. http://dx.doi.org/10.1177/0883073814538510.
7. Ames BN. Low micronutrient intake may accelerate the degenerative diseases of aging through allocation of scarce micronutrients by triage. *Proc Natl Acad Sci USA* 2006;**103**(47):17589–94.
8. Dutta D, Calvani R, Bernabei R, Leeuwenburgh C, Marzetti E. Contribution of impaired mitochondrial autophagy to cardiac aging mechanisms and therapeutic opportunities. *Circ Res* 2012;**110**(8):1125–38.
9. Sivitz WI, Yorek MA. Mitochondrial dysfunction in diabetes: from molecular mechanisms to functional significance and therapeutic opportunities. *Antioxid Redox Signal* 2010;**12**(4):537–77.
10. Thompson MM, Manning HC, Ellacott KL. Translocator protein 18 kDa (TSPO) is regulated in white and brown adipose tissue by obesity. *PLoS One* 2013;**8**(11): e79980.
11. Prabakaran S, Swatton JE, Ryan MM, Huffaker SJ, Huang JJ, Griffin JL, Wayland M, Freeman T, Dudbridge F, Lilley KS, Karp NA. Mitochondrial dysfunction in schizophrenia: evidence for compromised brain metabolism and oxidative stress. *Mol Psychiatry* 2004;**9**(7):684–97.

12. Scaini G, Rezin GT, Carvalho AF, Streck EL, Berk M, Quevedo J. Mitochondrial dysfunction in bipolar disorder: evidence, pathophysiology and translational implications. *Neurosci Biobehav Rev* 2016;**68**:694–713.
13. Maiese K. Forkhead transcription factors: new considerations for Alzheimer's disease and dementia. *J Transl Sci* 2016;**2**(4):241.
14. Hu Q, Wang G. Mitochondrial dysfunction in Parkinson's disease. *Transl Neurodegener* 2016;**5**(1):1.
15. Zsurka G, Kunz WS. Mitochondrial dysfunction and seizures: the neuronal energy crisis. *Lancet Neurol* 2015;**14**(9):956–66.
16. Krzywanski DM, Moellering DR, Fetterman JL, Dunham-Snary KJ, Sammy MJ, Ballinger SW. The mitochondrial paradigm for cardiovascular disease susceptibility and cellular function: a complementary concept to Mendelian genetics. *Lab Invest* 2011;**91**(8):1122–35.
17. Filler K, Lyon D, Bennett J, McCain N, Elswick R, Lukkahatai N, Saligan LN. Association of mitochondrial dysfunction and fatigue: a review of the literature. *BBA Clin* 2014;**1**:12–23.
18. Bhatti MT. Retinitis pigmentosa, pigmentary retinopathies, and neurologic diseases. *Curr Neurol Neurosci Rep* 2006;**6**(5):403–13.
19. Chapman TP, Hadley G, Fratter C, Cullen SN, Bax BE, Bain MD, Sapsford RA, Poulton J, Travis SP. Unexplained gastrointestinal symptoms: think mitochondrial disease. *Dig Liver Dis* 2014;**46**(1):1–8.
20. Johnson JM, Lai SY, Cotzia P, Cognetti D, Luginbuhl A, Pribitkin EA, Zhan T, Mollaee M, Domingo-Vidal M, Chen Y, Campling B. Mitochondrial metabolism as a treatment target in anaplastic thyroid cancer. *Semin Oncol* December 2015;**42**(6):915–22. WB Saunders.
21. Gueven N, Nadikudi M, Daniel A, Chhetri J. Targeting mitochondrial function to treat optic neuropathy. *Mitochondrion* 2016. http://dx.doi.org/10.1016/j.mito.2016.07.013.
22. Ponizovskiy MR. The changes of energy interactions between nucleus function and mitochondria functions causing transmutation of chronic inflammation into cancer metabolism. *Crit Rev Eukaryot Gene Expr* 2016;**26**(2).
23. Lonsdale D. Dysautonomia, a heuristic approach to a revised model for etiology of disease. *Evid Based Complement Alternat Med* 2009;**6**(1):3–10.
24. Bettendorff L, Sluse F, Goessens G, Wins P, Grisar T. Thiamine deficiency-induced partial necrosis and mitochondrial uncoupling in neuroblastoma cells are rapidly reversed by addition of thiamine. *J Neurochem* 1995;**65**(5):2178–84.
25. Hernández-Aguilera A, Fernández-Arroyo S, Cuyàs E, Luciano-Mateo F, Cabre N, Camps J, Lopez-Miranda J, Menendez JA, Joven J. Epigenetics and nutrition-related epidemics of metabolic diseases: current perspectives and challenges. *Food Chem Toxicol* 2016;**96**:191–204.
26. van der Wijst MG, Rots MG. Mitochondrial epigenetics: an overlooked layer of regulation? *Trends Genet* 2015;**31**(7):353–6.
27. Chinnery PF. Mitochondrial disorders overview. *GeneReviews®* 2014.
28. Khan NA, Govindaraj P, Meena AK, Thangaraj K. Mitochondrial disorders: challenges in diagnosis & treatment. *Indian J Med Res* 2015;**141**(1):13.
29. Rossignol R, Faustin B, Rocher C, Malgat M, Mazat JP, Letellier T. Mitochondrial threshold effects. *Biochem J* 2003;**370**(3):751–62.
30. Hajjar C, Sampuda KM, Boyd L. Dual roles for ubiquitination in the processing of sperm organelles after fertilization. *BMC Dev Biol* 2014;**14**(1):1.
31. Stewart JB, Chinnery PF. The dynamics of mitochondrial DNA heteroplasmy: implications for human health and disease. *Nat Rev Genet* 2015;**16**(9):530–42.
32. Wallace DC, Chalkia D. Mitochondrial DNA genetics and the heteroplasmy conundrum in evolution and disease. *Cold Spring Harb Perspect Biol* 2013;**5**(11):a021220.

33. Lanza IR, Zabielski P, Klaus KA, Morse DM, Heppelmann CJ, Bergen HR, Dasari S, Walrand S, Short KR, Johnson ML, Robinson MM. Chronic caloric restriction preserves mitochondrial function in senescence without increasing mitochondrial biogenesis. *Cell Metab* 2012;**16**(6):777–88.
34. Sweet RL, Zastre JA. HIF1-α-mediated gene expression induced by vitamin B. *Int J Vitam Nutr Res* 2013;**83**(3):188–97.
35. Inouye K, Katsura E. Etiology and pathology of beriberi. In: Shimazono N, Katsura E, editors. *Thiamine and beriberi*. Tokyo: Igaku Shoin Ltd; 1965. p. 1–28.
36. Ishimaru T, Yata T, Hatanaka-Ikeno S. Hemodynamic response of the frontal cortex elicited by intravenous thiamine propyldisulphide administration. *Chem Senses* 2004;**29**(3):247–51.
37. Lindenbaum GA, Larrieu AJ, Carroll SF, Kapusnick RA. Effect of cocarboxylase in dogs subjected to experimental septic shock. *Crit Care Med* 1989;**17**(10):1036–40.
38. Semenza GL. Oxygen sensing, hypoxia-inducible factors, and disease pathophysiology. *Annu Rev Pathol Mech Dis* 2014;**9**:47–71.
39. Ke Q, Costa M. Hypoxia-inducible factor-1 (HIF-1). *Mol Pharmacol* 2006;**70**(5): 1469–80.
40. Briston T, Yang J, Ashcroft M. HIF-1α localization with mitochondria: a new role for an old favorite? *Cell Cycle* 2011;**10**(23):4170–1.
41. Zhan L, Wang W, Zhang Y, Song E, Fan Y, Wei B. Hypoxia-inducible factor-1alpha: a promising therapeutic target in endometriosis. *Biochimie* 2016;**123**:130–7.
42. Deng W, Feng X, Li X, Wang D, Sun L. Hypoxia-inducible factor 1 in autoimmune diseases. *Cell Immunol* 2016;**303**:7–15.
43. Martin PR, Singleton CK, Hiller-Sturmhofel S. The role of thiamine deficiency in alcoholic brain disease. *Alcohol Res Health* 2003;**27**(2):134–42.
44. Casteels M, Sniekers M, Fraccascia P, Mannaerts GP, Van Veldhoven PP. The role of 2-hydroxyacyl-CoA lyase, a thiamin pyrophosphate-dependent enzyme, in the peroxisomal metabolism of 3-methyl-branched fatty acids and 2-hydroxy straight-chain fatty acids. *Biochem Soc Trans* 2007;**35**(5):876–80.
45. Wanders RJ, Komen J, Kemp S. Fatty acid omega-oxidation as a rescue pathway for fatty acid oxidation disorders in humans. *FEBS J* 2011;**278**(2):182–94.
46. Moore RO, Yontz FD. Effect of thiamine deficiency in rats on adipose tissue lactate dehydrogenase isozyme distribution. *J Nutr* 1969;**98**:325–9.
47. Giacalone M, Martinelli R, Abramo A, Rubino A, Pavoni V, Iacconi P, Giunta F, Forfori F. Rapid reversal of severe lactic acidosis after thiamine administration in critically ill adults a report of 3 cases. *Nutr Clin Pract* 2015;**30**(1):104–10.
48. Marrs C. Micronutrient deficiencies and mitochondrial dysfunction. In: Greenblatt JM, Brogan K, editors. *Integrative therapies for depression: redefining models for assessment, treatment and prevention*. CRC Press; 2015. p. 73–95.
49. Pieczenik SR, Neustadt J. Mitochondrial dysfunction and molecular pathways of disease. *Exp Mol Pathol* 2007;**83**(1):84–92.
50. Hroudová J, Fišar Z, Raboch J. Mitochondrial functions in mood disorders. In: Kocabasoglu N, editor. *Mood disorders*. 2013. p. 101–43. Available from: http://www.intechopen.com/books/mood-disorders/mitochondrial-functions-in-mood-disorders.
51. Atamna H, Newberry J, Erlitzki R, Schultz CS, Ames BN. Biotin deficiency inhibits heme synthesis and impairs mitochondria in human lung fibroblasts. *J Nutr* 2007;**137**(1):25–30.
52. Dröge W. Free radicals in the physiological control of cell function. *Physiol Rev* 2002;**82**(1):47–95.
53. Jones DP, Lemasters JJ, Han D, Boelsterli UA, Kaplowitz N. Mechanisms of pathogenesis in drug hepatotoxicity putting the stress on mitochondria. *Mol Interv* 2010; **10**(2):98.

54. Crane FL. Biochemical functions of coenzyme Q10. *J Am Coll Nutr* 2001; **20**(6):591–8.
55. Wollin SD, Jones PJ. α-Lipoic acid and cardiovascular disease. *J Nutr* 2003; **133**(11):3327–30.
56. Figueroa-Méndez R, Rivas-Arancibia S. Vitamin C in health and disease: its role in the metabolism of cells and redox state in the brain. *Front Physiol* 2015;**6**.
57. Chow CK, Ibrahim W, Wei Z, Chan AC. Vitamin E regulates mitochondrial hydrogen peroxide generation. *Free Radic Biol Med* 1999;**27**(5):580–7.
58. Ganji SH, Qin S, Zhang L, Kamanna VS, Kashyap ML. Niacin inhibits vascular oxidative stress, redox-sensitive genes, and monocyte adhesion to human aortic endothelial cells. *Atherosclerosis* 2009;**202**(1):68–75.
59. Kucharska J. Vitamins in mitochondrial function. In: Gvozdjáková A, editor. *Mitochondrial medicine: mitochondrial metabolism, diseases, diagnosis and therapy*. Springer Science & Business Media; 2008. p. 367–84.
60. Bao BY, Ting HJ, Hsu JW, Lee YF. Protective role of 1α, 25-dihydroxyvitamin D3 against oxidative stress in nonmalignant human prostate epithelial cells. *Int J Cancer* 2008;**122**(12):2699–706.
61. Marí M, Morales A, Colell A, García-Ruiz C, Fernández-Checa JC. Mitochondrial glutathione, a key survival antioxidant. *Antioxid Redox Signal* 2009;**11**(11):2685–700.
62. Puskas F, Gergely P, Banki K, Perl A. Stimulation of the pentose phosphate pathway and glutathione levels by dehydroascorbate, the oxidized form of vitamin C. *FASEB J* 2000;**14**(10):1352–61.
63. Wu G, Fang YZ, Yang S, Lupton JR, Turner ND. Glutathione metabolism and its implications for health. *J Nutr* 2004;**134**(3):489–92.
64. Muñoz A, Costa M. Nutritionally mediated oxidative stress and inflammation. *Oxid Med Cell Longevity* 2013;**2013**.
65. Vimokesant S, Kunjara S, Rungruangsak K, Nakornchai S, Panijpan B. Beriberi caused by antithiamin factors in food and its prevention. *Ann NY Acad Sci* 1982; **378**(1):123–36.
66. Bettendorff L, Wins P. Thiamin diphosphate in biological chemistry: new aspects of thiamin metabolism, especially triphosphate derivatives acting other than as cofactors. *FEBS J* 2009;**276**(11):2917–25.
67. Meshalkina LE, Kochetov GA, Hubner G, Tittmann K, Golbik R. New function of the amino group of thiamine diphosphate in thiamine catalysis. *Biochemistry* 2009; **74**(3):293–300.
68. Bettendorff L. Personal communication.
69. Lonsdale D, Faulkner WR, Price JW, Smeby RR. Intermittent cerebellar ataxia associated with hyperpyruvic acidemia, hyperalaninemia, and hyperalaninuria. *Pediatrics* 1969;**43**(6):1025–34.
70. Bonnefont JP, Chretien D, Rustin P, Robinson B, Vassault A, Aupetit J, Charpentier C, Rabier D, Saudubray JM, Munnich A. Alpha-ketoglutarate dehydrogenase deficiency presenting as congenital lactic acidosis. *J Pediatr* 1992;**121**(2):255–8.
71. Fernhoff PM, Lubitz D, Danner DJ, Dembure PP, Schwartz HP, Hillman R, Bier DM, Elsas LJ. Thiamine response in maple syrup urine disease. *Pediatr Res* 1985; **19**(10):1011–6.
72. Salem HM. Glyoxalase and methylglyoxal in thiamine-deficient rats. *Biochem J* 1954;**57**(2):227.
73. Rabbani N, Thornalley PJ. Glyoxalase in diabetes, obesity and related disorders. *Semin Cell Dev Biol* May 2011;**22**(3):309–17. Academic Press.
74. Thornalley PJ, Jahan I, Ng R. Suppression of the accumulation of triosephosphates and increased formation of methylglyoxal in human red blood cells during hyperglycaemia by thiamine in vitro. *J Biochem* 2001;**129**(4):543–9.

75. Lonsdale D, Faulkner WR, Price W, Smeby RR. Pyruvic acidemia with hyperalaninemia: vitamin B 1 dependency. *J Pediatr* 1969;**74**(5):827–8.
76. Kochetov GA, Solovjeva ON. Structure and functioning mechanism of transketolase. *Biochim Biophys Acta, Proteins Proteomics* 2014;**1844**(9):1608–18.
77. Bubber P, Ke ZJ, Gibson GE. Tricarboxylic acid cycle enzymes following thiamine deficiency. *Neurochem Int* 2004;**45**(7):1021–8.
78. Porpaczy Z, Sümegi B, Alkonyi I. Association between the α-ketoglutarate dehydrogenase complex and succinate thiokinase. *Biochim Biophys Acta, Protein Struct Mol Enzymol* 1983;**749**(2):172–9.
79. Rutter J, Winge DR, Schiffman JD. Succinate dehydrogenase–assembly, regulation and role in human disease. *Mitochondrion* 2010;**10**(4):393–401.
80. Rustin P, Munnich A, Rotig A. Succinate dehydrogenase and human diseases: new insights into a well-known enzyme. *Eur J Hum Genet* 2002;**10**(5):289–91.
81. Briere JJ, Favier J, Gimenez-Roqueplo AP, Rustin P. Tricarboxylic acid cycle dysfunction as a cause of human diseases and tumor formation. *Am J Physiol Cell Physiol* 2006;**291**(6):C1114–20.
82. Koslik HJ, Hamilton G, Golomb BA. Mitochondrial dysfunction in Gulf war illness revealed by 31Phosphorus magnetic resonance spectroscopy: a case-control study. *PLoS One* 2014;**9**(3):e92887.
83. Dodds MG. *Analysis of mitochondrial metabolic defects*. 2001.
84. Mkrtchyan G, Aleshin V, Parkhomenko Y, Kaehne T, Di Salvo ML, Parroni A, Contestabile R, Vovk A, Bettendorff L, Bunik V. Molecular mechanisms of the non-coenzyme action of thiamin in brain: biochemical, structural and pathway analysis. *Sci Rep* 2015;**5**.
85. McKenna MC. Glutamate dehydrogenase in brain mitochondria: do lipid modifications and transient metabolon formation influence enzyme activity? *Neurochem Int* 2011;**59**(4):525–33.
86. Hazell AS, Butterworth RF, Hakim AM. Cerebral vulnerability is associated with selective increase in extracellular glutamate concentration in experimental thiamine deficiency. *J Neurochem* 1993;**61**(3):1155–8.
87. Gandhi A. *Vitamin B6 metabolism and regulation of pyridoxal kinase*. 2009.
88. Smith AJ, Stone TW, Smith RA. Neurotoxicity of tryptophan metabolites. *Biochem Soc Trans* 2007;**35**(5):1287–9.
89. Minz B. *Sur la libération de la vitamine B1 par le tronc isolé du nerf pneumogastrique soumis à l'excitation électrique*. 1938. éditeur inconnu.
90. Cooper JR, Pincus JH. The role of thiamine in nervous tissue. *Neurochem Res* 1979;**4**(2):223–39.
91. Iwata H, Yabushita Y, Doi T, Matsuda T. Synthesis of thiamine triphosphate in rat brain in vivo. *Neurochem Res* 1985;**10**(6):779–87.
92. Cooper JR, Itokawa Y, Pincus JH. Tbiamine-triphosphate deficiency in subacute necrotizing encephalomyelopathy. *Science* 1969;**164**(3875):74–5.
93. Cooper JR, Pincus JH, Itokawa Y, Piros K. Experiences with phosphororibosyl transferase inhibition in subacute necrotizing encephalomyelopathy. *N Engl J Med* 1970;**283**:793–5.
94. Lake NJ, Compton AG, Rahman S, Thorburn DR. Leigh syndrome: one disorder, more than 75 monogenic causes. *Ann Neurol* 2016;**79**(2):190–203.
95. Banka S, de Goede C, Yue WW, Morris AA, Von Bremen B, Chandler KE, Feichtinger RG, Hart C, Khan N, Lunzer V, Mataković L. Expanding the clinical and molecular spectrum of thiamine pyrophosphokinase deficiency: a treatable neurological disorder caused by TPK1 mutations. *Mol Genet Metab* 2014;**113**(4):301–6.
96. Bettendorff L, Michel-Cahay C, Grandfils C, Rycker CD, Schoffeniels E. Thiamine triphosphate and membrane-associated thiamine phosphatases in the electric organ of *Electrophorus electricus*. *J Neurochem* 1987;**49**(2):495–502.

97. Bettendorff L, Kolb HA, Schoffeniels E. Thiamine triphosphate activates an anion channel of large unit conductance in neuroblastoma cells. *J Membr Biol* 1993;**136**(3):281–8.
98. Makarchikov AF, Lakaye B, Gulyai IE, Czerniecki J, Coumans B, Wins P, Grisar T, Bettendorff L. Thiamine triphosphate and thiamine triphosphatase activities: from bacteria to mammals. *Cell Mol Life Sci* 2003;**60**(7):1477–88.
99. Aasheim ET. Wernicke encephalopathy after bariatric surgery: a systematic review. *Ann Surg* 2008;**248**(5):714–20.
100. Hediger MA, Clémençon B, Burrier RE, Bruford EA. The ABCs of membrane transporters in health and disease (SLC series): introduction. *Mol Aspects Med* 2013;**34**(2):95–107.
101. Ganapathy V, Smith SB, Prasad PD. SLC19: the folate/thiamine transporter family. *Pflügers Arch* 2004;**447**(5):641–6.
102. Zhao R, Goldman ID. Folate and thiamine transporters mediated by facilitative carriers (SLC19A1-3 and SLC46A1) and folate receptors. *Mol Aspects Med* 2013;**34**(2):373–85.
103. Scharfe C, Hauschild M, Klopstock T, Janssen AJ, Heidemann PH, Meitinger T, Jaksch M. A novel mutation in the thiamine responsive megaloblastic anaemia gene SLC19A2 in a patient with deficiency of respiratory chain complex I. *J Med Genet* 2000;**37**(9):669–73.
104. Ricketts CJ, Minton JA, Samuel J, Ariyawansa I, Wales JK, Lo IF, Barrett TG. Thiamine-responsive megaloblastic anaemia syndrome: long-term follow-up and mutation analysis of seven families. *Acta Paediatr* 2006;**95**(1):99–104.
105. Mikstiene V, Songailiene J, Byckova J, Rutkauskiene G, Jasinskiene E, Verkauskiene R, Lesinskas E, Utkus A. Thiamine responsive megaloblastic anemia syndrome: a novel homozygous SLC19A2 gene mutation identified. *Am J Med Genet A* 2015;**167**(7):1605–9.
106. Pérez-Dueñas B, Serrano M, Rebollo M, Muchart J, Gargallo E, Dupuits C, Artuch R. Reversible lactic acidosis in a newborn with thiamine transporter-2 deficiency. *Pediatrics* 2013;**131**(5):e1670–5.
107. Lonsdale D. Sudden infant death syndrome requires genetic predisposition, some form of stress and marginal malnutrition. *Med Hypotheses* 2001;**57**(3):382–6.
108. Lonsdale D. Thiamine and magnesium deficiencies: keys to disease. *Med Hypotheses* 2015;**84**(2):129–34.
109. Naviaux RK. Metabolic features of the cell danger response. *Mitochondrion* 2014;**16**:7–17. http://dx.doi.org/10.1016/j.mito.2013.08.006. ISSN:1567-7249.
110. Miller WL. Steroid hormone synthesis in mitochondria. *Mol Cell Endocrinol* 2013;**379**:62–73.
111. O'Rourke B, Cortassa S, Aon MA. Mitochondrial ion channels: gatekeepers of life and death. *Physiology* 2005;**20**:303–15. http://dx.doi.org/10.1152/physiol.00020.2005.
112. Kroemer G, Galluzzi L, Brenner C. Mitochondrial membrane permeabilization in cell death. *Physiol Rev* 2007;**87**:99–163.
113. Moos WH, Maneta E, Pinkert CA, Irwin MH, Hoffman ME, Faller DV, Steliou K. Epigenetic treatment of neuropsychiatric disorders: autism and schizophrenia. *Drug Dev Res* 2016;**77**.
114. Lonsdale D, Shamberger RJ, Audhya T. Treatment of autism spectrum children with thiamine tetrahydrofurfuryl disulfide: a pilot study. *Neuroendocrinol Lett* 2002;**23**(4):303–8.
115. Lonsdale D. Thiamine tetrahydrofurfuryl disulfide: a little known therapeutic agent. *Med Sci Monit* 2004;**10**(9):RA199–203.
116. Boles RG, Williams JC. Mitochondrial disease and cyclic vomiting syndrome. *Dig Dis Sci* 1999;**44**(8 Suppl.):103S–7S.

117. Boles RG, Lovett-Barr MR, Preston A, Li BU, Adams K. Treatment of cyclic vomiting syndrome with co-enzyme Q10 and amitriptyline, a retrospective study. *BMC Neurol* 2010;**10**(1):1.
118. Parikh S, Saneto R, Falk MJ, Anselm I, Cohen BH, Haas R. A modern approach to the treatment of mitochondrial disease. *Curr Treat Options Neurol* 2009;**11**(6):414–30.
119. Tarnopolsky MA. The mitochondrial cocktail: rationale for combined nutraceutical therapy in mitochondrial cytopathies. *Adv Drug Deliv Rev* 2008;**60**(13):1561–7.
120. Ames BN, Elson-Schwab I, Silver EA. High-dose vitamin therapy stimulates variant enzymes with decreased coenzyme binding affinity (increased Km): relevance to genetic disease and polymorphisms. *Am J Clin Nutr* 2002;**75**(4):616–58.
121. Xu L, Shi R. Weigh and wait: the prospect of mitochondrial gene replacement. *Hum Fertil* 2016:1–8.
122. O'Keefe JH, Gheewala NM, O'Keefe JO. Dietary strategies for improving post-prandial glucose, lipids, inflammation, and cardiovascular health. *J Am Coll Cardiol* 2008;**51**(3):249–55.
123. Fairfield KM, Fletcher RH. Vitamins for chronic disease prevention in adults: scientific review. *JAMA* 2002;**287**(23):3116–26. http://dx.doi.org/10.1001/jama.287.23.3116.
124. Via M. The malnutrition of obesity: micronutrient deficiencies that promote diabetes. *ISRN Endocrinol* 2012;**2012**:103472. http://dx.doi.org/10.5402/2012/103472.
125. Manore MM. Effect of physical activity of thiamine, riboflavin and vitamin B6 requirements. *Am J Clin Nutr* 2000;**72**:598s–606s.
126. Constantini MW, et al. High prevalence of vitamin D deficiency in athletes and dancers. *Clin J Sport Med* 2010;**20**:368–71.
127. Lovell G. Vitamin D status in females in elite gymnastics. *Clin J Sport Med* 2008;**18**:159–61.
128. Frank LL. Thiamin in clinical practice. *J Parenter Enteral Nutr* 2015;**39**(5):503–20.
129. Manzanares W, Hardy G. Thiamine supplementation in the critically ill. *Curr Opin Clin Nutr Metab Care* 2011;**14**(6):610–7.
130. Schnall PL, Dobson M, Landsbergis P. Globalization, work, and cardiovascular disease. *Int J Health Serv* 2016. http://dx.doi.org/10.1177/0020731416664687.
131. Centers for Disease Control, Prevention. *Chronic diseases: the leading causes of death and disability in the United States*. 2015. p. 16. http://www.cdc.gov/chronicdisease/overview/index.htm.
132. Suls J, Green PA, Davidson KW. A biobehavioral [corrected] framework to address the emerging challenge of multimorbidity. *Psychosom Med* 2016;**78**(3):281–9.
133. Davis DR, Epp MD, Riordan HD. Changes in USDA food composition data for 43 garden crops, 1950 to 1999. *J Am Coll Nutr* 2004;**23**(6):669–82.
134. Worthington V. Nutritional quality of organic versus conventional fruits, vegetables, and grains. *J Altern Complement Med* 2001;**7**(2):161–73.
135. Daniell E, Ryan EP. *The nutrigenome and gut microbiome: chronic disease prevention with crop phytochemical diversity*. INTECH Open Access Publisher; 2012.
136. Marler JB, Wallin JR. *Human health, the nutritional quality of harvested food and sustainable farming systems*. Bellevue: Nutrition Security Institute; 2006.
137. Samsel A, Seneff S. Glyphosate's suppression of cytochrome P450 enzymes and amino acid biosynthesis by the gut microbiome: pathways to modern diseases. *Entropy* 2013;**15**(4):1416–63.
138. Myers JP, Antoniou MN, Blumberg B, Carroll L, Colborn T, Everett LG, Hansen M, Landrigan PJ, Lanphear BP, Mesnage R, Vandenberg LN. Concerns over use of glyphosate-based herbicides and risks associated with exposures: a consensus statement. *Environ Health* 2016;**15**(1):1.
139. Trusts PC. *Record high antibiotics sales for meat and poultry production*. 2011.

140. Schneider SA. Beyond the food we eat: animal drugs in livestock production. *Duke Environ Law Policy Forum* February 2015;**25**(227).
141. Ponnampalam EN, Mann NJ, Sinclair AJ. Effect of feeding systems on omega-3 fatty acids, conjugated linoleic acid and trans fatty acids in Australian beef cuts: potential impact on human health. *Asia Pac J Clin Nutr* 2006;**15**(1):21.
142. Leheska JM, Thompson LD, Howe JC, Hentges E, Boyce J, Brooks JC, Shriver B, Hoover L, Miller MF. Effects of conventional and grass-feeding systems on the nutrient composition of beef. *J Anim Sci* 2008;**86**(12):3575–85.
143. Thorsteinsdottir TR, Haraldsson G, Fridriksdottir V, Kristinsson KG, Gunnarsson E. Broiler chickens as source of human fluoroquinolone-resistant *Escherichia coli*, Iceland. *Emerg Infect Dis* 2010;**16**(1):133–6.
144. Goettsch W, Van Pelt W, Nagelkerke N, Hendrix MGR, Buiting AGM, Petit PL, Sabbe LJM, Van Griethuysen AJA, De Neeling AJ. Increasing resistance to fluoroquinolones in *Escherichia coli* from urinary tract infections in The Netherlands. *J Antimicrob Chemother* 2000;**46**(2):223–8.
145. Peters R. The biochemical lesion in vitamin B1 deficiency: application of modern biochemical analysis in its diagnosis. *Lancet* 1936;**227**(5882):1161–5.
146. Nardone R, Höller Y, Storti M, Christova M, Tezzon F, Golaszewski S, Trinka E, Brigo F. Thiamine deficiency induced neurochemical, neuroanatomical, and neuropsychological alterations: a reappraisal. *Sci World J* 2013;**2013**.
147. Vimokesant SL, Nakornchai S, Dhanamitta S, Hilker DM. Effect of tea consumption on thiamin status in man. *Nutr Rep Int* 1974;**9**(5).
148. World Health Organization. *Thiamine deficiency and its prevention and control in major emergencies* Report no: WHO/NHD/99.13. Geneva: Department of Nutrition for Health and Development, WHO; 1999.
149. Vimokesant SL, Hilker DM, Nakornchai S, Rungruangsak K, Dhanamitta S. Effects of betel nut and fermented fish on the thiamin status of northeastern Thais. *Am J Clin Nutr* 1975;**28**(12):1458–63.
150. Lonsdale D. A review of the biochemistry, metabolism and clinical benefits of thiamin(e) and its derivatives. *Evid Based Complement Alternat Med* 2006;**3**(1):49–59.
151. Kimura R. Taxonomic considerations on the *Clostridium thiaminolyticum* Kimura et Liao. *Vitamins* 1964;**30**:29–32.
152. Edwin EE, Lewis G. Section E. Diseases of dairy cattle. Thiamine deficiency, with particular reference to cerebrocortical necrosis. *J Dairy Res* 1971;**38**(1):79–90.
153. Edwin EE, Lewis G. The implication of ruminal thiaminase in cerebrocortical necrosis. *Proc Nutr Soc* 1971;**30**(1):7A.
154. Edwin EE, Jackman R. A rapid radioactive method for determination of thiaminase activity and its use in the diagnosis of cerebrocortical necrosis in sheep and cattle. *J Sci Food Agric* 1974;**25**(4):357–68.
155. Pill AH, Davies ET, Collings DF, Venn JAJ. The experimental reproduction of lesions of cerebrocortical necrosis in a calf. *Vet Rec* 1966;**78**:737–8.
156. Brin M. The antithiamine effects of amprolium in rats on tissue transketolase activity. *Toxicol Appl Pharmacol* 1964;**6**(4):454–8.
157. Bodey GP, Rodriguez S, Fainstein V, Elting LS. Clostridial bacteremia in cancer patients. A 12-year experience. *Cancer* 1991;**67**(7):1928–42.
158. Neustadt J, Pieczenik SR. Medication-induced mitochondrial damage and disease. *Mol Nutr Food Res* 2008;**52**(7):780–8.
159. Meyer JN, Leung MC, Rooney JP, Sendoel A, Hengartner MO, Kisby GE, Bess AS. Mitochondria as a target of environmental toxicants. *Toxicol Sci* 2013;**134**(1):1–17.
160. Cass H. A practical guide to avoiding drug-induced nutrient depletion. *Nutr Rev Arch* 2013.
161. Will Y, Dykens J. Mitochondrial toxicity assessment in industry – a decade of technology development and insight. *Expert Opin Drug Metab Toxicol* 2014;**10**(8):1061–7.

162. Linus Pauling Institute: Micronutrient Information Center. http://lpi.oregonstate.edu/infocenter/.
163. University of Maryland Medical Center:Vitamins. http://umm.edu/health/medical/reports/articles/vitamins.
164. http://naturaldatabase.therapeuticresearch.com/ce/ceCourse.aspx?pc=08-40&cec=0&pm=5.
165. https://www.statista.com/statistics/326883/leading-prescriptions-dispensed-in-the-us-diabetes-market/.
166. Liang X, Chien HC, Yee SW, Giacomini MM, Chen EC, Piao M, Hao J, Twelves J, Lepist EI, Ray AS, Giacomini KM. Metformin is a substrate and inhibitor of the human thiamine transporter, THTR-2 (SLC19A3). *Mol Pharm* 2015;**12**(12):4301–10.
167. Reinstatler L, Qi YP, Williamson RS, Garn JV, Oakley GP. Association of biochemical B12 deficiency with metformin therapy and vitamin B12 supplements the national health and nutrition examination survey, 1999–2006. *Diabetes Care* 2012;**35**(2):327–33.
168. De Jager J, Kooy A, Lehert P, Wulffelé MG, Van der Kolk J, Bets D, Verburg J, Donker AJ, Stehouwer CD. Long term treatment with metformin in patients with type 2 diabetes and risk of vitamin B-12 deficiency: randomised placebo controlled trial. *BMJ* 2010;**340**:c2181.
169. Xu L, Huang Z, He X, Wan X, Fang D, Li Y. Adverse effect of metformin therapy on serum vitamin B12 and folate: short-term treatment causes disadvantages? *Med Hypotheses* 2013;**81**(2):149–51.
170. Wessels B, Ciapaite J, van den Broek NM, Nicolay K, Prompers JJ. Metformin impairs mitochondrial function in skeletal muscle of both lean and diabetic rats in a dose-dependent manner. *PLoS One* 2014;**9**(6):e100525.
171. Braun B, Eze P, Stephens BR, Hagobian TA, Sharoff CG, Chipkin SR, Goldstein B. Impact of metformin on peak aerobic capacity. *Appl Physiol Nutr Metab* 2008;**33**(1):61–7.
172. Sharoff CG, Hagobian TA, Malin SK, Chipkin SR, Yu H, Hirshman MF, Goodyear LJ, Braun B. Combining short-term metformin treatment and one bout of exercise does not increase insulin action in insulin-resistant individuals. *Am J Physiol Endocrinol Metab* 2010;**298**(4):E815–23.
173. Andrzejewski S, Gravel SP, Pollak M, St-Pierre J. Metformin directly acts on mitochondria to alter cellular bioenergetics. *Cancer Metab* 2014;**2**(1):1.
174. http://www.statista.com/statistics/242668/top-diabetes-drugs-in-the-us-based-on-prescriptions-dispensed-2011-2012/.
175. Fleming JC, Tartaglini E, Steinkamp MP, Schorderet DF, Cohen N, Neufeld EJ. The gene mutated in thiamine-responsive anaemia with diabetes and deafness (TRMA) encodes a functional thiamine transporter. *Nat Genet* 1999;**22**(3):305–8.
176. Giacco F, Brownlee M. Oxidative stress and diabetic complications. *Circ Res* 2010;**107**(9):1058–70.
177. Thornalley PJ, Babaei-Jadidi R, Al Ali H, Rabbani N, Antonysunil A, Larkin J, Ahmed A, Rayman G, Bodmer CW. High prevalence of low plasma thiamine concentration in diabetes linked to a marker of vascular disease. *Diabetologia* 2007;**50**(10):2164–70.
178. Larkin JR, Zhang F, Godfrey L, Molostvov G, Zehnder D, Rabbani N, Thornalley PJ. Glucose-induced down regulation of thiamine transporters in the kidney proximal tubular epithelium produces thiamine insufficiency in diabetes. *PLoS One* 2012;**7**(12):e53175.
179. Golomb BA, Evans MA. Statin adverse effects. *Am J Cardiovasc Drugs* 2008;**8**(6):373–418.
180. Thorp VJ. Effect of oral contraceptive agents on vitamin and mineral requirements. *J Am Diet Assoc* 1980;**76**(6):581–4.
181. Tyrer LB. Nutrition and the pill. *J Reprod Med* 1984;**29**(7 Suppl.):547–50.

182. Wan L, O'Brien P. Molecular mechanism of 17α-ethinylestradiol cytotoxicity in isolated rat hepatocytes. *Can J Physiol Pharmacol* 2013;**92**(1):21–6.
183. Pratt LA, Brody DJ, Gu Q. Antidepressant use in persons aged 12 and over: United States, 2005-2008. *NCHS Data Brief* 2011.
184. Maher RL, Hanlon J, Hajjar ER. Clinical consequences of polypharmacy in elderly. *Expert Opin Drug Saf* 2014;**13**(1):57–65.
185. Comer JS, Olfson M, Mojtabai R. National trends in child and adolescent psychotropic polypharmacy in office-based practice, 1996-2007. *J Am Acad Child Adolesc Psychiatry* 2010;**49**(10):1001–10.
186. Merikangas KR, He JP, Rapoport J, Vitiello B, Olfson M. Medication use in US youth with mental disorders. *JAMA Pediatr* 2013;**167**(2):141–8.
187. Mitchell AA, Gilboa SM, Werler MM, Kelley KE, Louik C, Hernández-Díaz S, Study NBDP. Medication use during pregnancy, with particular focus on prescription drugs: 1976-2008. *Am J Obstet Gynecol* 2011;**205**(1):51-e1.
188. Ward BW. Multiple chronic conditions among US adults: a 2012 update. *Prev Chronic Dis* 2014;**11**.
189. Natural medicines comprehensive database: drug influences on nutrient levels and depletion. http://naturaldatabase.therapeuticresearch.com/ce/ceCourse.aspx?pc=08-40&cec=0&pm=5.
190. McCormick LM, Buchanan JR, Onwuameze OE, Pierson RK, Paradiso S. Beyond alcoholism: Wernicke-Korsakoff syndrome in patients with psychiatric disorders. *Cogn Behav Neurol* 2011;**24**(4):209.
191. Peixoto F. Comparative effects of the roundup and glyphosate on mitochondrial oxidative phosphorylation. *Chemosphere* 2005;**61**(8):1115–22.
192. Olufunso OO, Babunmi EA, Bassir O. Effect of glyphosate on rat liver mitochondria in vivo. *Bull Environ Contam Toxicol* 1979;**22**(1):357–64.
193. http://www.theecologist.org/News/news_round_up/2987365/almost_all_germans_contaminated_with_glyphosate.html.
194. Kruger M, et al. Detection of glyphosate residues in animals and humans. *J Environ Anal Toxicol* 2014;**4**:210. http://dx.doi.org/10.4172/2161-0525.1000210.
195. Shehata AA, et al. The effect of glyphosate on potential pathogens and beneficial members of poultry microbiota in vitro. *Curr Microbiol* 2013;**66**(4):350–8. http://dx.doi.org/10.1007/s00284-012-0277-2.
196. Sorenson MT, Poulsen HD, Hojberg O. *Memorandum on "the feeding of genetically modified glyphosate resistant soy products to livestock"*. Danish Centre for Food and Agriculture; 2014.
197. Swanson NL, Leu A, Abrahamson J, Wallet B. Genetically engineered crops, glyphosate and the deterioration of health in the United States of America. *J Org Syst* 2014;**9**(2):6–37.
198. Benbrook B. Impacts of genetically engineered crops on pesticide use in the U.S. – the first sixteen years. *Environ Sci Eur* 2012;**24**:24. http://dx.doi.org/10.1186/2190-4715-24-24.
199. Attene-Ramos MS, Huang R, Sakamuru S, Witt KL, Beeson GC, Shou L, Schnellmann RG, Beeson CC, Tice RR, Austin CP, Xia M. Systematic study of mitochondrial toxicity of environmental chemicals using quantitative high throughput screening. *Chem Res Toxicol* 2013;**26**(9):1323–32.
200. Golomb BA, Allison M, Koperski S, Koslik HJ, Devaraj S, Ritchie JB. Coenzyme Q10 benefits symptoms in Gulf war veterans: results of a randomized double-blind study. *Neural Comput* 2014;**26**(11):2594–651.
201. Rayhan RU, Stevens BW, Raksit MP, Ripple JA, Timbol CR, Adewuyi O, VanMeter JW, Baraniuk JN. Exercise challenge in Gulf war illness reveals two subgroups with altered brain structure and function. *PLoS One* 2013;**8**(6):e63903.

202. Golomb BA. Acetylcholinesterase inhibitors and Gulf war illnesses. *Proc Natl Acad Sci USA* 2008;**105**(11):4295–300.
203. Harari YN. *Sapiens: a brief history of humankind*. Random House; 2014.
204. Gorman GS, Elson JL, Newman J, Payne B, McFarland R, Newton JL, Turnbull DM. Perceived fatigue is highly prevalent and debilitating in patients with mitochondrial disease. *Neuromuscul Disord* 2015;**25**(7):563–6.
205. Platt BS. Thiamine deficiency in human beriberi and in Wernicke's encephalopathy. In: *Thiamine deficiency*. Boston: Little, Brown and Company; 1967. p. 135–43.
206. Inouye K, Katsura E. Clinical signs and metabolism of beriberi patients. In: *Beriberi and thiamine*. Tokyo: Igaku Shoin Ltd; 1965. p. 29–63.
207. Rawles JM, Weller RO. Familial association of metabolic myopathy, lactic acidosis and sideroblastic anemia. *Am J Med* 1974;**56**(6):891–7.
208. Wolf PL, Levin MB. Shōshin beriberi. *N Engl J Med* 1960;**262**(26):1302–6.
209. McIntyre N, Stanley NN. Cardiac beriberi: two modes of presentation. *Br Med J* 1971;**3**(5774):567–9.
210. Lonsdale D, Shamberger RJ. The potential value of red cell transketolase in the metabolic evaluation of disease. *Cleve Clin Q* 1978;**45**(3):267.
211. Lonsdale D, Shamberger RJ. Red cell transketolase as an indicator of nutritional deficiency. *Am J Clin Nutr* 1980;**33**(2):205–11.
212. Williams RD, Mason HL, Power MH, Wilder RM. Induced thiamine (vitamin B1) deficiency in man: relation of depletion of thiamine to development of biochemical defect and of polyneuropathy. *Arch Intern Med* 1943;**71**(1):38–53.
213. Kramer J, Goodwin JA. Wernicke's encephalopathy: complication of intravenous hyperalimentation. *JAMA* 1977;**238**(20):2176–7.
214. Lonsdale D. Wernicke's encephalopathy and hyperalimentation. *JAMA* 1978;**239**(12):1133.
215. Lonsdale D, Cooper JR. Thiamine metabolism in disease. *CRC Crit Rev Clin Lab Sci* 1975;**5**(3):289–313.
216. Bennett T, Evans D, Hampton JR, Hosking DJ. Abnormal cardiovascular reflexes in subjects with autonomic neuropathy. *J Physiol* 1975;**246**(2):47P.
217. Frank HJ, Frewin DB, Robinson SM, Wise PH. Cardiovascular responses in diabetic dysautonomia. *Aust N Z J Med* 1972;**2**(1):1–7.
218. Blass JP, Gleason P, Brush D, et al. Thiamine and Alzheimer's disease. *Arch Neurol* 1988;**45**:833–5.
219. Meador KJ, Lorig D, Nichols M, et al. Preliminary findings of high dose thiamine in dementia of Alzheimer's type. *J Geriatr Psychiatry Neurol* 1993;**6**:222–9.
220. Mastrogiacoma F, Bettendorff L, Grisar T, Kish SH. Brain thiamine, its phosphate esters and its metabolizing enzymes in Alzheimer's disease. *Ann Neurol* 1996;**39**:585–91.
221. Henderson GI, Schenker S. Reversible impairment of cerebral DNA synthesis in thiamine deficiency. *J Lab Clin Med* 1975;**86**:77–90.
222. Vortmeyer AO, Hagel C, Laas R. Hypoxia-ischemia and thiamine deficiency. *Clin Neuropathol* 1993;**12**(4):184–90.

CHAPTER 4

# Evaluation and Treatment of Thiamine Metabolism in Clinical Practice

## Contents

| | |
|---|---|
| When to Consider Thiamine Deficiency | 107 |
| How to Evaluate Thiamine Status in Clinical Care | 108 |
|     Thiamine Deficiency in the Office | 109 |
|     In Acute or Emergent Care: Consider Wernicke's | 109 |
|     Thiamine Deficiency Versus Dependency | 109 |
| Laboratory Measures to Evaluate Thiamine | 110 |
| Measuring Thiamine Functionally | 111 |
|     Transketolase Activity | 111 |
|     Thiamine Pyrophosphate Effect | 112 |
|     Supporting Research for TKA and TPPE | 112 |
|     Patterns of Transketolase Activity | 113 |
|     Thiamine in Leigh's Disease | 113 |
| Alternative Observations That Point to Thiamine Deficiency | 114 |
|     Blood or Urine Pyruvate | 114 |
|     Lactate | 115 |
|     Cerebral Lactate Doublets Using Mass Spectrometry | 115 |
|     Urinary Creatine, Creatinine, and Uric Acid | 116 |
|         *Creatine and Creatinine Patterns in Clinical Care* | *116* |
|         *Hyperuricuria* | *119* |
|     Urinary Amino Acids | 120 |
|         *Transamination* | *121* |
|         *Transmethylation* | *121* |
|     Urine Amino Acids in Thiamine Deficiency and Functional Autonomic Disturbances | 122 |
|         *Aminoaciduria* | *122* |
|         *Urinary Keto Acids* | *123* |
|     Pulling It All Together: Urinary Lactate, Pyruvate, and Amino Acid Ratios in Reye's Syndrome | 123 |
|         *Points of Consideration* | *126* |
| Nonlaboratory Methods to Evaluate Thiamine Deficiency and Autonomic Function | 126 |
|     Asymmetrical Pulse Pressure and Orthostatic Hyper- or Hypotension | 127 |
|     Cerebellar Functioning: Gait, Balance, and Cognitive Affective Control | 127 |
|         *Assessing Gait and Balance* | *128* |
|         *Other Clues of Cerebellar Dysfunction* | *129* |

*Thiamine Deficiency Disease, Dysautonomia, and High Calorie Malnutrition*
ISBN 978-0-12-810387-6
http://dx.doi.org/10.1016/B978-0-12-810387-6.00004-6

© 2017 Elsevier Inc.
All rights reserved.

Cognitive Decrements With Impaired Mitochondrial Oxidation 129
Fatigue, Hypersomnia, and Anorexia as Markers of Insufficient ATP 129
Thiamine Therapy: Beyond the RDA 130
  Thiamine Dosing 131
  Thiamine Derivatives for Clinical Care 132
    *Thiamine Tetrahydrofurfuryl Disulfide* 132
  Clinical Evaluation TTFD 133
    *The Effect of TTFD on Blood Pressure in SHR* 134
  Thiamine Dependency 136
IV Thiamine for Acute and Chronic Cases 137
  Additional Nutrients 138
  Paradoxical Reactions to IV Thiamine and Other Nutrients 138
Thiamine in Clinical Care: Treating Functional and Genetic Disturbances 139
  Pyruvate Dehydrogenase Deficiency 140
  Intermittent Cerebellar Ataxia With Pyruvate Dehydrogenase Deficiency 141
    *Cognitive Testing* 144
    *Long-Term Progress* 145
    *Points of Consideration* 145
Nutrient Interactions 146
  Thiamine-Responsive Hypoglycemia With Biotin: Connections With Transamination 147
  Beriberi With Methylation Issues Leading to Folate and B12 Deficiencies 147
  Thiamine-Responsive Megaloblastic Anemia: Problems With Methylation 148
  Thiamine-Responsive Febrile Lymphadenopathy: Interplay With Folate and Vitamin B12 149
    *Points of Consideration* 149
  Nutrient-Responsive Complex Regional Pain Syndrome 151
Conclusion 152
References 152

The present medical model demands a diagnosis in essentially descriptive terms; one that must be filtered first through the physician's clinical perception and then through some mechanism of technological confirmation, lab tests, imaging, etc. If either of these two requirements is not met, the presenting illness is deemed psychosomatic or effectively nonexistent. This is to the great detriment of the patients whose diseases yield uneasily, if at all, to modern diagnostic parameters, e.g., those involving mitochondria and disturbed autonomic function. These disease processes, as we have shown repeatedly, not only breach normative clinical classification systems but are refractory to most modes of conventional testing as well, particularly in the earlier stages.

    Over half a century ago the notion of biochemical lesions emerged, suggesting that "pathological disturbances might be initiated by changes in biochemistry…" and that medicine ought to "…concentrate the research upon the initial enzymatic changes in the diseased tissues rather than wait upon the developments leading to the tissue damage visible with the microscope."[1] The idea was to find aberrant biochemical patterns before the more visible lesions appeared. It is a notion that all but lost favor over the decades since, but one we ascribe wholeheartedly. Nutrient deficiencies, because of their role in oxidative metabolism and a host of other enzymatic reactions, evoke biochemical lesions. The pathological cascades initiated as a result become manifest long before anatomical lesions appear and more conventional testing admits.

This chapter elucidates laboratory and other methods to evaluate the thiamine deficiency–induced biochemical lesions, when to consider thiamine deficiency in clinical care, and how to treat it once identified. We explore the possibility of developing megadose thiamine as a therapeutic approach where there is clinical and laboratory evidence of mitochondrial dysfunction. Attention is drawn to those human disorders such as diabetes and brain diseases that are now known to be associated with abnormal thiamine metabolism.

## WHEN TO CONSIDER THIAMINE DEFICIENCY

Among the first questions to be answered is "when should I consider thiamine deficiency?" Our response is "always." Thiamine and nutrient status should be considered as a core component of modern health care. Thiamine is not a magic cure-all, but its position atop the pyruvate pathway makes it critical to human health and survival. When we recognize the myriad dietary, pharmaceutical, and environmental exposures capable of depleting thiamine and impairing mitochondrial functioning, it becomes clear that thiamine deficiency is more, not less, likely in both chronic and acute care. The research bears this out:

- Up to 76% of diabetics (type 1 and type 2) are thiamine deficient[2] because of altered kidney[3] and pancreatic[4] thiamine transporter function. Glucose regulation[5] and the side effects of hyperglycemia[6,7] improve with thiamine supplementation.
- At least 29% of obese patients are thiamine deficient; postbariatric thiamine deficiencies have been reported in as many as 49% of the patients.[8]
- Approximately 40% of community dwelling elderly are thiamine deficient, while 48% of elderly patients in acute care[9] may be thiamine deficient.
- Fifty-five percent of cancer patients have been found thiamine deficient.[10]

- An unknown number of critical care patients are thiamine deficient. Thiamine deficiency in critical care, whether in children or adults, is associated with a 50% increase in all-cause mortality.[11] Conversely, thiamine supplementation in cases of lactic acidosis critical care patients, where the association of thiamine deficiency is not often recognized in the emergency room, is a promising treatment.[12]
- A random sampling of 500 patients admitted to the emergency room over a 3-day period in the United Kingdom found that 20% of the patients were thiamine deficient.[13]
- Thirty-three percent of congestive heart failure patients are thiamine deficient.[14]
- Thirty-eight percent of pregnant women may be thiamine deficient,[15] more severely so with hyperemesis gravidarum. Thiamine deficiency during pregnancy is associated with maternal and fetal death.[16]
- Thirty percent of psychiatric patients demonstrate significant nutrient deficiencies, including thiamine.[17]
- Infection spurs thiamine deficiency.[18]
- Adverse medication and vaccine reactions often induce thiamine deficiency.[19]

If we know that thiamine is integral to mitochondrial functioning and its absence leads to a host of symptoms that may ultimately result in brain damage, heart failure, and death, and if we know that a good percentage of the population is thiamine deficient, particularly the chronically and acutely ill, should not we be assessing thiamine status as a matter of course? And, more importantly, should not we be supplementing thiamine in these and other populations as well? It is entirely possible, given thiamine's role in oxidative metabolism and mitochondrial functioning as a whole, that the presenting crisis is in some way related to thiamine status. Whether thiamine is the cause or the effect of the illness should not matter. That thiamine will improve outcomes is all that counts.

## HOW TO EVALUATE THIAMINE STATUS IN CLINICAL CARE

With the practice of medicine today governed by advanced technology, thiamine deficiency, however, hardly crosses the mind of the modern physician, so how can a given patient ever be considered in the differential diagnosis? The limited time for a given consultation and the preoccupation with electronic recording require some ideas that can provide clues.

## Thiamine Deficiency in the Office

A quick check on diet history: ask specific questions concerning the ingestion of sweets, including cakes, desserts, and carbonated drinks, as well as the routine question concerning alcohol. This particularly applies to the diet of children[20]:

1. The more polysymptomatic the history, the more likely it is to be mitochondrial in nature. For the combination of sweet ingestion and mitochondrial disease, think thiamine deficiency.
2. Postural orthostatic tachycardia syndrome is a common presentation of thiamine deficiency in adults and variable forms of emotional and behavior problems in children. Dysautonomia represents the most definitive presentation of beriberi in its early stages.[19]

## In Acute or Emergent Care: Consider Wernicke's

Wernicke's encephalopathy, a more serious form of thiamine deficiency, is well recognized in name but not in practice. Indeed, the triad of neurological symptoms (oculomotor irregularities, ataxia, and memory and mental status changes) has been taught in medical schools for generations and can be identified easily by most first-year medical students (and any undergraduate psychology student). In practice, however, thiamine deficiency is so far afield from clinical suspicions that even in its most severe forms clinical diagnosis is missed in 80% of adult cases.[21] In pediatric populations, thiamine deficiency is missed in up to 58% of cases.[22] Those numbers reflect a disturbing lack of clinical acuity partly because Wernicke's triad inadequately describes the symptomology (only 16% of confirmed Wernicke's patients exhibit all three symptom components[21]), but mostly because we simply do not look for deficiencies in thiamine or other nutrients in clinical care. Thiamine deficiency, it appears, is rarely suspected or assessed either clinically or medically, even in chronic alcoholics, but especially in nonalcoholics. In light of the sheer commonness of thiamine deficiency in the acute setting, the role of thiamine in mitochondrial functioning, and the subsequent risks associated with deficiency, we believe thiamine testing and supplementation ought to be considered as a standard of care.

## Thiamine Deficiency Versus Dependency

Thiamine dependency represents a more severe and often more chronic form of thiamine deficiency, involving a genetic abnormality in the binding of the cofactor to the enzyme. Even if the clinical expression is recognized, the failure of moderate thiamine replacement doses would easily lead to the conclusion that thiamine metabolism was not involved, leading the practitioner to cease with thiamine replacement. With thiamine dependency, massive doses of thiamine are required, often for extended periods of time. When clinical and/or laboratory evidence points to thiamine deficiency, but symptoms remain refractory to supplementation, thiamine dependency ought to be considered and dosing adapted accordingly.

## LABORATORY MEASURES TO EVALUATE THIAMINE

Once one suspects thiamine deficiency, the question becomes "should lab evaluation be sought, and if so, which tests?" The answer is yes, testing should be sought. However, accurate testing is not always available and so the clinician may be faced with the prospect of treating the patient blindly and looking for clinical clues to confirm thiamine response. Since thiamine is water soluble and nontoxic, the treatment-response method is acceptable, even warranted in cases where severe thiamine deficiency is suggested. Certainly, the physician can treat a given patient with megadoses of thiamine if the clinical evidence suggests the possibility. Over 40 years, Dr. Lonsdale has treated hundreds of patients and has never seen any toxicity.

Currently, there are five methods to measure thiamine status, each with varying degrees of sensitivity and specificity[23]:
- Blood thiamine
- Urinary thiamine excretion
- Pyruvate and lactate
- Whole blood high-performance liquid chromatography (HPLC)
- Erythrocyte transketolase activity (ETKA)/thiamine pyrophosphate effect (TPPE)

Most common among them is the determination of free thiamine concentrations in blood or plasma. This method is used by most of the major laboratories. Unfortunately, the concentration of thiamine measured in blood or plasma is usually normal even with advanced thiamine deficiency and at most reflects the recent intake of thiamine. Since blood contains only 0.8% of total body free thiamine, determination of free thiamine in blood does not reflect tissue levels.[24] Similarly, the excretion of thiamine is not particularly accurate, reflecting only the intake of thiamine immediately preceding the testing.

Since thiamine is required for pyruvate metabolism, elevated pyruvate and lactate can be indicative of thiamine deficiency, particularly when there are no other options for thiamine testing. However, these too are problematic, particularly when thiamine status is marginal. Nevertheless, when direct determination is unavailable, indirect measures may be useful.

Whole blood HPLC represents one of the newest methods of testing and can be used to measure thiamine, thiamine diphosphate (the biologically active form of thiamine), and its esters in the erythrocytes. HPLC provides a more sensitive determination of thiamine stores than either of the aforementioned blood or urinary methods. This method allows for the separation and measurement of free thiamine and its phosphate esters.[25] Because thiamine esters decline before unphosphorylated or phosphorylated thiamine does, this method is arguably more sensitive to early thiamine deficiency.[26] HPLC, however, is costly and not readily available.

Among the available tests we believe the most sensitive measure of thiamine status is the ETKA/TPPE. The pair of tests assesses functional thiamine usage and accurately reflects thiamine stores at the tissue level.[27,28] The remainder of this chapter will focus on transketolase testing, as we believe that is it the most accurate method available to date.

## MEASURING THIAMINE FUNCTIONALLY

To detect thiamine deficiency, particularly in the early stages, it is important to understand how thiamine is used inside the cells. Thiamine and magnesium are cofactors for the enzyme transketolase that occurs twice in the pentose phosphate pathway, also called the hexose monophosphate shunt (HMPS). Recall also that thiamine must be transported into the cell and into the mitochondria by way of solute carrier protein transporters and then phosphorylated to be activated. Either process can be compromised, yielding normal circulating thiamine concentrations but deficient intracellular and intramitochondrial thiamine. Understanding this process allows us to measure thiamine more accurately and more functionally. Since the HMPS exists in erythrocytes, they can be used to ascertain the activity of transketolase by measuring the concentration of its product per unit time.[29] Transketolase testing is done in two parts.

### Transketolase Activity

First, the baseline activity is recorded in international units per liter of blood per unit time and is reported as transketolase activity (TKA). In the laboratory used by Dr. Lonsdale, which is now closed, the normal range had been ascertained from individuals who were asymptomatic and ostensibly healthy (42–86 mU/L/min).

## Thiamine Pyrophosphate Effect

TKA is repeated after the addition of thiamine pyrophosphate (TPP) to the reaction medium. If the activity of the enzyme increases, it is taken as evidence that the enzyme was not saturated with its cofactor. It is reported as the percentage increase over baseline activity as indicated by what is called the TPPE. The normal range was accepted as 0%–18%. By controlling for thiamine, it is possible that this test might be used for magnesium deficiency, but to our knowledge this has not been done. It is suggested that any practitioner wishing to expand his or her practice to include detection of thiamine deficiency should approach the medical laboratory that he or she uses. The methodology was published by Massod et al.[30]

## Supporting Research for TKA and TPPE

Over the course of Dr. Lonsdale's clinical practice, TKA and TPPE were performed on 1011 patients between 1983 and 1986. Either TKA or TPPE or both were abnormal in 283 patients (28%). Out of the total number of patients with these abnormal findings, 36 were selected as representative and the clinical presentation correlated with subsequent laboratory testing after thiamine supplementation. This strongly suggests that widespread marginal nutritional deficiency exists in the United States and deserves more attention than it is presently receiving.[31]

From this work, Dr. Lonsdale came to the conclusion that thiamine deficiency may exist in a mild asymptomatic form, thus providing the wide range of acceptable or normal TPPE on a sliding scale. Perhaps a TPPE of 15% may give rise to thiamine deficiency symptoms in one individual, whereas 18% might be asymptomatic in another. Dr. Lonsdale's experience showed that in many instances the TKA would be in the normal range when the TPPE was increased, but still within the acceptable range. If this test result is then considered to be normal, it might give rise to rejection of thiamine deficiency as the definitive cause of the patient's symptoms. In other situations, the TKA was in the normal range and the TPPE was well over the acceptable range of 18%, clearly indicating thiamine deficiency. After therapy with thiamine, the TKA would increase within the normal range and the TPPE would decrease, often to zero, indicating full saturation of the enzyme. If the enzyme is fully saturated with thiamine, a strictly normal TPPE would be zero. We are presently aware that some laboratories are performing TKA without the TPPE. Thus we would expect that symptoms occurring because of thiamine deficiency would be misdiagnosed as caused by other factors when the TKA is in the normal range.

Wells et al. found that TKA would be over the normal range in vitamin B12 megaloblastic anemia but not in that caused by folate deficiency, thus differentiating the two different etiologies.[32]

Other laboratory studies that are often abnormal in thiamine deficiency include inflammatory markers, fibrinogen, and hypersensitive C-reactive protein (CRP). Increased triglycerides are virtually definitive as an indication of sugar ingestion.[19] In animal studies, sucrose and fructose have been shown to decrease insulin sensitivity with a potential association with induced hypertriglyceridemia.[33] Changes in the white cell count may include eosinophilia.[34]

## Patterns of Transketolase Activity

1. Sometimes the TKA is low while the TPPE is normal and this would suggest that there is some abnormality in the enzyme.[35]
2. In most cases of thiamine deficiency, in our experience the TPPE is increased, sometimes remarkably so, and the TKA is in the normal range.
3. In a more severe deficiency state, the TKA is low, but in the normal range, and the TPPE is high.

Correlating the patient's symptoms with a fall in the TPPE and a rise in TKA (remaining within the normal range) is an excellent way of proving the clinical effect of thiamine supplementation. This can be complicated since the enzyme complex is also dependent on magnesium.[36] Magnesium depletion aggravates the clinical effects of thiamine deficiency.[37] Magnesium and calcium deficiency affect the distribution of thiamine in rat brain.[38] An increase in TKA was found in B12-deficient patients but not in those where the anemia was caused by folate deficiency.[39,40]

## Thiamine in Leigh's Disease

In 1969 Cooper and associates published their finding of thiamine triphosphate (TTP) deficiency in Leigh's disease, also known as subacute necrotizing encephalomyelopathy (SNE).[41] The pathophysiology of this disease is similar, but not identical, to that of Wernicke's disease. Their diagnosis depended upon finding a substance in urine that reportedly inhibited the formation of TTP.[42] The substance was never identified and this important research was eventually discontinued for lack of funding.

Urine from several polysymptomatic patients, clinically suspected of thiamine deficiency symptoms, but with normal transketolase tests, was sent to Cooper's laboratory and was reported positive for this test. Each responded to thiamine supplementation. None of these patients could be considered to be examples of Leigh's disease.[43] It was the only laboratory study ever reported to indicate TTP deficiency and there is presently no known clinically available method of depicting this vitally important link in our knowledge of thiamine metabolism in the brain. Although SNE is now considered the most common pediatric presentation of mitochondrial disease,[44] thiamine pyrophosphokinase, the enzyme that synthesizes TPP, has been implicated as one of the mutations that causes it and it is considered to be a treatable condition.[45] All of this information begs the question whether mitochondrial dysfunction is always genetically determined or whether it can be acquired as a result of prolonged cofactor deficiency, environmental trauma, "recreational" drugs, or even from prescription drugs.

## ALTERNATIVE OBSERVATIONS THAT POINT TO THIAMINE DEFICIENCY

Many clinicians have difficulty perceiving that biochemical reactions are in a continuously dynamic state. Blood and urine metabolites change in concentration constantly, and together they reflect total function of the organism. By the same token, the changes presumably reflect the stage of evolution of a disease, and a given metabolite may be low, normal, or increased in the same disease, in the same patient, at different times. Not infrequently a clinical diagnosis is based upon laboratory observations without sufficiently considering these factors. For this reason it is important to understand some of the corresponding changes in biochemistry that may point to thiamine deficiency. Ideally, these methods would be used in association with transketolase testing and thus afford the clinician a more complete picture of the patient's disease process and functional deficits that could be used to guide treatment. However, when the more sensitive thiamine testing methods are not available, thiamine deficiency may be arrived at inferentially by combining clinical suspicion with indirect measures of thiamine activity. It should be noted that these methods are not as sensitive as transketolase testing and if negative cannot rule out thiamine deficiency. Again, we should point out, however, that thiamine, even at high doses, makes empirical treatment of thiamine deficiency without testing feasible and safe.

### Blood or Urine Pyruvate

An increase in blood and urine pyruvate is well recognized in thiamine deficiency because pyruvate is blocked at the pyruvic dehydrogenase and lactate is derived from it.[46] Case Example 4.1 illustrates the role of thiamine in treating lactic acidosis.[47]

**Case Example 4.1 Lactic Acidosis in a 4-Year-Old Boy**
A 4-year-old boy was reported with medulloblastoma who presented with lactic acidosis after hypovitaminotic parenteral nutrition given to him for septic shock. The authors discuss the difference between type A (hypoxic) and type B (pseudo-hypoxic) lactic acidosis, pointing out that type B is an underrecognized clinical entity. This patient was given intravenous thiamine that rapidly normalized the lactate level, which then remained stable, thus demonstrating that thiamine deficiency can produce lactic acidosis.

## Lactate

Lactate is a fuel used readily in the body in response to changing metabolic needs (exertion and stressors[48]) and efficiencies (oxygen usage, nutrient cofactor availability). In a grossly oversimplified manner, the extent to which one produces and utilizes lactate during training indicates one's overall fitness. In a similar manner, lactate production and utilization are key indicators of overall mitochondrial functioning. Where the chief complaint is excessive fatigue and/or excessive postexertional fatigue, lactic acidosis may differentiate the underlying cause from other disabling dysautonomic syndromes.[49] Although measures of lactate are common in critical care where lactic acidosis presents a very real risk, thiamine deficiency is often not considered as the underlying cause.

## Cerebral Lactate Doublets Using Mass Spectrometry

Just as excess lactate and tolerance thresholds in the muscles represent overall fitness in the face of increased metabolic demands, so too does brain lactate. The connection between lactate and mitochondrial functioning was only recently discovered and remains hotly debated.[50] For a long time it was believed that lactate remained outside the mitochondrion. Now, evidence suggests that mitochondria can convert lactate to ATP and that lactate is shuttled in and out of mitochondria to be used when needed.[51] Although arguably a more expensive, technically sophisticated, and a less direct measure of thiamine deficiency, mass resonance spectrometry (MRS) is emerging as a valuable tool to visualize cerebral lactate utilization.[50]

The lactate molecule has two weakly coupled signals or resonances. When viewed on the MRS, the lactate doublet presents as a double peak in the signal algorithm indicating the switch from aerobic to anaerobic metabolism.[52] In patients with genetic mitochondriopathies, researchers have been able to delineate the regional differences in brain lactate corresponding to the neurological and clinical symptomatology associated with each mitochondriopathy. Cerebral lactate doublets have been recognized in autism,[53] aging[49] (although mechanisms remain contended[54]), and other mitochondrial disease processes and may become a useful tool to evaluate the degree and scope of neurological involvement in dysautonomic syndromes with or without thiamine deficiency.

## Urinary Creatine, Creatinine, and Uric Acid

A singular need in evaluating nutritional and biochemical adequacy is a relatively simple method by which energy metabolism might be measured easily in patients. If such a tool were readily available and could be used repetitively for monitoring therapeutic progress it would have to be noninvasive, and it would be more valuable if a standard clinical laboratory were able to perform the studies. Such a concept is roughly similar to that which is used by an engineer in evaluating the running qualities of highly complicated machinery. An analogy might be considered in the use of an ammeter in the automobile. There is no such thing as a "normal" position for the needle in this instrument. The central line marks the division between a charging and a discharging state of the battery. This analogy seemingly has little to do with the complicated machinery of the human body, or perhaps in more finite terms a single cell, but it is the cumulative action of all the cells in the body that represents the total energy metabolism of the organism and therefore it should be possible to monitor collective cellular metabolism in some way similar to that used by the engineer.

### Creatine and Creatinine Patterns in Clinical Care

We have attempted to use the unique biochemical relationship of creatine to creatinine in the body as a means of obtaining this kind of general information. Creatine is synthesized in liver and kidney when the amidine group of arginine is transferred to the nitrogen of glycine to form ornithine and guanidinoacetic acid. Methylation then proceeds, first by the reaction of methionine and ATP in the presence of an activating enzyme to form S-adenosyl methionine, which then transfers the methyl group to guanidinoacetic acid by the action of guanidinoacetate methylpherase to form creatine and S-adenosyl homocysteine. The formation of creatine therefore requires ATP, which is essentially a test of oxidative metabolism and is also dependent upon the presence of methionine and the rate of formation of S-adenosyl methionine.[55]

The methyl group of creatine is nonlabile and its nitrogen is not used as a source of protein synthesis. Creatine may therefore be considered to be an end product of metabolism of glycine, arginine, and methionine. Creatine is then carried in the blood and 95% is subsequently found in muscle. The remaining 5% is located in the brain and testes.[56] There is evidence for an active transport across the muscle cell plasma membrane, and it is then phosphorylated to form phosphocreatine by the reaction creatine + ATP = phosphocreatine and ADP. This reversible reaction is the means for provision of ATP as required at the contractile site in muscle, and equilibrium of the reaction is influenced by the concentration of magnesium ions. Creatine, generated during muscular activity, may play a role in energy production through a regulatory feedback mechanism.[57] Formation of creatinine appears to be almost exclusively from phosphocreatine,[55] is nonenzymatic, and in normal health represents the final product of creatine metabolism. Fig. 4.1 illustrates the synthesis, transport, and utilization of creatine and its excretory relationship with creatinine.

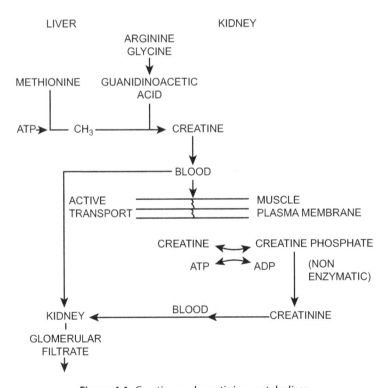

Figure 4.1 Creatine and creatinine metabolism.

Creatinine is found in large concentrations in the urine, as compared with only very small amounts of creatine. By examining urinary concentrations of creatine and creatinine it becomes possible therefore to derive information about a number of metabolic and physiologic states. A high concentration of both creatine and creatinine in normal ratio would indicate a fast metabolic turnover as compared with low concentrations, which would indicate the opposite. High urinary concentrations of creatine with relatively low creatinine might indicate several possibilities.

Overproduction of creatine in liver and kidney overwhelms the plasma membrane transport system or its "trapping" to form phosphocreatine in the muscle cell. At the time,[56] the mechanism was not known. We now know that creatine requires a transporter, and transporter deficiency prevents creatine entry into tissue and results in a significant intellectual impairment, epilepsy, and aphasia.[58] Lack of transporter function would lead to increased renal clearance. Loss of creatine from muscle cells because of abnormal leakage through plasma membrane is implicated in muscle dystrophy.

Because of Dr. Lonsdale's clinical experience in identifying a patient with defective pyruvate decarboxylation,[59] it became usual practice for him to obtain a 24-h urine in a day-and-night 12-h collection to ascertain whether there were any differences in creatinine and creatine. It was often surprising to see radical changes between the two, which suggested that this form of nitrogenous excretion was also affected by circadian rhythm. Although concentrations varied grossly from patient to patient and also in repeated studies on the same patient, the ratio of creatine to creatinine remained remarkably constant in healthy children, but quite disparate in unhealthy children.

Variation in this ratio may be quite a useful indicator of metabolic inefficiency in the absorption mechanism and hence be interpreted as providing indirect evidence of cell membrane activity. If the test is repeated in a patient under treatment, the patient can act as his/her own control. In some cases the ratio of creatine to creatinine can be plotted as a graph and the trend of the ratio can be easily portrayed. As described, the biochemistry is relatively simple, and it is by taking advantage of these metabolic limitations that it promises to be useful in providing information about the basic lesion that may be common to a number of diseases.

### Creatinuria in Adults

Creatinuria has been noted in beriberi as well as in experimentally induced thiamine deficiency. An observation in rats showed that creatinuria occurred as a result of protein calorie deficiency caused by experimental starvation. When anorexia was caused by thiamine deprivation, the creatinuria occurred much sooner and was statistically in greater concentration, suggesting that abnormal membrane physiology was involved in these two differently stimulated mechanisms. Creatinuria disappeared in beriberi patients with bed rest before thiamine had been discovered. TTP, which may have a role in membrane physiology, remains as the outstanding mystery of thiamine metabolism.

### Creatinuria in Children

In children, creatinuria is regarded as physiologic, and since we know that metabolism is fast in childhood, it is of possible value in calibrating the rate of that metabolism in the normal versus abnormal state. Clark and associates[60] published normal values many years ago and little or no work has been done since in using this information to study disease. The ratio of creatine to creatinine in urine of children is higher, but gradually diminishes to adult proportions at the age of approximately 18 years. The range for both creatine and creatinine is wide, but the ratio appears to be fairly constant in normal health, according to Clark et al. The ratio in the first 2 years is frequently greater than 1.0, but decreases to less than 0.1 in the adult. We have studied the urine by measuring both metabolites in a 12-h day and a 12-h night collection, presenting the data as total concentration of each, the ratio, and the concentration per unit of body weight. In general, creatinuria suggests a failure to absorb creatine into cells or to trap it as creatine phosphate.[56] Since it is the source of available ATP in muscles, they turn to anaerobic energy, a much less efficient form. This will be illustrated with case studies in Chapter 5.

Iwata and associates found higher tissue concentrations of catecholamines and depressed activity of monoamine oxidase in thiamine-deficient rats.[61–63] Ochoa showed that anaerobic conditions resulted in destruction of cocarboxylase.[64] Inasmuch as thiamine deficiency results in pseudohypoxia, it is possible that it might set up a vicious cycle, resulting in further destruction of TPP when anaerobic metabolism has been induced.

### *Hyperuricuria*

Hyperuricuria, an excess of uric acid in the urine, may be observed in some patients with thiamine deficiency. Hyperuricuria without hyperuricemia would presumably reflect rapid renal clearance of excessive uric acid from the blood. Dr. Lonsdale encountered a mentally retarded female child with hyperuricuria. The reader might recall that the Lesch–Nyhan syndrome is sex linked, only occurring in males.[65] Profound acidosis and increased concentrations of urinary uric acid in early infancy were repeatedly detected in this child. Blood uric acid was found to be elevated on only one or two occasions. Compulsive lip biting, as seen in Lesch–Nyhan syndrome and commonly associated with hyperuricemia, was so severe that teeth had to be removed to relieve the constant trauma. Concentration of red cell hypoxanthine-guanine phosphoribosyl transferase, the sex-linked enzyme deficiency responsible for causing Lesch–Nyhan syndrome, was normal as expected. Accumulation of pyruvate in serum after intravenous glucose suggested defective entry of pyruvate to the citric acid cycle.[66] Although she responded metabolically to administration of thiamine supplementation, the clinical effect was minimal, although she became easier to handle as a patient. Hyperuricuria, which disappeared after thiamine was administered, was thought to be caused by a compensatory activity of the HMPS, inducing de novo biosynthesis through activation of phosphoribosyl-pyrophosphate degradation.[67] It is of interest that one of the thiamine-responsive cases of maple syrup urine disease had unexplained hyperuricacidemia.[68] A logical explanation might be proposed that defective phosphorylation of thiamine was responsible for an effect in the decarboxylating components of branched-chain dehydrogenase and pyruvate dehydrogenase (PDH) at the same time. Hence overproduction of uric acid could have been a metabolic phenomenon similar to that seen in the child with compulsive lip biting just described.

## Urinary Amino Acids

Dr. Lonsdale's practice employed amino acid screening for many years using standard methods[69–71] and a wide experience of a number of inborn errors of metabolism was acquired.[72–76] Before we proceed, a quick review of theoretical biochemistry is warranted. Specifically, understanding how transamination and transmethylation relate to the process of oxidative metabolism will provide a foundation for understanding how cellular function creates and uses energy. The citric acid cycle and electron transport system produce energy and are the equivalent of an internal combustion engine. Transamination and transmethylation consume it for cellular construction and function and are the equivalent of a transmission. (Note: transulfuration is the equivalent of an "exhaust pipe" and really does not fulfill the analogy.)

## Transamination

Nitrogen balance is the key to growth, metabolic stability, and eventual physical decline. A child must be in a state of positive balance to grow and develop, and part of this is achieved by the transfer of nitrogen from transamination. It is dependent upon the presence of transaminases, which require a variable organization of cofactors and physical environment for their normal function. Most alpha amino acids have their amino group removed as the first stage of their metabolic breakdown. The amino group is transaminated to a keto acid, forming another amino acid. A keto acid may be further broken down by a decarboxylating enzyme to become an organic acid, which is then oxidized in a series of steps, or it may become reaminated to form the original parent amino acid. Thus nitrogen is transferred and cellular protein is synthesized or dietary protein is used as fuel. The mechanism of transamination in brain involves glutamic and aspartic acids as the two almost exclusively involved amino acids in this process.[77] Both play other important roles. Glutamic acid is used, for example, to synthesize gamma-amino butyric acid, a neurotransmitter that has an anticonvulsive action,[78] and is essential to the activation of choline acetylase,[79] as well as having an important effect on cation metabolism.[80] Aspartic acid is important in the elimination of free ammonia and in the ornithine urea cycle.[78] Deletion of either of these amino acids in the brain would have serious consequences.

## Transmethylation

The one carbon pool represents a group of compounds capable of transferring a methyl group to another compound and thus adding an additional carbon atom. Methionine is the most important methyl donor. Oxidative metabolism synthesizes ATP, which is required to form $S$-adenosyl methionine (SAM) from methionine, and energy is therefore consumed. The labile methyl group is then passed on to a number of receptor compounds and homocysteine is formed. Homocysteine may be transulfurated or remethylated back to methionine to complete the cycle. This remethylated step, like the formation of choline from ethanolamine, requires folate as methyl donor and is also one of the two enzymatic steps dependent upon vitamin B12. Formation of choline is an important methylation reaction in its endogenous synthesis, although diet is the main source of this metabolite, which is central in phospholipid synthesis and the formation of acetylcholine. Although choline deficiency in humans seldom, if ever, occurs, the effects seen in experimental animals are well known.[81]

We have used transmethylation, being an energy-consuming pathway, as being analogous to a transmission in a car where energy is converted into function. To complete the analogy, any breakdown in the linked stages of energy synthesis or energy consumption must affect the whole organism. Since it is obviously never complete, because that would be lethal, the loss of efficiency and its distribution within the body therefore decides how the disease will be expressed. The whole process is initiated by pyruvic dehydrogenase, where thiamine deficiency has been shown to have produced disease for thousands of years.

## Urine Amino Acids in Thiamine Deficiency and Functional Autonomic Disturbances

As will be discussed later in this chapter, we mention here a case of intermittent cerebellar ataxia that initiated Dr. Lonsdale's interest in energy metabolism and its relationship with thiamine.[59] In this particular case, it was discovered that the patient had gross differences in urinary excretion of pyruvate, alpha ketoglutarate, and some amino acids by day as compared with night. Although the night and day differences in urinary pyruvate and alpha ketoglutarate were initially thought to be associated with diet, it was eventually thought possible that it reflected disturbed circadian rhythm, since healthy children receiving a similar diet did not demonstrate such wide differences in their urinary concentrations of these metabolites.[66]

The urinary amino acid concentrations in the case cited revealed day and night differences for alanine, glutamic acid, and aspartic acid. Generally speaking, there appears to be some relationship between the nutritional state as a whole and urinary amino acid concentrations. Dr. Lonsdale observed gross changes in urinary amino acid chromatograms from treated phenylketonuria patients.[82] In some instances it was corrected by increasing the phenylalanine intake after finding the serum phenylalanine to be too low. In other cases the serum chromatogram became normal after increasing the calories through carbohydrate or phenylalanine-low formula.

### *Aminoaciduria*

In attempting to assess patients who might be metabolically abnormal and responsive to nutritional therapy, Dr. Lonsdale found that some of the selected patients excreted unusually low concentrations of urinary amino acids (oligoaminoaciduria). After supplementary nutrient therapy began, the pattern would change to hyperaminoaciduria. Subsequently, the urinary amino acid concentrations became normal. These changes are seemingly nonspecific and may reflect only the degree of nitrogen balance since the whole range of amino acids either increased or decreased.

The phenomenon may possibly be likened to the pattern of hydrocarbons in the exhaust pipe from an internal combustion engine, reflecting the efficiency of the engine. Obviously, it is considerably complicated by factors that may be primarily genetic or secondarily acquired, such as renal tubular absorption. For example, renal tubular hyperaminoaciduria in galactosemia clears when a galactose-free diet is provided to the patient.[83] On the other hand, it may well be that urinary amino acid relationships may be much more important than this relatively simplistic suggestion. Perhaps by studying a disease where there is some evidence of defective energy metabolism, some clues might be found. There have been some attempts to do this in Reye's syndrome, a condition in which mitochondrial changes have suggested an abnormality of this nature.[84] A change in the ratio of branched-chain to aromatic amino acids has been reported in the disease[85] and increased concentrations of homovanillic acid have suggested a relationship between brain catecholamines and cerebral ischemia.[86]

### Urinary Keto Acids

Urinary keto acid concentrations, like amino acids, have not proved to be very helpful in determining the exact nature of metabolic abnormality in most cases. The method used was originally reported to be the determination of pyruvic acid,[87] but it is not specific and will recognize the presence of other organic acids. Now that mass spectrometry is available, this methodology is insufficient, but 2D paper chromatography reveals the presence of pyruvic acid and alpha ketoglutarate[88] and each has a distinctive color reaction if the paper is dipped in sodium hydroxide, followed by diazotized sulfanilic acid. In selected cases therefore it was possible to observe semi-quantitative determinations of these two metabolites.

## Pulling It All Together: Urinary Lactate, Pyruvate, and Amino Acid Ratios in Reye's Syndrome

Although it is now known that most cases of Reye's syndrome are caused by giving a child aspirin, there are still occasional reports of this syndrome appearing without an etiology being recognized. Research reported here was initiated because of a rising belief that energy metabolism was an important key to many, if not all, diseases. There was therefore reason to look for evidence.[89]

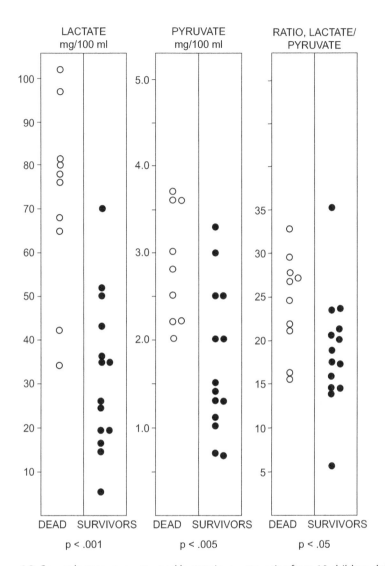

**Figure 4.2** Serum lactate, pyruvate, and lactate/pyruvate ratios from 10 children dying from Reye's syndrome compared with 14 survivors.

In a group of patients with Reye's syndrome under the care of physicians at Rainbow Babies and Children's Hospital, Cleveland, Ohio, urine was examined for amino acids and total keto acids and blood was examined for concentrations of ammonia and pyruvic and lactic acids. In Figs. 4.2 and 4.3 these concentrations are compared in the patients who died with those who survived. The ratio of glycine to alanine was lower in urines from both groups of Reye's syndrome patients than in healthy controls, and there were

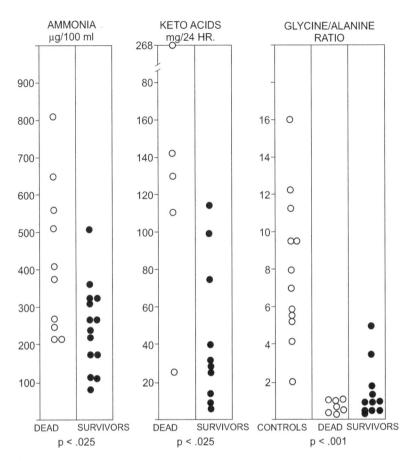

**Figure 4.3** Serum ammonia, urinary total keto acids, and glycine/alanine ratio from patients dying of Reye's syndrome.

statistically significant differences between nonsurvivors and those who survived for serum lactate, pyruvate, and ammonia as well as keto acids. There were 24 patients in all, but not all of them had urine collections completed, and this explains the discrepancy in the number of evaluations as shown.

The absolute concentrations of both glycine and alanine in urine were usually much increased in these patients, but a lower glycine-to-alanine ratio suggested that the alanine increase was disproportionately greater than that of glycine, indicating that there was a greater alanine production, or renal loss, in Reye's syndrome urines than in urines from healthy individuals. This was irrespective of whether concentrations of glycine and alanine were in their normal or abnormal individual ranges, respectively. Normally, pyruvate, lactate, and alanine are in equilibrium and a defect in pyruvate metabolism results in a proportional increase in the concentrations of all three substances in the plasma.[90] Since lactate can be metabolized only by conversion back to pyruvate—and this occurs especially readily in aerobic tissue, such as the heart and kidney—the rise in alanine concentration supports the interpretation of hypoxic tissue in Reye's syndrome. This suggested evidence of a hypoxic tissue state, which was more severe in the patients who died, compared with the survivors.

The two survivors with the highest glycine/alanine ratio were the mildest and least affected children of the 11 children tested.

*Points of Consideration*
The difference in serum ammonia and urinary keto acids between survivors and nonsurvivors in Reye's syndrome certainly seems to suggest that this disease is an example of energy failure affecting brain metabolism. Little can be said about the glycine/alanine ratios except to say that it appeared to reflect the severity of the disease. It is included here as an interesting observation.

It is apparent that the primary defect in Reye's syndrome is a breakdown of the normal mechanisms for energy production or utilization, and that the various enzyme defects described in the disease have this mechanism in common. The amino acid pattern produced by salicylates[91] turned out to be that seen in Reye's syndrome, now thought to be a mitochondrial disease in which aspirin may or may not be a related agent.[92] A breakdown of energy metabolism suggests an acquired mitochondrial dysfunction, perhaps in association with genetic risk.

## NONLABORATORY METHODS TO EVALUATE THIAMINE DEFICIENCY AND AUTONOMIC FUNCTION

Details concerning the heterogeneous clinical expression of thiamine deficiency are demonstrated in a number of case reports in Chapter 5. It is invariably polysymptomatic and it is almost certain that many cases are misdiagnosed as psychosomatic. Should the patient's symptoms be recognized as those of dysautonomia, modern technological studies confirming this diagnosis are likely to be ascribed solely to a genetic disposition. TPP plays a role in nerve structure and function and brain metabolism. Signs and symptoms of this deficiency include peripheral neuropathy, ataxia, and ocular changes such as nystagmus. More advanced symptoms include confabulation, memory loss, and psychosis, sometimes resulting in Wernicke's encephalopathy or Wernicke–Korsakoff syndrome. Clinical scenarios include unexplained heart failure, renal failure with dialysis, alcoholism, starvation, and hyperemesis gravidarum. Bariatric surgery may increase the risk for thiamine deficiency, especially in those patients who are given intravenous dextrose without thiamine repletion. An understanding of its role as a potential therapeutic agent for diabetes, some inborn errors of metabolism, and neurodegenerative diseases warrants further research.[93] Dr. Lonsdale has noted the presence of inflammatory markers such as hypersensitive CRP and fibrinogen in transketolase-positive thiamine-deficient patients, sometimes indicating associated inflammation. This has been borne out by animal studies.[94] In light of the heterogeneity of symptoms, we thought it was important to highlight some of the lesser recognized signs of dysautonomic function that can be evaluated clinically.

## Asymmetrical Pulse Pressure and Orthostatic Hyper- or Hypotension

As discussed in Chapter 2, the brain stem and associated sympathetic and parasympathetic nerves associated with autonomic regulation of the heart are deeply affected by thiamine deficiency and the subsequent derailment of oxidative metabolism. Even in the earliest stages in polysymptomatic patients, heart dysfunction may be observed by the astute clinician simply by auscultation. Consider a quick assessment of left versus right brachial pulse pressures. Pulse pressures in the left arm are often greater than the right with thiamine deficiency. Similarly, a quick assessment in changes in blood pressure across different positions, lying, sitting, standing, and sitting again, may also indicate thiamine deficiency, particularly if other etiologies have been ruled out. An overly large increase or decrease, particularly with corresponding dizziness, is a good indicator of potential thiamine deficiency.

## Cerebellar Functioning: Gait, Balance, and Cognitive Affective Control

The cerebellum is responsible for the rate, force, rhythm, and accuracy of motor movements but also fulfills the same role for mental and cognitive processes. In that regard, in much the same way cerebellar damage evokes issues with balance, muscle tone, body perception, and voluntary movement, it also induces similar alterations in cognitive function, attention, and mood regulation.[95] To accomplish these tasks, the cerebellum consumes enormous amounts of ATP. The energy consumed by the Purkinje cells alone, the sole output neurons of the cerebellum,[96] is estimated at $\sim 10^{11}$ ATP molecules per second for each Purkinje cell.[97] With an estimated 15 million Purkinje cells in the cerebellum,[98] the sheer volume of energy consumption is staggering, particularly if one considers that Purkinje cells consume only 15% of the total ATP of the cerebellum.[99] In light of these energy requirements it is not difficult to imagine how decrements in mitochondrial oxidative metabolism might disturb cerebellar signaling and yield the telltale motor and cognitive changes.

Gait and balance together with cognitive and affective disturbances are obvious in advanced thiamine deficiency disorders such as beriberi and Wernicke's encephalopathy.[100] Increasingly, researchers have recognized that when there are mitochondrial disturbances, whether genetic or acquired, the cerebellum is affected.[101] Earlier in the disease process, however, cerebellar ataxias and/or cognitive and affective changes[102] are rarely recognized, mostly because they are not assessed. The measurement of gait impairment thus becomes a powerful marker of incipient pathology,[103] one that can be easily and quickly conducted in the physician's office or at home.

### Assessing Gait and Balance

Compared with the healthy controls, individuals with mitochondrial damage or disease present with reduced gait speed, take smaller steps, and show a greater step time with a large degree of width and length variability.[101] The telltale drunken sailor gait is often present, although it may be subtle at first. Individuals with the largest illness load and longer disease trajectories perform most poorly. Basic cerebellar function can be assessed easily and quickly by simply watching the patient walk and perform other organized movements. These measures may also be used to monitor treatment response. Have the patient walk normally and heel to toe. Observe the patient walking away and toward you.

Look at:
- Pace (step velocity and step length)
- Rhythm (step time)
- Variability (step length and step time variability)
- Asymmetry (step time asymmetry)
- Postural stability (step width, step width variability and step length asymmetry)

Look for:
- A wide-based gait
- Unsteady, irregular, uncertain, and variable length step patterns (Note: with mild disturbances, these changes may be subtle and may wax and wane.)
- Loss of muscle tone, muscle weakness, fatigability

## Other Clues of Cerebellar Dysfunction
Other common indications of cerebellar dysfunction include:
- Scanning speech–overly enunciated word patterns
- Nystagmus
- Tremors

## Cognitive Decrements With Impaired Mitochondrial Oxidation
Like the measurement of gait and balance, simple in-office cognitive assessments of learning and memory can unmask what may be subtle changes in the early stages of thiamine deficiency. More often than not patients will report sensing the decline in cognitive capacity and report things such as "cognitive fuzziness," "forgetfulness," and difficulties with "reading," "speaking," or "word finding." Their symptoms will often be misdiagnosed when conventional laboratory studies and/or imaging tests are negative or inconclusive.

Reduced oxidative capacity affects central nervous system function globally and therefore will impact all aspects of cognitive ability to some degree or another. This means that the clinician should expect to see changes in executive capacity (planning, attention, verbal fluency, reasoning, and working memory), visuospatial organization and memory, language capacity (expressive and receptive), personality, and psychiatric function (psychosis).[102] In rodent studies, learning and memory are impacted well before lesions are visible.[104] We should expect no less in humans. Common cognitive difficulties expressed by patients with newer onset/functional mitochondrial damage include difficulty finding words (naming and fluency), understanding written text, decreased attention span, visual and verbal memory deficits, and an overall decline in cognitive ability.[105]

## Fatigue, Hypersomnia, and Anorexia as Markers of Insufficient ATP
Over half a century ago, Hans Selye recognized fatigue, the increased need for sleep, and reduced appetite as key indicators of what he termed "sickness behaviors." It was a prescient observation that has been all-but disregarded in modern medicine. Although not diagnostic of a particular disease process, these behaviors indicate insufficient oxidative metabolism. Whether the diminished ATP is a result of inherently impaired mitochondria or an insufficient capacity relative to an illness or stressor is not clear. What is clear, however, is that reduced ATP triggers neurally mediated compensatory

reactions that fall under the rubric of dysautonomia. Top among these reactions is the reallocation of energy resources by the hypothalamic orexin/hypocretin neurons.

The orexin/hypocretin neurons (same nuclei, different names) are the brain's ATP and glucose sensors. Responsible for maintaining wakefulness, arousal, and feeding initiation, these neurons require five to six times the amount ATP to fire.[106] When ATP is low, firing diminishes or ceases and fatigue, sleep, and anorexia ensue. Similarly, when glucose concentrations are elevated firing diminishes significantly (via an ATP-dependent, inward rectifying $K^+$ channel[107]). Ablation[108] and/or mutation of these neurons induces narcolepsy and cataplexy[109] as well as hypophagia.[108]

With illness and/or depleted energy stores, these neurons induce sleep and reduce feeding. The sleepiness, fatigue, malaise, and anorexia common with most pathogenic illnesses and also mitochondrial distress are the result of a reallocation of resources mediated by the orexin/hypocretin system. These neurons also modify pain (dynorphin receptors colocated on orexin/hypocretin neurons), digestion (via the neuropeptide galanin),[84] and cortical spreading depression in migraines[110,111] and epileptogenesis,[112] among other functions. Low cerebrospinal fluid concentrations of these hormones have been implicated in major depression and suicidal thoughts.[113]

From this system of neurons we can see that wakefulness and feeding are key components of healthy mitochondria. When energy resources are low, sleep and loss of appetite would be expected. Consider new-onset sleep disorders, whether hypersomnia or narcolepsy, related to the orexin/hypocretin system. Similarly, consider the connection between excessive sleep, low motivation, loss of pleasure, and depressed mood as linking back to orexin/hypocretin through modulation of the serotonin in the dorsal raphe nucleus and dopamine via connections in the ventral tegmental area. Whether arrived at clinically or mechanistically, one should suspect depleted mitochondria underlying this constellation of symptoms. With mitochondrial involvement, consider thiamine.

## THIAMINE THERAPY: BEYOND THE RECOMMENDED DAILY ALLOWANCE

The use of pharmacological doses of vitamins is relatively new. It has been generally thought that their replacement requires only the recommended daily allowance (RDA), assuming that the deficiency has been clinically recognized. We have emphasized previously that thiamine is required in huge doses for months in the treatment of beriberi. If there was normoglycemia, the patient quickly responded. If there was hyperglycemia, the response was slower and if there was hypoglycemia, there was sometimes no response. Platt described a beriberi patient who stopped breathing after receiving an injection of thiamine and was resuscitated with epinephrine[114]; this is a very good reason for recognizing the symptoms of thiamine deficiency as early as possible, because the potential dangers of treatment are associated with chronicity.[93]

Although the necessity for using megadoses is unknown, we believe that the activity of the enzymes that depend on thiamine gradually deteriorates with long-term malnutrition and the cofactor is used to restore that activity by its stimulation. From clinical experience there is no doubt that physiological doses are useless. When there is no clinical response to a low dose, a physician may be misled into thinking that the proposed diagnosis of deficiency is wrong and ascribe the symptoms to other causes. The potential role of megadose thiamine in diabetes is an emerging clinical benefit that needs further research.[115] Magnesium is a cofactor with thiamine and should always be supplemented in an appropriate megadose. Since no micronutrient works on its own, a well-rounded multivitamin should also be used as a supplement.

## Thiamine Dosing

In most cases, irrespective of age, 100–150 mg of thiamine hydrochloride a day by mouth would be effective. Over many years of clinical use, Dr. Lonsdale never saw any toxicity. However, there have been a few case reports of anaphylactic-like allergic reactions to thiamine[116,117] and so clinical observation is always warranted. Nevertheless, Dr. Lonsdale has utilized very high doses of thiamine, and Case Example 4.2 demonstrates both the need and the tolerability of thiamine. Response can be expected sometimes

### Case Example 4.2 High-Dose Thiamine Therapy

A child was referred to Dr. Lonsdale because her appearance suggested a chromosomal abnormality. This was perfectly normal but the transketolase activity was not, and at the age of 6 months the child was started on 150 mg of thiamine hydrochloride a day. The clinical response was dramatic, but as she grew, the mother would note recurrence of some symptoms and would automatically raise the dose without any medical consultation. Although never completely normal she went through high school where she participated in the marching band. She died at the age of 27 years from an infection. The dose of thiamine had been elevated to 7 g a day without showing any prior toxicity.

within days, but depending on the chronicity it may be several weeks. We have emphasized in Chapter 1 that it took that kind of dose as long as 6 months to show improvement in beriberi. In suspected pyruvate dehydrogenase deficiency (PDD) that leads to a range of clinical manifestations, mutation analysis is more sensitive and specific than enzymatic analysis as a first-line diagnostic test. Thiamine doses greater than 400 mg a day are often required for sustained response.[118]

## Thiamine Derivatives for Clinical Care

Although thiamine hydrochloride is the form of thiamine most readily available, a more effective formulation called thiamine tetrahydrofurfuryl disulfide (TTFD) is preferred. TTFD is the synthetic counterpart of allithiamine, the disulfide derivative of thiamine that occurs naturally in garlic and other plants of the allium species.

### Thiamine Tetrahydrofurfuryl Disulfide

Allicin, a compound that gives garlic its odor, is formed by enzymatic action during the grinding of fresh bulbs of garlic. Allicin conjugates with thiamine in an alkaline medium to form allithiamine [2′methyl-4′-aminopirymidyl-(5′) methylformamino-5-hydroxy-2-pentenyl-(3) allyl disulfide]. Originally thought to have lost the biologic effect of thiamine, animal studies proved that it was biologically more effective than the original thiamine. The vitamin B research committee of Japan then began to synthesize a number of allithiamine derivatives by substituting the S-alkyl radical of allithiamine by different alkyl groups. The hitherto completely unknown characteristics of allithiamine, vastly different from thiamine, became clear. Of these, thiamine propyl disulfide (TPD) proved to be the best substitute. It was easily reduced to thiamine in the presence of cysteine or glutathione. When given orally it was vigorously absorbed from the intestine. Unfortunately, TPD produced an overwhelming odor of garlic from the patient, leading to the synthesis of the most modern derivative, TTFD (Fursultiamine, Lipothiamine). Manufactured by Takeda Chemical Industries in Osaka, Japan, it was deliberately synthesized to obviate the garlic odor and is used as a prescription drug in Japan under the name Alinamin.

Among its thiamine-replacing benefits, TTFD was shown to protect mice from cyanide poisoning and prevented trichloroethylene or lead intoxication. The prosthetic group is removed at the cell membrane nonenzymatically and the thiazole ring of thiamine closes in the cytosol. A series of S-acylthiamine derivatives were also synthesized, but the prosthetic group has to be removed enzymatically.[119] S-Benzoylthiamine monophosphate

(Benfotiamine) is the one presently being used. A major difference between the derivatives is that TTFD crosses the blood–brain barrier, whereas Benfotiamine does not.[120]

Dr. Lonsdale held an independent investigator license for clinical use of TTFD from 1973 to 2013 and sent regular reports to the Food and Drug Administration, reporting the absence of toxicity and the benefits in hundreds of patients.[121]

Thiamine derivatives that are better absorbed and provide higher blood and tissue concentrations than thiamine hydrochloride have been considered to be improved forms of the vitamin for use in nutritional deficiency. Their advantage over thiamine hydrochloride in postulated vitamin-dependent disorders may be an important role, and there may be still another use in developing pharmacologic applications in several diseases for which therapy is still inadequate, toxic, or both.

As the role of the vitamin in biochemical processes is further elucidated, the therapeutic applicability of the newer alkyl derivatives of thiamine can be explored objectively. They are more likely to be of clinical value when metabolic or histologic abnormalities resemble those of athiaminosis, but where there is a metabolic derangement rather than a simple nutritional deficiency. Even in beriberi, the classical clinical prototype of thiamine deficiency, large doses of the vitamin are required for long periods,[122] although it is often mistakenly accepted that beriberi is readily reversible with small doses that are considered to fill physiologic need. Large doses have been given clinical trial where evidence exists for impaired absorption, utilization, or dependency. Severe thiamine deficiency may be found in the elderly,[123–125] alcoholism,[126,127] achlorhydria,[128] intestinal malabsorption,[129] and children with gastroenteritis.[130] Therapeutic attempts with thiamine hydrochloride have demonstrated inconsistent and unpredictable responses. The use of thiamine alone may result in the lack of therapeutic effect since its absorption and biochemical activation[131] are critical factors. Essential nutrients work together in complicated biochemical relationships.[132,133]

## Clinical Evaluation Thiamine Tetrahydrofurfuryl Disulfide

TPD, a derivative of thiamine, was tested in the treatment of SNE.[134] TPD was reportedly superior to thiamine hydrochloride in the treatment of alcoholics with neurologic complications.[135] TTFD produced clinical remission in Leigh's disease, although some of the patients became resistant to its pharmacologic effects for unknown reasons.[136] An attempt to identify antibodies to TTFD was unsuccessful.[137] Four infants with repeated life-threatening apnea and abnormal brain stem–evoked potential tests obtained clinical remission with TTFD. It has shown some benefit in the treatment of polyneuropathy.[138] It has also shown benefit in preventing exercise-induced fatigue[139] and some improvement in Alzheimer's disease.[140]

An uncontrolled pilot study showed that TTFD improved the clinical situation in 8 out of 10 autistic children.[141] It has been hypothesized that the action of TTFD in different clinical situations is simply because it stimulates energy metabolism that may be a common etiology in many different diseases.[121] Abnormal TKA in psychiatric patients[142,143] may be primary or secondary to poor nutrition, but several patients experienced marked clinical improvement after thiamine supplementation, and TTFD might be a more powerful therapeutic agent if absorption mechanisms are compromised.

Because of Dr. Lonsdale's experience with dysautonomic function and a report in the literature concerning the relationship of adrenergic mechanisms in hypertension,[144] an experiment was performed using TTFD to ascertain whether it might have an effect on blood pressure in spontaneously hypertensive rats (SHRs).

### The Effect of TTFD on Blood Pressure in Spontaneously Hypertensive Rats

The SHR rat is used in models of primary hypertension. The animal becomes hypertensive early in life and blood pressure continues to increase with age, often resulting in a cardiovascular event. Over the course of 4 months, blood pressure and body weight of two groups of SHR rats were monitored: the control group was fed normally and the TTFD group was given increasing doses of TTFD from 5 to 15 mg.

Of the 13 TTFD-supplemented rats, 5 showed a definite TTFD response (Figs. 4.4 and 4.5). In contrast to the control group, which showed a 20–25 mm Hg increase in blood pressure across the experiment, blood pressures of the TTFD animals remained stable. The results suggested that TTFD had a biologic effect on blood pressure in some of these genetically abnormal rats.

It was not clear whether the response was time or dose related or some combination of both. Neither was it clear by what mechanism(s) thiamine affected the regulation of the blood pressure. It has been suggested that the hypertensive mechanism in SHR is adrenergic in nature,[144] and this would support the evidence that TTFD is cholinergic in action. It was shown that it had a biologic effect on audiogenically seizure-prone mice weanlings of

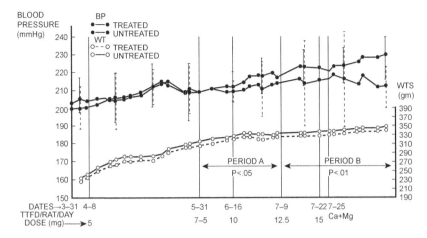

**Figure 4.4** Thiamine treatment in spontaneously hypertensive rats demonstrating statistically significant prevention of expected hypertension. *TTFD*, thiamine tetrahydrofurfuryl disulfide; *WTS*, weights of animals.

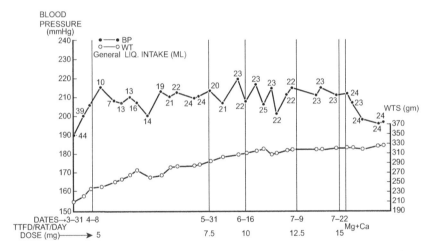

**Figure 4.5** Thiamine treatment in the record of a single TTFD treated SHR rat whose normal rise in blood pressure was clearly prevented. *SHR*, spontaneously hypertensive rats; *TTFD*, thiamine tetrahydrofurfuryl disulfide.

the DBA/J2 strain[101] and this was also thought to be cholinergic in nature. It is therefore hypothesized that the antihypertensive effect of TTFD in this rat experiment was caused by its stimulation of cholinergic action to a point where it produced a homeostatic balance between the genetically determined adrenergic dominance and parasympathetic activity.

Dr. Lonsdale had concluded that the rising blood pressure in SHR may be caused by sympathetic action initiated by genetically determined hypoxia or pseudohypoxia. It therefore seemed possible that TTFD might have an effect on preventing the rise in blood pressure. More recently, Taylor et al. wrote that obstructive apnea during sleep elevates the set point for efferent sympathetic outflow during wakefulness. Such resetting is attributed to hypoxia-induced regulation or peripheral chemoreceptors and brain stem sympathetic function.[145] Focal ischemia models have been established in divergent substrains of SHR.[146]

Prolonged Thiamine Deficiency in Animals
Animal experiments have thrown some light on the effects of dietary thiamine deprivation. The usual clinical effects in rats are fairly well known, involving anorexia, gradually increasing weakness, weight loss, and death. Some workers have observed muricidal behavior[147] and persistent penile erection,[148] suggesting that aggressive functional variations might occur, perhaps in reference to the proportion of other nutrients in the diet. Skelton reported the general adaptation syndrome in rats experimentally deprived of thiamine and suggested that the vitamin had a bearing on stress resistance.[149,150] The effects of nonspecific stress were studied in dogs by inducing shock from hemorrhage. Thiamine-fortified animals withstood bleeding better than the controls, and copious intestinal hemorrhage, which occurred in controls, was not observed in those receiving thiamine.[151]

Methylglyoxal has been reported in urine from thiamine-deficient rats.[152,153] Glyoxalases, enzymes that are ubiquitous in many animal and plant tissues, synthesize D-lactate from methylglyoxal[154] and this may represent an atavistic pathway activated by prolonged anaerobic metabolism.

Liang[155] reported glyoxylic aciduria in athiaminotic rats, suggesting that this represented abnormal glycine metabolism.

## Thiamine Dependency

As will be discussed more fully later in this chapter, a case of intermittent cerebellar ataxia in a 6-year-old boy initiated Dr. Lonsdale's interest in energy metabolism, its relationship with thiamine, and the notion of nutrient dependency.[59] Briefly, the child experienced recurrent periods of cerebellar ataxia that were self-limiting but appeared to be initiated by a stressor, such as an inoculation, an illness, or head trauma. Careful examination of the boy's metabolic status revealed thiamine deficiency. From the experimental facts it became evident that the child's health was dependent upon high doses of thiamine to function. Upward of 600 mg daily were administered to prevent episodes of ataxia. If he encountered some form of infection, mild head trauma, or inoculation, the dose had to be doubled to avoid ataxia. Here, and in many other cases, huge doses of the vitamin are required to accomplish the physiologic effect.

Thiamine, along with magnesium, is the cofactor to many important enzymes that preside over energy metabolism. If the bonding mechanism of thiamine is genetically compromised, its concentration has to be increased enormously by supplementation to prevent the inevitable symptoms of deficiency. This is referred to as vitamin dependency. What is perhaps not understood sufficiently is that prolonged vitamin deficiency appears to affect this bonding mechanism, suggesting that with chronic deficiency dependency may emerge. For example, it has long been known that to cure chronic beriberi, megadoses of thiamine are required for months.[114] Dr. Lonsdale hypothesizes that the megadoses of thiamine given by supplementation to a patient with long-term symptoms arising from previously unrecognized deficiency appear to reactivate the inefficient enzyme. It is as though the enzyme has to be repeatedly exposed to megadoses of its cofactor to stimulate it and restore its lost function. Perhaps this explains why genetically determined dependency and long-term dietary deficiency both require pharmaceutical doses of thiamine. The practitioner may easily view the lack of clinical response from low doses of the vitamin as evidence that the patient's symptoms are a result of another cause.

## IV THIAMINE FOR ACUTE AND CHRONIC CASES

There are many instances when IV thiamine and nutrient replacement are preferential to oral supplementation; these include the following:
- In acute medical care settings when severe deficiency is suspected, e.g., any of the conditions listed previously;
- If there is severe anorexia resulting from the deficiency;
- With chronic illness associated with long-term deficiency;
- When nutrient malabsorption is compromised by gastrointestinal damage or dysfunction[156];
- Following some surgical procedures[157];
- Hyperemesis gravidarum[158];
- Prolonged obesity prior to surgery.[159]

## Additional Nutrients

Thiamine is never given alone, either orally or intravenously. It is always regarded as a member of a complex team. The problem is clinical perspective. It is always preferable to prove that there is thiamine deficiency, but Dr. Lonsdale found that thiamine deficiency was just part of many diseases and that the underlying etiology was really mitochondrial in nature. For example, a patient with thrombocytopenic purpura that failed to respond to conventional treatment responded to intravenous water-soluble vitamins that included thiamine. Ten infusions at intervals of a few days were required to produce the remission and there were no side effects or evidence of toxicity. An elderly lady suffered repeated febrile episodes every 2 weeks after she attended square dancing. Not only did she have an abnormal transketolase, but also she had a marked increase in hemoglobin and circulating red cells, the kind of hemoconcentration associated with living at altitude. She responded to intravenous vitamins containing thiamine and the febrile episodes ceased. It was concluded that thiamine deficiency had resulted in pseudohypoxia in the brain stem and that the febrile episodes were an imitation of mountain sickness.[160]

Although thiamine deficiency seemed to dominate the clinical picture in Dr. Lonsdale's practice, other micronutrient deficiencies are often present. In patients with long-standing symptoms it became necessary to offer a spectrum of water-soluble vitamins given intravenously. For example, a girl of 18 years of age returned from school and went white water rafting with friends. She was thrown out of the boat by the surge and when she returned home her fatigue was so great that she could barely raise her head from the pillow in bed. A diagnosis of acute mononucleosis was made elsewhere. Two infusions of the formula shown in Table 4.1 completely relieved the fatigue and she was able to return to school immediately in good health. The doses of vitamins used intravenously are shown in the table.

## Paradoxical Reactions to IV Thiamine and Other Nutrients

When water-soluble vitamins are given intravenously for the first time the patient often complains of fatigue, sometimes with headache, on the following day only. Thereafter there is often rapid clinical improvement. This is never a serious threat, although it is often mistaken by the patient as "side effects." For this reason it is necessary to reassure the patient that this may take place. Curiously enough it was almost always a prediction of clinical success and was termed "paradox" for reference purposes since it would be unexpected by the patient. Over a period of many years, hundreds if not

Table 4.1 Nutritional IV for Thiamine Replacement

| | |
|---|---|
| Sterile water | 500 mL |
| Magnesium chloride | 2 g (10 mL) |
| Potassium chloride | 5 meq (2.5 mL) |
| Dexpanthenol | 500 mg (2 mL) |
| Folic acid | 10 mg (1 mL) |
| Manganese chloride | 1 mg (0.5 mL) |
| Zinc chloride | 10 mg (1 mL) |
| Chromium | 40 µg (2.5 mL) |
| Ascorbic acid | 20 g (40 mL) |
| Adenosine 5′-monophosphate | Per order |
| Procaine 2% vitamin B complex 100 | 5 mL |
| Pyridoxine hydrochloride | 100 mg (1 mL) |
| Methylcobalamin | 0.1 mL |
| Vitamin B complex 100 | 2 mL |
|    Thiamine hydrochloride | 100 mg per mL |
|    Riboflavin 5′-phosphate sodium | 2 mg per mL |
|    Pyridoxine hydrochloride | 2 mg per mL |
|    Dexpanthenol | 2 mg per mL |
|    Niacinamide | 100 mg per mL |

thousands of nutritional IVs were given without a single toxicity reaction and many different diseases were successfully treated. The rationale is simple: healing is a natural process requiring the consumption of cellular energy.

Of all the nutritional IVs that Dr. Lonsdale gave to patients this paradoxical response was only severe in one patient. This was a retired physician who had been found to have a benign brain tumor and had been treated with a shunt to permit the flow of cerebrospinal fluid. His major symptom was extreme fatigue and he was offered treatment with the formula in Table 4.1. Over the next 48 h he vomited repeatedly. On the assumption that the dose was too great for him, their concentration was reduced. The same episode of repeated vomiting occurred again. The mechanism remains unknown.

## THIAMINE IN CLINICAL CARE: TREATING FUNCTIONAL AND GENETIC DISTURBANCES

Dr. Lonsdale's interest in thiamine began as a result of his experience with the case of thiamine-dependent PDH, details of which are given later. The clinical presentation of this child's symptoms was an exact imitation of childhood beriberi, leading to library research to acquire a thorough knowledge of how this ancient, extremely polysymptomatic disease was expressed.[46] Being a pediatrician at that time in a multispecialty clinic, a common referral was children with various forms of learning disability and behavioral problems, attention deficit, and hyperactivity, often associated with obesity. Diet history repeatedly revealed an excess of sugary "junk," on an ad libitum basis. Many adolescents were polysymptomatic and had frequently been diagnosed previously as psychosomatic disease.[161] Erythrocyte transketolase studies confirmed thiamine deficiency. Efforts to correct diet had variable success but in nearly every case symptoms disappeared and transketolase normalized with supplements of thiamine and magnesium. In a few cases, as exemplified in a case report, it was necessary to use TTFD after a failure with thiamine hydrochloride.[162] The effectiveness of TTFD is because of its penetration into cells without the necessity of a thiamine transporter.

In 1982 Dr. Lonsdale entered a private practice specializing in nutrient therapy and many of the adult patients had symptoms indicating changes in autonomic function where thiamine deficiency was proved. Noting that dysautonomia had been commonly associated in the medical literature with various organic diseases, it strongly suggested that some form of mitochondrial dysfunction led to dysautonomia and might be the forerunner of the organic disease.[163]

For the remainder of the chapter we will present case studies to illustrate the heterogeneity of conditions associated with thiamine deficiency and the patterns of response. We will also discuss the need for micronutrients besides thiamine. We begin with the case that spurred his lifelong interest in thiamine deficiency and dependency syndromes.

## Pyruvate Dehydrogenase Deficiency

PDD disorders represent a class of inborn errors in the PDH enzyme complex. The disease is considered rare in the general population but among the more common disorders of mitochondrial metabolism. The cardinal symptom is an abnormal and potentially life-threatening build up of lactic acid with nausea and vomiting, severe breathing difficulties, and heart rhythm irregularities. Symptoms emerge in infancy and/or early childhood depending upon which mutation is involved. As the disease progresses, significant neurological sequelae are expected, including intellectual disability, seizures, and motor development difficulties with hypotonia and ataxia.

Recall from the previous chapter that the PDH complex sits atop the tricarboxylic acid/citric acid cycle effectively controlling the conversion of

carbohydrates to ATP. Recall also that thiamine is a critical cofactor in PDH and thus can not only initiate mitochondrial damage when deficient, but also, as the following case suggests, ameliorate mitochondrial dysfunction in the face of other deficiencies. It should be noted that when Dr. Lonsdale first encountered this child with PDH deficiency in the 1960s, our understanding of the disease process was limited. At the time it was assumed to be genetic in origin but DNA studies were still in the future. The following case[164] illustrates two key features of thiamine usage in clinical care:
- Thiamine can be used to compensate for genetic errors in oxidative metabolism.
- Stressors, whether they be dietary (sugar) or illness related, enhance the need for additional nutrients to compensate.

## Intermittent Cerebellar Ataxia With Pyruvate Dehydrogenase Deficiency

A 6-year-old boy with intermittent cerebellar ataxia was referred to the Cleveland Clinic, Cleveland, and came under Dr. Lonsdale's care. There were two boys in this family, both of whom showed malfunction of PDH in fibroblast tissue culture cells. It appeared to be the decarboxylating mechanism that was at fault. Both boys were clinically improved when they supplemented their diet with thiamine hydrochloride in large doses.

The older boy, J.V., was studied in detail, beginning at the age of 6 years. Whenever he had an infection, a head injury, or inoculation, he was prone to experience a self-limiting episode of cerebellar ataxia, involving loss of balance, slurred speech, and disorientation, and he would also have frightening delusions. The late winter and early spring were particularly "stressful" times, and he found it necessary to double or triple the daily dose of thiamine at these times when beginning to notice symptoms of "infection." The daily preventive dose of thiamine hydrochloride was set at 600 mg. A particularly bad episode that lasted for 11 days is described next. Details of the episode were published.[59]

Each morning the ataxia and neurologic signs were improved, but deteriorated during the day, so that he was unable to walk by evening. After several days he gradually began to improve, although no treatment was given and he did not receive any vitamin supplement. Each one of these multiple attacks appeared to leave his general condition and neurologic health a little worse. He was having difficulties in school, had visuomotor incoordination, and had early signs of optic atrophy. They were typical of

recurrent episodes of childhood beriberi, which is more acute and fulminating than adult forms of the disease. Studies revealed the following data:
1. Urine, in day and night 12h consecutive collections, revealed large amounts of alanine, pyruvate, and alpha ketoglutarate. These concentrations were much greater during the day than the night.[65]
2. Urinary concentrations of glutamic acid and aspartic acid were consistently low until the patient began to improve clinically. This is shown in Figs. 4.6 and 4.7.
3. It was also striking that the glutamic and aspartic acid concentrations rose by day and fell by night during the phase of clinical recovery, coinciding with the diurnal oscillation demonstrated by alanine. This was more obvious for glutamate than aspartate.

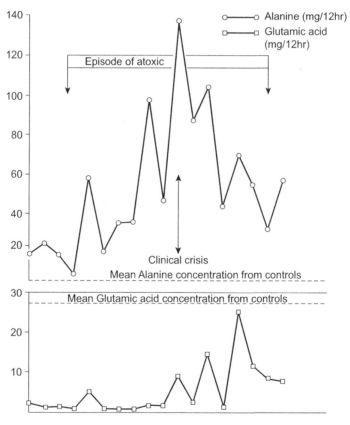

**Figure 4.6** *Ion exchange in urine amino acids: alanine and glutamic acid.* Alternating day and night 12-h concentrations of alanine and glutamic acid in urine of a child during ataxic episode caused by partially defective decarboxylation of pyruvate. Higher values are those of day specimens and lower ones of night specimens. *Reproduced with permission from* Pediatrics;*84:129–34. Copyright 1969 by the AAP.*

Evaluation and Treatment of Thiamine Metabolism in Clinical Practice    143

4. Urine was examined and reported to contain a substance reported to inhibit the formation of TTP in the brain.[165] This substance has never been identified.
5. Since low activity of the decarboxylating component of PDH was demonstrated, the child was given an experimental trial with massive doses of thiamine hydrochloride. Repeated examination of urine revealed much lower concentrations of alanine and pyruvate.
6. His clinical improvement was matched by increased ability to perform a Bender–Gestalt test. This test, performed in March, showed marked improvement in the following December (Figs. 4.8 and 4.9).

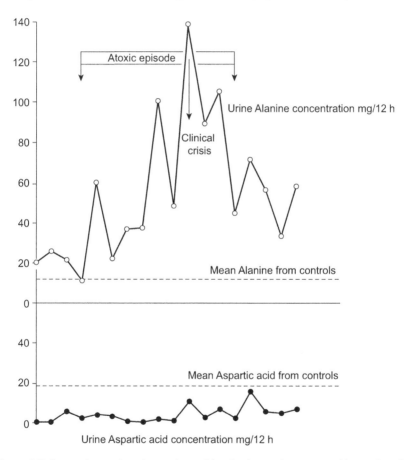

**Figure 4.7 *Ion exchange in urine amino acids: alanine and asparate.*** Alternating day and night 12-h concentrations of alanine and aspartate in the same urines as represented in Fig. 4.6. Higher values are those of day specimens and lower ones of night specimens. Oscillation of higher and lower day/night concentrations of aspartate began at the time of clinical climax. *Reproduced with permission from* Pediatrics;**84**:129–34. Copyright 1969 by the AAP.

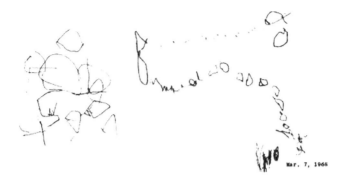

**Figure 4.8** Bender–Gestalt test performed by a child with pyruvate decarboxylase deficiency after recovery from an ataxic episode.

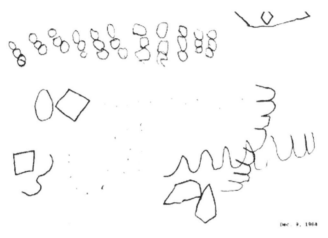

**Figure 4.9** Bender–Gestalt test performed by the same child after 9 months of continuous therapy with 600 mg/day thiamine hydrochloride.

## Cognitive Testing

Cognitive measures of baseline deficits and treatment responsiveness are useful indicators to assess change. In a 6-year-old boy in the late 1960s this meant the Bender–Gestalt test. The test was used to evaluate aspects of visual motor maturity and memory. The test consists of nine figures, each on its own 3 × 5 card. The subject is shown each figure and asked to copy it onto a piece of blank paper. Fig. 4.8 shows the patient's effort before treatment had begun, demonstrating his perceptual difficulties. Fig. 4.9 shows a repeat of the Bender–Gestalt test 9 months after continuing treatment with thiamine. Although still somewhat crude it clearly shows an improvement in visual perception and coordination.

## Long-Term Progress

After administering the megadoses of thiamine, this boy's health remained remarkably stable without any more episodes of ataxia. He graduated successfully from high school. All evidence of optic atrophy disappeared. He recognized subjective changes in his own reaction to infections such as colds or "flu," describing these as "funny feelings" or "nervousness," and he found that he could abolish symptoms by temporarily increasing the dose of thiamine supplement. The dose of 600 mg might be increased to 1200 or 1800 mg, invariably aborting an episode of ataxia.

Another illustration of this boy's inability to react to environmental stress was demonstrated early in his treatment program. He entered an air-conditioned store from a 90°F outside temperature. He became unconscious and began asthmatic wheezing that he had never previously experienced. The same thing happened in the family car when the air conditioning was turned on. His brother, who had the same defect, had only experienced one minor episode of ataxia. In adolescence he suffered a relatively minor head injury that caused him to become unconscious, again attesting to the fact that his ability to meet stress was compromised. He was taken to the nearest emergency room and his mother called Dr. Lonsdale to notify me of the situation. A call to the emergency room to request that an injection of thiamine be given to the boy was met with ridicule.

## Points of Consideration

This case history represents an uncommon condition. An acquired biochemical effect may be induced relatively easily by nutritional depletion of vital cofactors and masquerade as "encephalitis" unless the mechanisms by which adaptation occurs are kept in mind. Since most physicians do not believe that such deficiencies can occur in well-developed societies, the diagnosis of acute beriberi, or other nutritional depletion disease, is unlikely to be contemplated.

A good example of such energy depletion might be suggested by exercise or "stress"-induced asthma, as this patient experienced with a sudden change of ambient temperature. Dr. Lonsdale has recognized several other incidents where the reaction of the patient appears to be that generally ascribed to infection. If no evidence of bacterial cause is discerned it is usually assumed that a virus is the cause, whereas it is suggested here that such clinical presentations may be caused by a brain-directed response to a relatively trivial stress insult of a noninfectious variety when there is thiamine deficiency. Thiamine-responsive febrile lymphadenopathy is discussed later in this chapter.

Attempts were made to identify the biochemical mechanisms involved in this devastating disease that could be largely prevented by so simple means. Several possibilities existed, including those that have been considered in reference to thiamine-deficient metabolism. In this case, however, there were several facts that considerably complicated the issues, and their possible interpretation:
1. There was evidence of depletion in the mechanism of PDH, the means of entry of pyruvate into the citric acid cycle.
2. Evidence existed for a possible defect in the synthesis of brain-dependent TTP.
3. Study of one episode revealed a series of biochemical changes proved to be caused by blocked entry of pyruvate into the citric acid cycle. This, resulting in abnormal accumulation of pyruvate, might result in an acceleration of transamination with consequently increased synthesis of alanine, alpha ketoglutarate, and oxaloacetate. Glutamate and aspartate are the principle participants in all brain transamination reactions, and it is possible that they were "siphoned" away from their normal role in nitrogen balance. This hypothesis could explain the low concentrations of urinary glutamate and aspartate in the early stage of the ataxic episode, and their "circadian" rise in the later stages, during clinical recovery.
4. Initially, it was considered that the daytime increases in concentrations of the urinary metabolites were related to dietary intake. However, the presence in urine of the TTP inhibitory substance suggested another possibility. Although its role is still conjectural, it certainly has a part to play in neurological function and may have influenced the mechanisms of circadian rhythm. A similar situation is seen later in this work in discussion of the fluctuations seen in urinary creatine and creatinine that were identified in a child with learning disability.

## NUTRIENT INTERACTIONS

Although the majority of our focus has been on thiamine, additional vitamin and mineral deficiencies often coexist with thiamine deficiency. Sometimes thiamine replacement unmasks latent nutrient deficiencies. The reader must bear in mind that the use of therapeutic megadose vitamins is still in its infancy. At the time of Dr. Lonsdale's work there were no readily available laboratory tests to prove deficiency of other noncaloric nutrients and today, although specialty nutrient testing labs exist, nutrient testing is still woefully underutilized in clinical care. Because of this, Dr. Lonsdale always gave his patients supplementary magnesium and a well-rounded multivitamin when using megadose thiamine therapy. The following case reports illustrate this concept.

## Thiamine-Responsive Hypoglycemia With Biotin: Connections With Transamination

Thiamine-responsive hypoglycemia has been reported in a child. Curiously, the metabolic block was in pyruvate carboxylase, which is biotin dependent. The authors attempted to explain this by pointing out evidence that the concentration of acetyl-CoA, produced by activity of PDH, has a stimulating effect on the activity of pyruvate carboxylase.[166] This is logical, since the combination of oxaloacetate and acetyl-CoA is the first step in entry of citrate to the citric acid cycle. Hence it was assumed that this was a thiamine-dependent stimulation of carboxylase by this indirect method. It is possible that biotin supplementation might have been effective. It is helpful to point out that phosphoenolpyruvate to pyruvate is a unidirectional step. Therefore alanine, normally transaminated to pyruvate, must then be carboxylated to oxaloacetate and converted to phosphoenol pyruvate by carboxykinase to enter the Embden–Meyerhof pathway to gluconeogenesis. This is the so-called anaplerotic form of gluconeogenesis.

## Beriberi With Methylation Issues Leading to Folate and B12 Deficiencies

Correcting a long-standing thiamine deficiency may unmask other nutrient deficiencies. The following case illustrates the integration of oxidative metabolism in reference to transmethylation.[46]

The patient was a middle-aged woman who had suffered for 5 years from a condition that was progressive but unrecognized by physicians. Gross edema, foot and wrist drop, ophthalmoplegia, and recurrent episodes of unconsciousness were not recognized as beriberi until she suffered a severe incident of life-threatening apnea, requiring tracheostomy. Red cell TKA was low, and the urine contained large amounts of pyruvate and other keto acids. Thiamine supplementation resulted in slow neurological recovery. This was accompanied, however, by a progressive anemia and ethanolamine was found in large concentrations in the urine. Ethanolamine receives a labile methyl group from folate in the endogenous synthesis of choline. It was therefore hypothesized that ethanolamine wastage occurred as a result of folate deficiency and serum folate was found to be abnormally low.

A supplement of folate was provided and a rapid reticulocyte response and correction of the anemia gave evidence that this was a correct interpretation. It was of some interest that the anemia was not megaloblastic in character. After 2 years of folate and thiamine therapy she developed vitamin B12 deficiency, resulting in recurrence of severe neurologic symptoms, which were treated successfully with injections of cyanocobalamin. After the first of the vitamin B12 injections she developed fever and myositis, which lasted for several days before her general improvement commenced—a phenomenon that is not uncommonly seen when commencing parenteral nutrient therapy. Her neurologic state was considered to be partially induced, and her recovery retarded by a chronic addiction to cigarettes. This case illustrates quite well some of the potential biochemical relationships between vitamins.

## Thiamine-Responsive Megaloblastic Anemia: Problems With Methylation

A patient with sensorineural deafness, diabetes, hyperaminoacidura, and megaloblastic anemia was reported.[167] It was discovered that the anemia was responsive to thiamine, although at that time thiamine had no known documented hematopoietic action. Hypersegmentation of granulocytes had suggested folate deficiency, but megaloblastosis and anemia did not respond to either B12 or folate. The biochemical explanation for this was probably transporter deficiency, which will be discussed more thoroughly in subsequent chapters, but another explanation might also be hypothesized. For example, several patients have been described with deficiency of methionine-activating enzyme.[168] This enzyme catalyzes synthesis of SAM and requires ATP. It is a vital link in the important process of transmethylation, which increases the length of carbon chains. Also SAM has a negative feedback effect on 5.10-$N$-methylenetetrahydrofolate reductase, which methylates active folate. Deficiency of SAM results in continued activity of this enzyme and causes it to catalyze increased amounts of methylated (inactive) folate. This then "piles up" at the B12-dependent step, where the labile methyl group is normally transferred back from inactive folate to methionine. This step is catalyzed by 5-$N$-methyltetrahydrofolate methytransferase. When folate is demethylated it becomes "active" in its cofactor functions. This mechanism has been suggested from experimental studies.[169,170]

It is hypothesized that such a mechanism is capable of explaining a high serum folate concentration in the presence of hypersegmented neutrophils in this reported patient, a phenomenon that was observed in one of the children with methionine-activating enzyme deficiency.[167] Possible substrate inhibition of the B12-dependent step results in lack of active, and accumulation of inactive, folate. In the case of thiamine-responsive megaloblastic anemia, a similar explanation other than transporter deficiency could be hypothesized. If thiamine deficiency had resulted in a relative shortage of ATP, it might have caused inefficient SAM production, thus giving rise to loss of folate activity and megaloblastic anemia.

## Thiamine-Responsive Febrile Lymphadenopathy: Interplay With Folate and Vitamin B12

Another case report is of interest,[171] since the two children described had thiamine-responsive recurrent febrile lymphadenopathy. A proven (or often assumed) infection is invariably accepted as the etiology for this extremely common condition. One of the two unrelated boys was found to have abnormal red cell TKA, typical of TPP deficiency. Cessation of these recurrent episodes indicated that he responded to therapeutic doses of thiamine. The other boy in whom the TKA was normal was found to excrete the substance that is associated with inhibition of TTP synthesis.[68] Serum folate and B12 concentrations were found to be increased. Both of them decreased into the normal range and clinical remission occurred when this child received therapeutic doses of thiamine hydrochloride supplementation.

After a period of normal health, thiamine was discontinued. Another episode of fever, lymphadenopathy, extreme irritability, and night terrors recurred several weeks later. An episode of sleepwalking was accompanied by spontaneous urinary incontinence. Serum concentrations of folate and B12 were again increased, and thiamine supplementation was restarted. Within a few days the lymphadenopathy resolved and the serum concentrations of folate and B12 became normal. This child continued to take thiamine in the same dose and remained completely well until about a year later, when nocturnal symptoms began again. A high-potency multivitamin and mineral complex was prescribed and symptoms rapidly resolved.[171]

### *Points of Consideration*

These two cases of febrile lymphadenopathy deserve to be explained in biochemical terms, even though speculative. It is suggested that the mechanism is as follows. Both children were allowed unlimited sweets, including juice, carbonated beverages, and candy, time-honored "treats." Lymphadenopathy was well documented as one of the poorly understood effects seen in beriberi. One of the boys had a high pulse pressure with a diastolic pressure of zero and a femoral pulse audible by auscultation. Both of these findings are seen in beriberi in which autonomic neuropathy is typical. The fever and lymphadenopathy were considered to represent a centrally initiated "defense" response, which might or might not have been activated by viral or other infection as an additional "stress factor." The association of genetic risk, stress, and malnutrition will be discussed later in the book. The nocturnal disturbances were additional evidence of central nervous system irritation caused by pseudohypoxia increased sensitivity in the limbic system.[163]

This explanation is tentatively supported in one child by the presence of TTP inhibitory substance, suggesting that the brain was marginally deficient in TTP. The mechanism in the transketolase-positive child may have been similar, since TTP is synthesized from TPP and the abnormal erythrocyte transketolase had proved TPP deficiency. Alternatively, there may have been a defect in phosphorylation of the vitamin, resulting in the loss of both TPP and TTP.

It is a logical assumption that these reactions in both children were exact imitations of how the body reacts to the assault of an infecting organism. Irrespective of whether such an organism was or was not the initiating etiologic cause, the clinical manifestations would invariably be perceived as those of infection under most observational circumstances. Hence the use of an antibiotic would be the usual therapy chosen, as indeed it had been repeatedly in both cases before these investigations had been performed. The fact that a vitamin was preventive appears superficially to be completely illogical according to our present perception of this kind of disease. In fact, the supersensitive brain may be capable of reacting to virtually any "stressor" from the environment, in much the same way as the boy with intermittent ataxia when he entered the air-conditioned room. In dealing with the human "machine," in its environment, it is essential that we attempt to discern the nature of the defense, rather than assume that some unseen, undetected organism is responsible. To suspect this possibility in either one of these boys, a careful diet history was an essential.

Finally, a few words should be said about recurrence of symptoms in one of these children in whom corrective therapy was reestablished by providing a multivitamin. Vitamins each have their specific actions in a vast biochemical ecology, which is much like the food chain in nature. Each step is dependent upon the presence of one or more of the members of this nutritional team. It is this that creates major problems in reaching a better understanding of vitamin therapy. The double-blind study using a single agent is inadequate for this kind of patient. The clinical presentation of the biochemical lesion appears to be diverse and is the key to establishing a diagnosis. Having established the underlying biochemical etiology the patient becomes his own control by matching the laboratory changes to the clinical situation. Also it is probably true that different clinical presentations respond to the same vitamin or vitamins, because they will prove to have similar biochemical etiology. Finally, there is the important phenomenon of interaction as, for example, has long been known for the relationship between folate and B12.

## Nutrient-Responsive Complex Regional Pain Syndrome

Reflex sympathetic dystrophy,[172,173] now known as complex regional pain syndrome, may be responsive to therapeutic thiamine. It is a syndrome that represents a classic example of unusual sympathetic dominance in a limb after trauma. The trauma itself may be relatively trivial and the ensuing neurologic sequelae appear to be disproportionate in severity. The condition is sometimes mistaken with connective tissue disorder, neoplasm, or phlebitis and is occasionally considered to be psychosomatic. We hypothesize that the light trauma acts as a stress factor, related to genetic risk and/or marginal malnutrition.

An adolescent male received a whiplash injury to the cervical spine. He gradually developed increasing pain, numbness, and paresthesia in the left wrist, then the right. There was numbness in one wrist and the associated thumb and index finger, a characteristic of beriberi neuropathy that seemed to be an unlikely diagnosis in view of the history of trauma. He later developed glove anesthesia in both forearms and insensitivity to pinprick, also characteristic of beriberi. He experienced constant neck pain and headaches. Repeated roentgenology of the cervical spine and myelography had been performed elsewhere in a desperate effort to find a skeletal cause. These studies had not revealed any evidence of structural defect. One year after the accident he still had symptoms. On examination, both hands and forearms were cyanotic and cold to the touch. The femoral artery was easily audible by auscultation in the inguinal area, and the blood pressure was 150/30 mm Hg and was labile, all consistent with a diagnosis of beriberi. Gross white fingernail spots were seen, suggesting serious nutritional deficiency.[174] Diet history revealed an excess of sweets and cola. No treatment was given other than dietary instruction and supplementation with thiamine and a high-potency vitamin and mineral mix. General health began to improve and all neurologic symptoms had disappeared in 2 months. Both forearms were normal in color. Although red cell TKA was never outside normal range, it increased from 54.4 to 65.6 mU/L/min. TPPE decreased from 11.4% to 1.0%. Thus the trend of this test indicated thiamine response, only by comparison before and after treatment. The symptoms suggested that the trauma acted as a stress insult that triggered the neurologic symptoms of beriberi since peripheral neuropathy was the presenting feature. Today, it would be advisable to look for the possibility of single nucleotide polymorphisms in thiamine transporters that could present an additional risk from poor nutrition.

## CONCLUSION

We have provided evidence that thiamine deficiency is surprisingly common in the United States and that the clinical presentation is extremely variable. Activity of the autonomic nervous system is compromised, including an exaggeration of its normal asymmetric distribution. We have shown that thiamine deficiency and mild hypoxia produce the same effects in the brain stem and limbic system, giving rise to maladaptive autonomic dysfunction. A high index of clinical suspicion is required to avoid labeling the constellation of symptoms as psychosomatic.

Although genetically determined thiamine dependency is relatively rare, modern technology is increasingly efficient in recognizing it. There is also reason to believe that the enzymes that depend upon thiamine as their cofactor gradually deteriorate when high carbohydrate malnutrition is prolonged. To restore functional activity of the enzyme, pharmacological doses of the vitamin are required for weeks to months, as was shown in the treatment of beriberi by the early investigators. We have presented the methods of evaluating thiamine deficiency in the laboratory and recommend the use of ETKA and TPPE as the most definitive.

## REFERENCES

1. Peters R. Significance of biochemical lesions in the pyruvate oxidase system. *Br Med Bull* 1953;**9**(2):116–21.
2. Thornalley PJ, Babaei-Jadidi R, Al Ali H, Rabbani N, Antonysunil A, Larkin J, Ahmed A, Rayman G, Bodmer CW. High prevalence of low plasma thiamine concentration in diabetes linked to a marker of vascular disease. *Diabetologia* 2007;**50**(10):2164–70.
3. Larkin JR, Zhang F, Godfrey L, Molostvov G, Zehnder D, Rabbani N, Thornalley PJ. Glucose-induced down regulation of thiamine transporters in the kidney proximal tubular epithelium produces thiamine insufficiency in diabetes. *PLoS One* 2012;**7**(12):e53175.

4. Mee L, Nabokina SM, Sekar VT, Subramanian VS, Maedler K, Said HM. Pancreatic beta cells and islets take up thiamin by a regulated carrier-mediated process: studies using mice and human pancreatic preparations. *Am J Physiol Gastrointest Liver Physiol* 2009;**297**(1):G197–206.
5. vinh quoc Luong K, Nguyen LTH. The impact of thiamine treatment in the diabetes mellitus. *J Clin Med Res* 2012;**4**(3):153–60.
6. Yuka K. Effect of thiamine repletion on cardiac fibrosis and protein O-glycosylation in diabetic cardiomyopathy. *J Diabetes Metab* 2012. https://www.omicsonline.org/effect-of-thiamine-repletion-on-cardiac-fibrosis-and-protein-o-glycosylation-in-diabetic-cardiomyopathy-2155-6156.S7-001.php?aid=4725.
7. Babaei-Jadidi R, Karachalias N, Ahmed N, Battah S, Thornalley PJ. Prevention of incipient diabetic nephropathy by high-dose thiamine and benfotiamine. *Diabetes* 2003;**52**(8):2110–20.
8. Lakhani SV, et al. Small intestinal bacterial overgrowth and thiamine deficiency after Roux-en-Y gastric bypass surgery in obese patients. *Nutr Res* 2008;**28**:293–8.
9. Pepersack T, Garbusinski J, Robberecht J, Beyer I, Willems D, Fuss M. Clinical relevance of thiamine status amongst hospitalized elderly patients. *Gerontology* 1999;**45**(2):96–101.
10. Isenberg-Grzeda E, Shen MJ, Alici Y, Wills J, Nelson C, Breitbart W. High rate of thiamine deficiency among inpatients with cancer referred for psychiatric consultation: results of a single site prevalence study. *Psychooncology* 2016. http://dx.doi.org/10.1002/pon.4155.
11. Manzanares W, Hardy G. Thiamine supplementation in the critically ill. *Curr Opin Clin Nutr Metab Care* 2011;**14**(6):610–7.
12. Leite HP, de Lima LFP. Metabolic resuscitation in sepsis: a necessary step beyond the hemodynamic? *J Thorac Dis* 2016;**3**(2).
13. Jamieson CP, Obeid OA, Powell-Tuck J. The thiamin, riboflavin and pyridoxine status of patients on emergency admission to hospital. *Clin Nutr* 1999;**18**(2):87–91.
14. Hanninen SA, Darling PB, Sole MJ, Barr A, Keith ME. The prevalence of thiamin deficiency in hospitalized patients with congestive heart failure. *J Am Coll Cardiol* 2006;**47**(2):354–61.
15. Sanchez DJ, Murphy MM, Bosch-Sabater J, Fernandez-Ballart J. Enzymic evaluation of thiamin, riboflavin and pyridoxine status of parturient mothers and their newborn infants in a Mediterranean area of Spain. *Eur J Clin Nutr* 1999;**53**(1):27–38.
16. Bâ A. Alcohol and B1 vitamin deficiency-related stillbirths. *J Matern Fetal Neonatal Med* 2009;**22**(5):452–7.
17. Carney MW, Ravindran A, Rinsler MG, Williams DG. Thiamine, riboflavin and pyridoxine deficiency in psychiatric in-patients. *Br J Psychiatry* 1982;**141**(3):271–2.
18. Wijnia JW, Oudman E, van Gool WA, Wiersma AI, Bresser EL, Bakker J, van de Wiel A, Mulder CL. Severe infections are common in thiamine deficiency and may be related to cognitive outcomes: a cohort study of 68 patients with Wernicke-Korsakoff syndrome. *Psychosomatics* 2016;**57**(6).
19. Lonsdale D. Thiamine and magnesium deficiencies: keys to disease. *Med Hypotheses* 2015;**84**(2):129–34.
20. Hoffman R. Thiamine deficiency in the Western diet and dementia risk. *Br J Nutr* 2016;**116**(1):188–9. http://dx.doi.org/10.1017/S000711451600177X.
21. Harper CG, Giles M, Finlay-Jones R. Clinical signs in the Wernicke-Korsakoff complex: a retrospective analysis of 131 cases diagnosed at necropsy. *J Neurol Neurosurg Psychiatry* 1986;**49**(4):341–5.
22. Vasconcelos MM, Silva KP, Vidal G, Silva AF, Domingues RC, Berditchevsky CR. Early diagnosis of pediatric Wernicke's encephalopathy. *Pediatr Neurol* 1999;**20**(4):289–94.
23. World Health Organization. *Thiamine deficiency and its prevention and control in major emergencies*. Report no: WHO/NHD/99.13. Geneva: Department of Nutrition for Health and Development, WHO; 1999.

24. DiNicolantonio JJ, Niazi AK, Lavie CJ, O'Keefe JH, Ventura HO. Thiamine supplementation for the treatment of heart failure: a review of the literature. *Congest Heart Fail* 2013;**19**(4):214–22.
25. Lu J, Frank EL. Rapid HPLC measurement of thiamine and its phosphate esters in whole blood. *Clin Chem* 2008;**54**(5):901–6.
26. Talwar D, Davidson H, Cooney J, Jo'reilly DS. Vitamin B1 status assessed by direct measurement of thiamin pyrophosphate in erythrocytes or whole blood by HPLC: comparison with erythrocyte transketolase activation assay. *Clin Chem* 2000;**46**(5):704–10.
27. Boni L, Kieckens L, Hendricz A. An evaluation of a modified erythrocyte transketolase assay for accessing thiamine nutritional adequacy. *J Nutr Sci Vitaminol* 1980;**26**:507–14.
28. Jeyasingham MD, Pratt O, Burns A, et al. The activation of red blood cell transketolase in groups of patients especially at risk from thiamine deficiency. *Psychol Med* 1987;**117**:198–202.
29. Schenk G, Duggleby RG, Nixon PF. Properties and functions of the thiamin diphosphate dependent enzyme transketolase. *Int J Biochem Cell Biol* 1998;**30**(12):1297–318.
30. Massod MF, Mcguire SL, Werner KR. Analysis of blood transketolase activity. *Am J Clin Pathol* 1971;**55**(4):465–70.
31. Lonsdale D. Red cell transketolase studies in a private practice specializing in nutritional correction. *J Am Coll Nutr* 1988;**7**(1):61–7.
32. Wells DG, Baylis EM, Holoway L, Marks V. Erythrocyte-transketolase activity in megaloblastic anaemia. *Lancet* 1968;**292**(7567):543–5.
33. Laville M, Nazare JA. Diabetes, insulin resistance and sugars. *Obes Rev* 2009;**10**(s1):24–33.
34. Lonsdale D. Is eosinophilic esophagitis a sugar sensitive disease? *J Gastric Disord Ther* 2016;**2**(1):114. http://dx.doi.org/10.16966/2381-8689.
35. Blass JP, Gibson GE. Abnormality of a thiamine requiring enzyme in patients with the Wernicke-Korsakoff syndrome. *N Engl J Med* 1977;**297**:1367–70.
36. Eisinger J, Bagneres D, Arroyo P, et al. Effect of magnesium, high energy phosphates, piracetam and thiamine on erythrocyte transketolase. *Magnes Res* 1994;**7**:59–61.
37. Dyckner T, Elk B, Nyhlin H, Wester PO. Aggravation of thiamine deficiency by magnesium depletion. A case report. *Acta Scand* 1985;**218**:129–31.
38. Kimura M, Itokawa Y. Effects of calcium and magnesium deficiency on thiamine distribution in rat brain and liver. *J Neurochem* 1977;**28**:389–93.
39. Markannen T, Kalliomaki JL. Transketolase activity of blood cells in various clinical conditions. *Am J Med Sci* 1966;**252**(5).
40. Deleted in review.
41. Cooper JR, Itokawa Y, Pincus JH. Thiamine triphosphate deficiency in subacute necrotizing encephalomyelopathy. *Science* 1969;**164**(3875):74–5.
42. Cooper JR, Pincus JH, Itokawa Y, Piros K. Experiences with phosphoribosyl transferase inhibition in subacute necrotizing encephalomyelopathy. *N Engl J Med* 1970;**283**:793–5.
43. Lonsdale, unpublished observations.
44. Lake NJ, Compton AG, Rahman S, Thorburn DR. Leigh syndrome: one disorder, more than 75 monogenic causes. *Ann Neurol* 2016;**79**(2):190–203.
45. Banka S, de Goede C, Yue WW. Expanding the clinical and molecular spectrum of thiamine pyrophosphokinase deficiency: a treatable neurological disorder caused by TPK1 mutations. *Mol Genet Metab* 2014;**113**(4):301–6.
46. Lonsdale D, Cooper JR. Thiamine metabolism in disease. *CRC Crit Rev Clin Lab Sci* 1975;**5**(3):289–313.

47. Shah S, Wald E. Type B lactic acidosis secondary to thiamine deficiency in a child with malignancy. *Pediatrics* 2015;**135**(1):e221–4.
48. Jacobs RA, Meinild AK, Nordsborg NB, Lundby C. Lactate oxidation in human skeletal muscle mitochondria. *Am J Physiol Endocrinol Metab* 2013;**304**(7):E686–94. http://dx.doi.org/10.1152/ajpendo.00476.2012.
49. Ross JM, Öberg J, Brené S, Coppotelli G, Terzioglu M, Pernold K, Goiny M, Sitnikov R, Kehr J, Trifunovic A, Larsson NG. High brain lactate is a hallmark of aging and caused by a shift in the lactate dehydrogenase A/B ratio. *Proc Natl Acad Sci USA* 2010;**107**(46):20087–92. http://dx.doi.org/10.1073/pnas.1008189107.
50. Dienel GA. Brain lactate metabolism: the discoveries and the controversies. *J Cereb Blood Flow Metab* 2012;**32**(7):1107–38. http://dx.doi.org/10.1038/jcbfm.2011.175.
51. Cruz RSO, et al. Intracellular shuttle: the lactate aerobic metabolism. *Sci World J* 2012;**2012**:420984. http://dx.doi.org/10.1100/2012/420984.
52. Overgaard M, Rasmussen P, Bohm AM, Seifert T, Brassard P, Zaar M, Homann P, Evans KA, Nielsen HB, Secher NH. Hypoxia and exercise provoke both lactate release and lactate oxidation by the human brain. *FASEB J* 2012;**26**(7):3012–20.
53. Goh S, Dong Z, Zhang Y, DiMauro S, Peterson BS. Mitochondrial dysfunction as a neurobiological subtype of autism spectrum disorder: evidence from brain imaging. *JAMA Psychiatry* 2014;**71**(6):665–71.
54. f Kmp V. High brain lactate is not caused by a shift in the lactate dehydrogenase A/B ratio. *Biol* 2011;**240**:464–74.
55. Borsook H, Dubnoff JW. The hydrolysis of phosphocreatine and the origin of urinary creatinine. *J Biol Chem* 1947;**168**(2):493–510.
56. Fitch CD. Significance of abnormalities of creatine metabolism. In: *Pathogenesis of human muscular dystrophies*, vol. 404. Amsterdam: Excerpta Medica; 1977. p. 328–36.
57. Seraydarian MW, Artaza L. Regulation of energy metabolism by creatine in cardiac and skeletal muscle cells in culture. *J Mol Cell Cardiol* 1976;**8**(9):669–78.
58. Perna MK, Kokenge AN, Miles KN, Udobi KC, Clark JF, Pyne-Geithman GJ, Khuchua Z, Skelton MR. Creatine transporter deficiency leads to increased whole body and cellular metabolism. *Amino Acids* 2016;**48**(8):2057–65.
59. Lonsdale D, Faulkner WR, Price JW, Smeby RR. Intermittent cerebellar ataxia associated with hyperpyruvic acidemia, hyperalaninemia, and hyperalaninuria. *Pediatrics* 1969;**43**(6):1025–34.
60. Clark LC, Thompson HL, Beck EI, Jacobson W. Excretion of creatine and creatinine by children. *AMA Am J Dis Child* 1951;**81**(6):774–83. http://jamanetwork.com/journals/jamapediatrics/article-abstract/494968.
61. Iwata H, Nishikawa T, Watanabe K. Pharmacological studies on thiamine deficiency IV. Blood catecholamine content and blood pressure of thiamine deficient rats. *Experientia* 1969;**25**(3):283–4.
62. Iwata H, Watanabe K, Nishikawa T, Ohashi M. Effects of drugs on behavior, heart rate and catecholamine levels in thiamine-deficient rats. *Eur J Pharmacol* 1969;**6**(2):83–9.
63. Iwata H, Nishikawa T, Fujimoto S. Monoamine oxidase activities in tissues of thiamine-deficient rats. *J Pharm Pharmacol* 1969;**21**(4):237–40.
64. Ochoa S. Enzymic synthesis of cocarboxylase in animal tissues. *Biochem J* 1939;**33**(8):1262.
65. Seegmiller JE. Biochemical and genetic studies of an X-linked neurological disease (The Lesch-Nyhan syndrome). *Harvey Lect* 1970;**65**:175–92.
66. Lonsdale D, Price JW. Pyruvic aciduria in the detection of thiamine responsive encephalopathy. *Cleve Clin Q* 1972;**40**(2):79–88.
67. Fox IH, Kelley WN. Phosphoribosylpyrophosphate in man: biochemical and clinical significance. *Ann Intern Med* 1971;**74**(3):424–33.
68. Scriver CR, Clow CL, Mackenzie S, Delvin E. Thiamine-responsive maple-syrup-urine disease. *Lancet* 1971;**297**(7694):310–2.

69. O'Brien D. Manual of practical micro and general procedures in clinical chemistry. *Pediatrics* 1962;**30**.
70. Efron ML. Two-way separation of amino acids and other ninhydrin-reacting substances by high-voltage electrophoresis followed by paper chromatography. *Biochem J* 1959;**72**(4):691.
71. Piez KA, Morris L. A modified procedure for the automatic analysis of amino acids. *Anal Biochem* 1960;**1**(3):187–201.
72. Lonsdale D, Foust M. Normal mental development in treated phenylketonuria: report of ten cases. *Am J Dis Child* 1970;**119**(5):440–6.
73. Lonsdale D, Mercer RD, Faulkner WR. Maple syrup urine disease: report of two cases. *Am J Dis Child* 1963;**106**(3):258–66.
74. Lonsdale D, Barber DH. Maple-syrup-urine disease: report of a case, with a pedigree. *N Engl J Med* 1964;**271**(26):1338–41.
75. Gretter TE, Lonsdale D, Mercer RD, Robinson C, Shamberger RJ. Maple syrup urine disease variant. Report of a case. *Cleve Clin Q* 1972;**39**(3):129.
76. Lonsdale D, Faulkner WR. Two-dimensional chromatography to evaluate amino acid excretion. *Cleve Clin Q* 1965;**32**:5.
77. Fruton JD, Simmonds S. General metabolism of protein amino acids. In: *General biochemistry*. 2nd ed. London: John Wiley and Sons; 1960. p. p763.
78. McIlwain H, Bachelard HS. Chemical factors in chemical neurotransmission. In: *Biochemistry and the central nervous system*. 4th ed. London: J&A Churchill Ltd; 1971. p. p494.
79. Nachmansohn D, John HM, Waelsch H. Effect of glutamic acid on the formation of acetylcholine. *J Biol Chem* 1943;**150**(2):485–6.
80. McIlwain H, Bachelard HS. Metabolic, ionic and electrical phenomena in separated cerebral tissues: cerebral lipids. In: *Biochemistry and the central nervous system*. New York: Churchill Livingstone; 1985. p. 54–83.
81. Nagler AL, Dettbarn WD, Seifter E, Levenson SM. Tissue levels of acetyl choline and acetyl cholinesterase in weanling rats subjected to acute choline deficiency. *J Nutr* 1968;**94**:13–9.
82. Watts RWE, Chalmers RA, Lawson AM. Abnormal organic acidurias in mentally retarded patients. *Lancet* 1975;**305**(7903):368–72.
83. Darling S, Rtensen OM. Amino-aciduria in galactosaemia. *Acta Paediatr* 1954;**43**(4):337–41.
84. De Vivo DC. Reye syndrome: a metabolic response to an acute mitochondrial insult. *Neurology* 1978;**28**(2):105.
85. Rittenhouse J, Mason M, Baublis J. Aminoacid ratios in Reye's syndrome. *Lancet* 1979;**314**(8133):105–6.
86. Shaywitz BA, Venes J, Cohen DJ, Bowers MB. Reye syndrome monoamine metabolites in ventricular fluid. *Neurology* 1979;**29**(4):467.
87. Friedemann TE, Haugen GE. Pyruvic acid II. The determination of keto acids in blood and urine. *J Biol Chem* 1943;**147**(2):415–42.
88. Smith I, Smith MJ. Ketoacids. In: 2nd ed. Smith I, editor. *Chromatographic and electrophoretic techniques*, vol. 1. New York: Interscience Publishers; 1960.
89. Huckabee WE. Abnormal resting blood lactate: I. The significance of hyperlactatemia in hospitalized patients. *Am J Med* 1961;**30**(6):833–9.
90. Israels S, Haworth JC, Dunn HG, Applegarth DA. Lactic acidosis in childhood. *Adv Pediatr* 1975;**22**:267–303.
91. Ben-Ishay D. Aminoaciduria induced by salicylates. *J Lab Clin Med* 1964;**63**(6):924–32.
92. Schrör K. Aspirin and Reye syndrome. *Paediatr Drugs* 2007;**9**(3):195–204.
93. Frank LL. Thiamin in clinical practice. *J Parenter Enteral Nutr* 2015;**39**(5):503–20.

94. de Andrade JAA, Gayer CRM, de Almeida Nogueira NP, Paes MC, Bastos VLFC, Neto JDCB, Alves SC, Coelho RM, da Cunha MGAT, Gomes RN, Águila MB. The effect of thiamine deficiency on inflammation, oxidative stress and cellular migration in an experimental model of sepsis. *J Inflamm* 2014;**11**(1):1.
95. Schmahmann JD. Cerebellar cognitive affective syndrome and the neuropsychiatry of the cerebellum. In: *Handbook of the cerebellum and cerebellar disorders*. Netherlands: Springer; 2013. p. 1717–51.
96. Hong S, Negrello M, Junker M, Smilgin A, Thier P, De Schutter E. Multiplexed coding by cerebellar Purkinje neurons. *eLife* 2016;**5**:e13810.
97. Howarth C, Peppiatt-Wildman CM, Attwell D. The energy use associated with neural computation in the cerebellum. *J Cereb Blood Flow Metab* 2010;**30**(2):403–14.
98. Nairn JG, Bedi KS, Mayhew TM, Campbell LF. On the number of Purkinje cells in the human cerebellum: unbiased estimates obtained by using the "fractionator". *J Comp Neurol* 1989;**290**(4):527–32.
99. Howarth C, Gleeson P, Attwell D. Updated energy budgets for neural computation in the neocortex and cerebellum. *J Cereb Blood Flow Metab* 2012;**32**(7):1222–32.
100. Liong CC, Rahmat K, Mah JSY, Lim SY, Tan AH. Nonalcoholic Wernicke encephalopathy: an entity not to Be missed!. *Can J Neurol Sci* 2016:1–2.
101. Lax NZ, Hepplewhite PD, Reeve AK, Nesbitt V, McFarland R, Jaros E, Taylor RW, Turnbull DM. Cerebellar ataxia in patients with mitochondrial DNA disease: a molecular clinicopathological study. *J Neuropathol Exp Neurol* 2012;**71**(2):148–61.
102. Schmahmann JD. Disorders of the cerebellum: ataxia, dysmetria of thought, and the cerebellar cognitive affective syndrome. *J Neuropsychiatry Clin Neurosci* 2004;**16**(3):367–78.
103. Galna B, Newman J, Jakovljevic DG, Bates MG, Schaefer AM, McFarland R, Turnbull DM, Trenell MI, Gorman GS, Rochester L. Discrete gait characteristics are associated with m. 3243A> G and m. 8344A> G variants of mitochondrial disease and its pathological consequences. *J Neurol* 2014;**261**(1):73–82.
104. Zhao N, Zhong C, Wang Y, Zhao Y, Gong N, Zhou G, Xu T, Hong Z. Impaired hippocampal neurogenesis is involved in cognitive dysfunction induced by thiamine deficiency at early pre-pathological lesion stage. *Neurobiol Dis* 2008;**29**(2):176–85.
105. Mancuso M, et al. Mitochondria, cognitive impairment, and Alzheimer's disease. *Int J Alzheimer Dis* 2009;**2009**:951548. http://dx.doi.org/10.4061/2009/951548. 8 pp.
106. Liu ZW, Gan G, Suyama S, Gao XB. Intracellular energy status regulates activity in hypocretin/orexin neurones: a link between energy and behavioural states. *J Physiol* 2011;**589**(17):4157–66.
107. Girault EM, Yi CX, Fliers E, Kalsbeek A. Orexins, feeding, and energy balance. *Prog Brain Res* 2012;**198**:47–64.
108. Hara J, Beuckmann CT, Nambu T, Willie JT, Chemelli RM, Sinton CM, Sugiyama F, Yagami KI, Goto K, Yanagisawa M, Sakurai T. Genetic ablation of orexin neurons in mice results in narcolepsy, hypophagia, and obesity. *Neuron* 2001;**30**(2):345–54.
109. Hasegawa E, Yanagisawa M, Sakurai T, Mieda M. Orexin neurons suppress narcolepsy via 2 distinct efferent pathways. *J Clin Invest* 2014;**124**(2):604–16.
110. Lauritzen M, Dreier JP, Fabricius M, Hartings JA, Graf R, Strong AJ. Clinical relevance of cortical spreading depression in neurological disorders: migraine, malignant stroke, subarachnoid and intracranial hemorrhage, and traumatic brain injury. *J Cereb Blood Flow Metab* 2011;**31**(1):17–35.
111. Holland PR, Akerman S, Goadsby PJ. Orexin 1 receptor activation attenuates neurogenic dural vasodilation in an animal model of trigeminovascular nociception. *J Pharmacol Exp Ther* 2005;**315**(3):1380–5.
112. Rejdak K, Papuć E, Grieb P, Stelmasiak Z. Decreased cerebrospinal fluid hypocretin-1 (orexin A) in patients after repetitive generalized tonic–clonic seizures. *Epilepsia* 2009;**50**(6):1641–4.

113. Brundin L, Bjorkqvist M, Petersen A, Traskman-Bendz L. Reduced orexin levels in the cerebrospinal fluid of suicidal patients with major depressive disorder. *Eur Neuropsychopharmacol* 2007;**17**:573–9.
114. Platt BS. Thiamine deficiency in human beriberi and in Wernicke's encephalopathy. In: *Thiamine deficiency*. Boston: Little, Brown and Company; 1967. p. 135–43.
115. Thornalley PJ. The potential role of thiamine (vitamin B1) in diabetic complications. *Curr Diabetes Rev* 2005;**1**(3):287–98.
116. Fernandez M, Barcelöa M, Mu–toz C, Torrecillas M, Blanca M. Anaphylaxis to thiamine (vitamin B1). *Allergy* 1997;**52**(9):958–9.
117. Stephen JM, Grant R, Yeh CS. Anaphylaxis from administration of intravenous thiamine. *Am J Emerg Med* 1992;**10**(1):61–3.
118. van Dongen S, Brown RM, Brown GK, Thorburn DR, Boneh A. Thiamine-responsive and non-responsive patients with PDHC-E1 deficiency: a retrospective assessment. In: *JIMD reports*, vol. 15. Berlin Heidelberg: Springer; 2014. p. 13–27.
119. Fujiwara M. Absorption, excretion and fate of thiamine and its derivatives in [the] human body. In: *Thiamine and beriberi*. Tokyo: Igaku Shoin Ltd; 1965. p. 179–213.
120. Volvert ML, Seyen S, Piette M, Evrard B, Gangolf M, Plumier JC, Bettendorff L. Benfotiamine, a synthetic S-acyl thiamine derivative, has different mechanisms of action and a different pharmacological profile than lipid-soluble thiamine disulfide derivatives. *BMC Pharmacol* 2008;**8**(1):10.
121. Lonsdale D. Thiamine tetrahydrofurfuryl disulfide: a little known therapeutic agent. *Med Sci Monit* 2004;**10**(9):RA199–203.
122. Tanphaichitr V, Vimokesant SL, Dhanamitta S, Valyasevi A. Clinical and biochemical studies of adult beriberi. *Am J Clin Nutr* 1970;**23**:1017–26.
123. Griffiths IX, Brocklehurst JC, Scott DL, et al. Thiamine and ascorbic acid levels in the elderly. *J Clin Gerontol Geriatr* 1967;**9**:1–10.
124. Oldham HG. Thiamine requirements of women. *Ann NY Acad Sci* 1962;**98**:542–9.
125. Thomson AD. Thiamine absorption in old age. *Gerontol Clin* 1966;**8**(6):354–61.
126. Delaney RL, Lankford HG, Sullivan JF. Thiamine, magnesium and plasma lactate abnormalities in alcoholic patients. *Exp Biol Med* 1966;**123**(3):675–9.
127. Tomasulo PA, Kater RMH, Iber FL. Impairment of thiamine absorption in alcoholism. *Am J Clin Nutr* 1968;**21**:1341–4.
128. Brummer P, Markkanen T. Urinary excretion of thiamine and riboflavin in achlorhydria. *Acta Med Scand* 1960;**166**(1):75–7.
129. Thomson AD. The absorption of radio-active sulphur-labelled thiamine hydrochloride in control subjects and in patients with intestinal mal-absorption. *Clin Sci* 1966;**31**:167–79.
130. Truswell AS, Hansen JD, Konno T. Thiamine deficiency in children with severe gastroenteritis. *S Afr Med J* 1972;**46**:2083–4.
131. Matsuda T, Maeda S, Baba A, Iwata H. Existence of ascorbic acid as an activator of thiamine diphosphatase in rat brain. *J Neurochem* 1979;**32**(2):443–8.
132. Fujiwara M, Itokawa Y, Kimura M. Experimental studies on the relationships between thiamine and divalent cations, calcium and magnesium. In: *Thiamine*. NY: John Wiley and Sons; 1976. p. 63–80.
133. Weil ML, Menkes JH, Shaw KNF, Pincus JH. Pyridoxine responsive inhibition of thiamine metabolism. *Clin Res Cardiol* 1971;**19**:229.
134. Pincus JH, Cooper JR, Itokawa Y, Gumbinas M. Subacute necrotizing encephalomyelopathy: effects of thiamine and thiamine propyl disulfide. *Arch Neurol* 1971;**24**(6):511–7.
135. Von Yano R. Klinische Erfahrungen mit einem neuen Thiamin-Derivat bei Rheumatischen Erkrankungen. *Med Klin* 1964;**59**:1396–8.
136. Pincus JH, Cooper JR, Murphy JV, Rabe EF, Lonsdale D, Dunn HG. Thiamine derivatives in subacute necrotizing encephalomyelopathy. *Pediatrics* 1973;**51**(4):716–21.

137. Grode GA, Falb RD, Crowley JP, Truitt Jr EB. Observations on the development of antibodies to thiamine tetrahydrofurfuryl disulfide in rabbits. *Pharmacology* 1974;**11**(2):102–7.
138. Djoenaidi W, Notermans SLH. Thiamine tetraphydrofurfuryl disulfide in nutritional polyneuropathy. *Eur Arch Psychiatry Neurol Sci* 1990;**239**(4):218–20.
139. Suzuki M, Itokawa Y. Effects of thiamine supplementation on exercise-induced fatigue. *Metab Brain Dis* 1996;**11**(1):95–106.
140. Mimori Y, Katsuoka H, Nakamura S. Thiamine therapy in Alzheimer's disease. *Metab Brain Dis* 1996;**11**(1):89–94.
141. Lonsdale D, Shamberger RJ, Audhya T. Treatment of autism spectrum children with thiamine tetrahydrofurfuryl disulfide: a pilot study. *Neuroendocrinol Lett* 2002;**23**(4):303–8.
142. Carney MW, Williams DG, Sheffield BF. Thiamine and pyridoxine lack newly-admitted psychiatric patients. *Br J Psychiatry* 1979;**135**(3):249–54.
143. Schwartz RA, Gross M, Lonsdale D, Shamberger R. Transketolase activity in psychiatric patients. *J Clin Psychiatry* 1979;**40**(10):427–9.
144. Saavedra JM, Grobecker H, Axelrod J. Adrenaline-forming enzyme in brainstem: elevation in genetic and experimental hypertension. *Science* 1976;**191**(4226):483–4.
145. Taylor KS, Murai H, Millar PJ, Haruki N, Kimmerly DS, Morris BL, Tomlinson G, Bradley TD, Floras JS. Arousal from sleep and sympathetic excitation during wakefulness. *Hypertension* 2016. http://dx.doi.org/10.1161/HYPERTENSIONAHA.116.08212.
146. Yao H, Nabika T. Standards and pitfalls of focal ischemia models in spontaneously hypertensive rats: with a systematic review of recent articles. *J Transl Med* 2012;**10**(1):1.
147. Onodera K, Tadano T, Sakai K, Kisara K, Ogura Y. [Muricide induced by thiamine deficiency in the rats (author's transl)]. *Nihon Yakurigaku Zasshi Folia Pharmacol Jap* 1978;**74**(5):641–8.
148. Onodera K, Tadano T, Kisara K, Kimura Y, Ogura Y. Persistent erection in thiamine-deficient rats. *Andrologia* 1978;**10**(6):467–72.
149. Skelton FR. Some specific and non-specific effects of thiamine deficiency in the rat. *Exp Biol Med* 1950;**73**(3):516–9.
150. Selye H. The general adaptation syndrome and the diseases of adaptation. *J Clin Endocrinol Metab* 1946;**6**(2):117–230.
151. Govier WM, Greig ME. Studies on shock induced by hemorrhage. 5. The effect of cellular damage on the in vitro hydrolysis and synthesis of cocarboxylase by liver tissue. *J Pharmacol Exp Ther* 1943;**79**:240–5.
152. Salem HM. Glyoxalase and methylglyoxal in thiamine-deficient rats. *Biochem J* 1954;**57**(2):227.
153. Roser RL. Determination of urinary levels of methylglyoxal and thiamine in human subjects. 1978.
154. Racker E. The mechanism of action of glyoxalase. *J Biol Chem* 1951;**190**(2):685–96.
155. Liang CC. Studies on experimental thiamine deficiency. Trends of keto acid formation and detection of glyoxylic acid. *Biochem J* 1962;**82**(3):429.
156. Krajmalnik-Brown R, Ilhan ZE, Kang DW, DiBaise JK. Effects of gut microbes on nutrient absorption and energy regulation. *Nutr Clin Pract* 2012;**27**(2):201–14.
157. Restivo A, Carta MG, Farci AMG, Saiu L, Gessa GL, Agabio R. Risk of thiamine deficiency and Wernicke's encephalopathy after gastrointestinal surgery for cancer. *Support Care Cancer* 2016;**24**(1):77–82.
158. Yahia M, Najeh H, Zied H, Khalaf M, Salah AM, Sofienne BM, Laidi B, Hamed J, Hayenne M. Wernicke's encephalopathy: a rare complication of hyperemesis gravidarum. *Anaesth Crit Care Pain Med* 2015;**34**(3):173.
159. Kerns JC, Arundel C, Chawla LS. Thiamin deficiency in people with obesity. *Adv Nutr* 2015;**6**(2):147–53.
160. Villafuerte FC, Corante N. Chronic mountain sickness: clinical aspects, etiology, management, and treatment. *High Alt Med Biol* 2016;**17**(2):61–9.

161. Lonsdale D, Shamberger RJ. Red cell transketolase as an indicator of nutritional deficiency. *Am J Clin Nutr* 1980;**33**(2):205–11.
162. Lonsdale D. Hypothesis and case reports: possible thiamin deficiency. *J Am Coll Nutr* 1990;**9**(1):13–7.
163. Lonsdale D. Dysautonomia, a heuristic approach to a revised model for etiology of disease. *Evid Based Complement Alternat Med* 2009;**6**(1):3–10.
164. Blass JP, Avigan J, Uhlendorf BW. A defect in pyruvate decarboxylase in a child with an intermittent movement disorder. *J Clin Invest* 1970;**49**(3):423.
165. Deleted in review.
166. Brunette MG, Delvin E, Hazel B, Scriver CR. Thiamine-responsive lactic acidosis in a patient with deficient low-Km pyruvate carboxylase activity in liver. *Pediatrics* 1972;**50**(5):702–11.
167. Rogers LE, Porter FS, Sidbury JB. Thiamine-responsive megaloblastic anemia. *J Pediatr* 1969;**74**(4):494–504.
168. Gaull GE, Tallan HH, Lonsdale D, Przyrembel H, Schaffner F, Von Bassewitz DB. Hypermethioninemia associated with methionine adenosyltransferase deficiency: clinical, morphologic, and biochemical observations on four patients. *J Pediatr* 1981;**98**(5):734–41.
169. Chiao FF, Stokstad ELR. Effect of methionine on hepatic folate metabolism in rats fed a vitamin B12-and methionine-deficient diet. *Exp Biol Med* 1977;**155**(3):433–7.
170. Herbert V, Zalusky R. Interrelations of vitamin B12 and folic acid metabolism: folic acid clearance studies. *J Clin Invest* 1962;**41**(6):1263.
171. Lonsdale D. Recurrent febrile lymphadenopathy treated with large doses of vitamin B1: report of two cases. *Dev Pharmacol Ther* 1979;**1**(4):254–64.
172. Bonica JJ. Causalgia and other reflex sympathetic dystrophies. *Postgrad Med* 1973;**53**(6):143.
173. Bernstein BH, Singsen BH, Kent JT, Kornreich H, King K, Hicks R, Hanson V. Reflex neurovascular dystrophy in childhood. *J Pediatr* 1978;**93**(2):211–5.
174. Pfeiffer CC, Jenney EH. Fingernail white spots: possible zinc deficiency. *JAMA* 1974;**228**(2):157.

# CHAPTER 5

# Thiamine-Deficient Dysautonomias: Case Insights and Clinical Clues

## Contents

| | |
|---|---|
| Beriberi, Dysautonomia, and Thiamine Deficiency: Symptoms and Time Course | 163 |
|     Experimental Thiamine Deficiency in Healthy Humans | 163 |
|     Threshold and Tipping Points for Thiamine Deficiency | 164 |
| Functional Dysautonomia: Family Studies With Case Details | 165 |
|     Family 1: Night Terrors, Gastrointestinal Dysmotility, Hypopyrexia, and Other Dysautonomias | 165 |
|     *Points of Consideration* | *167* |
|     Family 2. Diet-Induced Thiamine Deficiency With Postural Orthostatic Tachycardia Syndrome and Pandysautonomia | 168 |
|     *Points of Consideration* | *170* |
|     Family 3. Reflex Sympathetic Dystrophy/Complex Regional Pain Syndrome | 170 |
|     *Points of Consideration* | *171* |
|     The Value of Family Histories in Complicated Cases | 172 |
| Pediatric Cases of Thiamine Responsive Dysautonomias | 172 |
|     Failure to Thrive in Thiamine-Deficient Infants | 172 |
|     *Points of Consideration* | *174* |
|     Slowed Growth in Thiamine-Deficient Children | 175 |
|     Anorexia and Thiamine Deficiency | 175 |
|     *Points of Consideration* | *176* |
|     Cyclic Vomiting | 177 |
|     *Points of Consideration* | *178* |
|     *Points of Consideration* | *180* |
|     Night Terrors, Sleepwalking, Hyperactivity, and Attentional Deficits | 181 |
|     *Points of Consideration* | *183* |
|     Recurrent Febrile Lymphadenopathy | 183 |
|     *Points of Consideration* | *185* |
|     *Points of Consideration* | *186* |
|     Hypoxias: Reye's Syndrome, Sudden Infant Death Syndrome, and Other Disorders of Altered Hemostasis | 187 |
|     *Points of Consideration* | *189* |
|     Variations in Presentation | 192 |
|     *Points of Consideration* | *192* |
|     Seizures | 196 |

*Thiamine Deficiency Disease, Dysautonomia, and High Calorie Malnutrition*
ISBN 978-0-12-810387-6
http://dx.doi.org/10.1016/B978-0-12-810387-6.00005-8

© 2017 Elsevier Inc.
All rights reserved.

| | |
|---|---|
| Pyridoxine, Thiamine, and Brain Inflammation | 196 |
| Reassessing Complicated Cases | 200 |
| Thiamine-Responsive Dysautonomias in Adults | 200 |
|     Cardiac Irregularity and Associated Symptoms | 201 |
|         *Points of Consideration* | *201* |
|         *Points of Consideration* | *203* |
|     Fatigue as the Presenting Complaint | 203 |
| Familial Dysautonomia and Epigenetics | 205 |
|     Familial Dysautonomia | 205 |
|     Molecular Components of Familial Dysautonomia | 206 |
| Conclusion | 207 |
| References | 208 |

Dysautonomia indicates a disruption in autonomic function and represents a class of conditions with different genotypes and phenotypes. As was outlined in the previous chapters, the autonomic system regulates involuntary responses of vital organs and basic organismal homeostasis and so, by definition individuals with dysautonomia do not regulate those functions well. In short, dysautonomia is a disorder of pathological exaggeration where adaptive processes manifest as either too much or too little. How and in what manner the autonomic system is disrupted, however, is contingent upon a number of variables involving a complex calculus of genetic, epigenetic, and lifestyle factors.

Dysautonomias can be primary and initiated by genetic aberrations in either nuclear DNA (nDNA) or mitochondrial DNA (mtDNA), secondary or functional, developing as a result of medications, environmental toxicants, and/or dietary and lifestyle considerations, or some combination thereof.[1] Both primary and secondary dysautonomias can present at birth or emerge later in childhood and even into adulthood. Though common, the mitochondrial components of dysautonomia[2] remain largely unrecognized.[3,4] Thiamine, because of its position atop the pyruvate pathway and its role in oxidative metabolism, has emerged as a key but underappreciated player in autonomic regulation. Inasmuch as energy homeostasis represents an indispensable component of organismal survival, it should not be unexpected that permutations in cellular bioenergetics would evoke compensatory mechanisms in autonomic regulation. Energy homeostasis, after all, represents the most basic of survival mechanisms under the regulatory influence of the autonomic system. It is from this perspective that we posit disturbed autonomic function is the prototypical example of mitochondrial impairment and, as a result, the collection of symptoms that should be investigated as potentially thiamine responsive.

Presented in this chapter is a collection of cases involving functional dysautonomias, where mitochondria and thiamine are implicated directly. The cases reflect those seen in Dr. Lonsdale's practice; some were published in medical journals while others were not. Most of the cases involve children because of Dr. Lonsdale's pediatric specialty.

## BERIBERI, DYSAUTONOMIA, AND THIAMINE DEFICIENCY: SYMPTOMS AND TIME COURSE

Before presenting the case studies, a review of the symptoms, their expression, and time course is in order. A pivotal study involving human subjects illustrates the polysymptomatic effect of thiamine deficiency.

### Experimental Thiamine Deficiency in Healthy Humans

A study of pure thiamine deficiency (as distinct from the nutritional aspects of beriberi) was performed in 1943.[5] We shall refer to this in some detail since it has great relevance to modern nutritional deficiencies. Severe thiamine deprivation resulted in depressed mental states, generalized weakness, giddiness, backache, soreness of muscles, insomnia, anorexia, nausea, vomiting, weight loss, poor muscular tone, low blood pressure, and bradycardia with the subjects at rest. On exertion, heart palpitation and precordial distress (pseudoangina) occurred. Tachycardia and sinus arrhythmia were observed. The investigators reported electrocardiographic changes and impairment of gastrointestinal motility.

Moderate, prolonged restriction of thiamine, but not of calories, resulted in emotional instability, reflected by irritability, moodiness, quarrelsome behavior, lack of cooperation, vague fears and agitation, mental depression, variable restriction of activity, and numerous somatic complaints, symptoms that are common in America today. The effects on one subject, a 48-year-old woman, were described in detail. After 120 days of this deprivation, blood pressure was between 90 and 98 and the diastolic between 50 and 60 mm Hg. Heart rate was 50–60 bpm and there was marked sinus arrhythmia. Pallor and giddiness were observed when standing from the sitting position, and rising from the squatting position could be accomplished only with assistance. The patellar tendon reflexes were hypoactive but could be increased through reinforcement, and the Achilles tendon reflex was absent. The comments of the authors included the statement that symptoms were suggestive of dysfunction of the central and peripheral nervous pathways preceded by months of gross signs of neurologic dysfunction.

The results are instructive, illustrating how commonplace are the early symptoms of thiamine deficiency. In fact, they are so commonplace that it is probable that they would be diagnosed as psychosomatic, particularly if the laboratory studies are negative. In 1965, Japanese researchers published the seminal work on thiamine deficiency.[6] In it, they report the time course, presentation, chemistry, and pathology of naturally occurring beriberi. Functional changes in the autonomic nervous system figure prominently in the disease.

## Threshold and Tipping Points for Thiamine Deficiency

Among the many difficulties in recognizing thiamine deficiency is included the nonlinear trajectory of symptoms. That is, symptoms may wax and wane over a period relative to dietary and other environmental factors until overt thiamine deficiency is reached. Even then, if thiamine concentrations are restored just minimally above a threshold, some improvement may be observed. In one of the more important animal studies delineating the time course of thiamine deficiency,[7] researchers noted that in thiamine-deprived rats, symptoms began with weight loss, progressive anorexia, hair loss, and drowsiness at about 2.5 weeks into the experiment. No neurological signs of thiamine deficiency were seen at that time. It was not until after 4.5 weeks of continuous thiamine deficiency that the researchers noted a rapid progression of symptoms and decline of health. Over the proceeding 5 days, overt symptoms appeared and progressed rapidly. These symptoms included lack of coordination when walking, impairment of the righting reflex, reluctance to walk, walking backward, walking in circles, imbalance, rigid posturing, and eventually a total loss of righting activity and severe drowsiness. One injection of thiamine returned the animals to normal neurological functioning.

As part of this study, brain thiamine and other markers of thiamine metabolism were measured to determine thiamine concentrations associated with symptoms and recovery. Neurological symptoms appeared when cerebral thiamine concentrations reached 20% of normal. Recovery began when those concentrations climbed to 26% of normal. This suggests that at least in rodents, 80% of normal brain thiamine stores must be depleted before overt neurological symptoms appear. Similarly, it does not appear to take much to correct that deficit. In this study, a mere 6% increase in thiamine concentration set the course for improvement. Note, however, that some symptoms developed much earlier; symptoms that included severe drowsiness, a reluctance to walk (lack of motivation), and imbalance (ataxia).

We now know that in individuals with appropriate nutrition prior to the total removal of thiamine from the diet, thiamine depletion occurs within $\pm 18$ days.[8] When we consider current dietary and environmental trends, it is likely that chronic and subclinical thiamine insufficiencies are present in broad swathes of the population. Arguably, this then predisposes individuals to more serious thiamine deficiency syndromes in the face of secondary or tertiary mitochondrial insults, such as the addition of a new medication, a vaccine, or an illness that precipitates further dietary decline.

From this perspective, it is easy to see why thiamine deficiency disorders are nonlinear, at least until a particular point. Different exposures and triggers may decrease thiamine periodically, even to the point where overt neurological symptoms present. When those exposures are removed and barring deficiencies in metabolism and diet, symptoms may abate, at least temporarily, and until the next threshold is crossed anew and thiamine deficiency becomes the medical emergency.

In contrast, the more persistent or chronic thiamine deficits that do not cross the 80% depletion threshold (or the human equivalent) may also wax and wane and show all the core neurological symptoms expected in overt Wernicke's disease, though to a much lesser degree. To the extent that persistent thiamine deficiency disables mitochondrial functioning and degrades oxidative metabolism, the molecular survival cascades that ensue initiate compensatory illnesses. Centrally, higher-order survival centers are invariably affected, as are disturbances in sympathetic/parasympathetic balance.

When dealing with more chronic and/or more severe thiamine deficiencies, particularly those where other illnesses and/or potential genetic abnormalities exist, thiamine dosing may require escalation before therapeutic effect is recognized. Similarly, as was discussed in Chapter 4, other nutrients are often required. It is important to recognize that the individual nature in which thiamine replacement must be approached.

## FUNCTIONAL DYSAUTONOMIA: FAMILY STUDIES WITH CASE DETAILS

Many case reports of dysautonomia have been reported in the literature over the last several decades. In isolation, these cases add little to our knowledge of etiology while obfuscating the prevalence of these conditions. When reviewed in totality, however, case reports reveal common clinical patterns and innumerable etiological clues. For example, the following series of case reports involving three families illustrates the diversity of phenotypic expression within and among family members. Among the constellation of symptoms, however, are common pathophysiological features. These include a maladaptive overresponse to stressors involving the autonomic system and a treatment response to thiamine and nutrient supplementation.

### Family 1: Night Terrors, Gastrointestinal Dysmotility, Hypopyrexia, and Other Dysautonomias

M.D., a white male, was first seen at the age of 6 months with diarrhea, fever, and abdominal pain. A similar event reportedly occurred at age 7 weeks and intermittent episodes of unexplained diarrhea occurred once a week. A milk-free diet was prescribed and stools became normal. One week later he had intermittent episodes of paroxysmal abdominal pain, screaming, and repeated bowel movements. This resolved spontaneously. At the age of 5 years he returned with a 2-year history of repeated episodes of hypopyrexia as low as 95°F. A personality change was noted before each episode and he would become more withdrawn. A typical attack started after a deep sleep in the early evening, during which time it was difficult or impossible to awaken him. He would then scream, sit up with widely dilated pupils, widespread piloerection, cyanosis of lips, and extremely shallow slow breathing. His mother had observed that the pupils would not constrict, even in bright light. He would be totally unreactive to communication and appear to be blind. Enuresis would occur during the episode and in the morning he would have no recollection of the event. These typical night terrors occurred in clusters of two or three nights and were often followed by fever for several days, each cycle recurring every few months.

At the time of a physical examination, a complex clinical presentation was observed while the patient was asleep. Widespread piloerection, bradycardia, virtually 100% abdominal respiration with no chest movement, a blood pressure of 76/20 mm Hg, and a brief episode of ovoid pupil in one eye were observed. Deep patellar knee reflexes were either unobtainable or would occur unpredictably with slow relaxation and he would exhibit an irritating cough on partial arousal without awakening. Facial pallor was marked and there was divergent strabismus and slow wandering movement of the eyes.

The pupils became pinpoint in size during the period of observation. Red cell transketolase activity (TKA) was 69.8 mU/L/min (normal 42.1–86.1) and the thiamine pyrophosphate percentage uptake or effect (TPPE) was 27.7% (normal 0%–17.4%), proving thiamine deficiency. He responded to vitamin therapy that included thiamine.

P.D., the 7-year-old sister of M.D., was examined because of a lifelong history of paroxysmal abdominal pain. Birth history revealed that her mother was toxemic in pregnancy and there had been some neonatal jaundice requiring phototherapy. Early development was normal. At the age of 6 weeks she had an acute episode of gastroenteritis and was chronically debilitated for a month. Following this she had chronic nasal congestion and repeated episodes of asthmatic bronchitis, mostly in the winter months. Paroxysms of abdominal pain started with apparent colic in the first year and had continued. Repeated vomiting occurred, and since the age of 4½ years she had been enuretic at night and sleep sweating was noted. She would frequently get up at night for a bowel movement. Stools were large and sometimes blocked the toilet.

Abdominal pains occurred up to two or three times a day, lasted about half an hour, caused her to cry sometimes, and occasional loud borborygmi were heard. She would become pale and her skin clammy and mottled in appearance. She frequently had a headache. She developed a rapid heart rate during the attack. There had been recent onset of night terrors and sleepwalking. Examination was normal except for marked blanching dermographia produced in the lower extremities by gentle stroking with the tip of a finger and sluggish deep patellar tendon reflexes, which became normal with reinforcement. The family history is seen in Fig. 5.1.

## *Points of Consideration*

In our present disease model, it is extremely difficult to see the two children as having similar functional events except on a purely psychological level of explanation. The functional nature is not in the least disputed. The mechanism is considered to be automatic and biologic and is regarded as

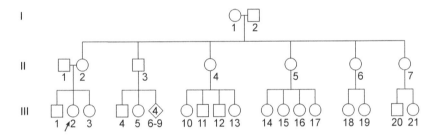

| I 2 Diabetes: lung cancer | III 4 Hyperactivity: dyslexia |
|---|---|
| II 2 Arthritis: Raynaud's disease: syncope | III 10 Hyperactivity: school problem |
| II 3 Hyperactive | III 11 Learning disability: dyslexia |
| II 4 Abdominal cancer: syncope | III 12 Behavior problem |
| II 5,6,7 Hyperactive: abdominal & chest pain | III 13 Hyperactivity |
| III 1 MD Case 1 | III 20 Recurrent bronchitis |
| III 2 Proband PD Case 2 | III 21 Chronic nasal congestion: rhinorrhea |
| III 3 Night terrors: enuresis: bruxism | |

Figure 5.1 Proband and pedigree analysis for Family 1.

a disordered response to stress. The abnormal TPPE in the first child is of interest. Recall that an accelerated uptake of thiamine pyrophosphate (TPP) by red cells is clearly indicative of its deficiency. Our experience indicates that the test has far-reaching implications. Although it is a specific indicator of nutritional deficiency, it can be abnormal because of genetic implications. In a patient with trisomy 21 and sleep apnea, in another patient with Prader–Willi syndrome dying of cor pulmonale, and a boy who had an epileptic fit in a swimming pool and suffered prolonged hypoxia of the brain, we have seen a similar effect upon this laboratory test. It may be an excellent indicator of hypoxic or pseudohypoxic stress, and this function may be more important than its purely nutritional implications.

The first child in this family had good evidence of a dysautonomic effect during sleep in particular. The most obvious feature was general piloerection, which is clinical proof of sympathetic activity. Widely dilated pupils and sweating are also sympathetic. On the other hand, pinpoint pupils represent evidence of parasympathetic activity, and suggest that the balance between the two systems is distorted or perhaps labile, so that there is a lack of a coordinated normal physiologic response. Toxemia in pregnancy is associated with thiamine deficiency[9] and may have had an effect on the second child while in utero.

Paroxysmal abdominal pain with borborygmi indicates overactive peristalsis, and this can be seen as evidence of an uncoordinated parasympathetic dominance or overshoot. The family history certainly does not indicate a specific familial disease unless the underlying mechanism is considered in terms of appropriate biochemistry and its relationship with the autonomic and endocrine responses engendered by stress. The family history suggests that there was an abnormal genetic background. Nevertheless, thiamine treatment remediated the children's symptoms. This indicates that even in the face of genetically influenced conditions, thiamine, because of its critical role in mitochondrial oxidative metabolism, is necessary for proper autonomic function.

## Family 2. Diet-Induced Thiamine Deficiency With Postural Orthostatic Tachycardia Syndrome and Pandysautonomia

D.M., 14 years and 9 months old, complained of "dizzy spells." He was a white male who was considered well until 3 weeks previously, when he suddenly experienced extreme fatigue while playing basketball. He was found to have pyrexia of 101°F, received an injection of penicillin, and was apparently well the next day. During the past year he had experienced minor episodes of dizziness on standing up and, in a recent episode, had "blacked out" completely, hitting his head as he fell. It was noticed that there was some wandering of the eyes and slight tremor of the hands while he was unconscious. He admitted to ingestion of 36 ounces of cola and one quart of iced tea a day, a one-half gallon of ice cream a week, and massive supplementation of most of his food with tomato ketchup. He had occasional cardiac palpitations and complained of pain in the chest at intervals.

On examination he was seen to be wearing tinted spectacles, and there was marked conjunctival injection. He admitted to photophobia. The heart rate was 60 bpm, the blood pressure 90/60 mm Hg, and the femoral pulse easily audible by auscultation. Deep patellar reflexes were hard to elicit, but were brisk with reinforcement, and there was marked dermographia of the lower extremities. He was told to change his diet drastically, removing all the high-calorie carbohydrate foods and beverages.

One year later he reported again because of recurrence of dizziness and admitted that he had reverted to his former dietary habits. During the year he had gained 6.4 kg in weight and 6.2 cm in height. The heart rate was 52 bpm with mild sinus arrhythmia, and deep patellar tendon reflexes were normal. Dermographia was present. A supplement of thiamine was given in a dose of 150 mg per day, and he was again cautioned about diet and referred to a dietician.

D.M.M., sister of D.M., was 12 years, 4 months old. She was seen because of an attack of numbness in the legs and general sweating. On a cool evening, while watching a ballgame, she had sudden onset of abdominal pain and profuse sweating. It was noted that she became pale and the episode lasted about half an hour. Subsequently, there were three or four similar attacks and at least one of them was associated with numbness in the legs. She was described as irritable, "mean—she wants to snap at you with every little thing," and she complained of chronic fatigue. She would return from school and go to bed, although she also had insomnia. She had chronic nasal congestion and her menstrual periods were associated with severe cramping. She admitted to consuming 32 ounces of cola and 32 ounces of iced tea every day.

On examination her heart rate was 68 bpm and blood pressure 134/40 mm Hg, with both systolic and diastolic lability. In discussing the situation with her mother it was noticed that the mother had obvious cyanosis of the feet and hands. She observed that her heart frequently "missed a beat" and that she had had these symptoms for years.

## Points of Consideration

In the light of modern knowledge, the transmission of abnormal mitochondrial genes would be expected as the etiology, extremely suggestive of thiamine deficiency as the underlying cause. At the time, it was not possible to test for this. The symptoms that they had in common were dysautonomic in character. The passing-out spells were typical of postural orthostatic tachycardia syndrome, probably including postural hypotension. Photophobia was noted as a chronic symptom as in pandysautonomia. The girl's symptoms would most likely have been classified as psychosomatic in origin elsewhere. The sweating was a typical sympathetic phenomenon and she had a moderately wide pulse pressure and lability of both the systolic and diastolic components. The mother had some of the elements of increased sympathetic tone giving her Raynaud's phenomenon, and there was apparently an associated cardiac autonomic effect as well.

Diet certainly played a part in these cases. Recall from Chapter 3 that excessive sugar intake and high-calorie malnutrition are associated not only with diminished thiamine intake but also disrupt thiamine metabolism itself, decreasing absorption and increasing excretion.[10] Thereafter the conversion of pyruvate to acetyl-CoA is limited, diminishing acetylcholine synthesis[11] and disrupting autonomic balance. Concurrently, the lack of thiamine impairs oxidative capacity, reducing ATP production and increasing reactive oxygen species (ROS), the inflammatory cascades,[12] and if sufficiently serious or chronic, the changes in hemostasis noted in thiamine deficiency induced pseudohypoxia.[13] In adults, these cascades may take years to fully foment and present with sufficient strength to be clinically recognizable, but in children and adolescents, where the energy demands to fuel growth and development are immense, the reactions become more prominent more quickly.

## Family 3. Reflex Sympathetic Dystrophy/Complex Regional Pain Syndrome

M.F. was a 10-year-old girl who had sprained her ankle 2 years previously. It was followed by swelling of the joint and great pain, which appeared to be out of proportion to the degree of injury. Subsequently, she experienced a series of quite trivial injuries, each of which caused swelling and pain. Plaster casts were applied on six different occasions over the 2-year period. She developed coldness of both feet and hands, and mottled vascularity of the legs, which was worse in the injured one. On examination, she had a mild systolic click and systolic murmur caused by mitral valve prolapse (MVP), and there was gliosis of the temporal side of both optic discs. Both legs were extremely cold to the touch, mottled in appearance, and there was marked epicritic painful sensation on stroking the skin over the repeatedly injured foot. The mother volunteered that she herself had suffered from a form of polyneuritis for years.

Dr. Lonsdale reports a similar case in an adolescent male. The case was discussed in detail in Chapter 3, but briefly the boy suffered an injury, which precipitated uncharacteristic symptoms of pain and swelling, neuropathies that improved with thiamine supplementation and dietary modification.

## *Points of Consideration*

The case of M.F. was typical of reflex sympathetic dystrophy, now referred to as complex regional pain syndrome,[14] which was well documented in the adult medical literature, but had only recently appeared in the pediatric equivalent at the time of Dr. Lonsdale's work. It did not explain coldness and dysautonomic function in the uninjured leg or the MVP, which is known to be associated in most subjects with autonomic dysfunction.[15] Many of the clinical features of patients with MVP can logically be attributed to abnormal autonomic neural function. The authors postulated an abnormal central modulation of baroreflexes as the best explanation at that time.[16] It is unknown whether the mother's symptoms were related to those of the child, but it suggested that there was a familial element. Perhaps the injuries represented repeated physical stresses that caused an abnormal autonomic response because of an inherited component. In this case, there was nothing to suggest a role from the diet.

It is not very surprising that we draw the conclusion that the patient is developing psychosomatic symptoms, which in some ill-defined way enable him/her to "hide away in terms of a physical illness that prevents the usual involvement in day-to-day activities." The denial of reality seems to be the cornerstone of such an explanation and implies a collapse of the patient's ability to cope. In essence, this is, of course, quite true and society "allows" physical illness but is still somewhat wary of a mental one.

The point at issue appears to be a most important one. The brain signals the body organs through the neuroendocrine system, which is directed by the hypothalamus—the computer. A carefully modulated signal gives rise to an appropriate response, but if the autonomic and endocrine systems are out of phase, dysautonomic symptoms would be expected. Thus there is nothing very revolutionary about the concept of dysautonomia, except that it appears more frequently than individual case reports would suggest. For example, abdominal epilepsy was entertained at one time as an appropriate diagnosis, even though it was always rejected by many physicians. Essentially, the patient complains of paroxysmal abdominal pain, often with borborygmi and sometimes in association with a bowel movement or a sensation of imminent bowel movement without any result. Surely this can be pictured as a parasympathetic signal causing contraction and peristalsis. The fact that it occurs paroxysmally seems to be very similar to neuronal discharge referred to as epilepsy. Why it occurs at any particular moment is as unclear as it is in epilepsy. Unless the cause of the pain can be observed at the time that it occurs, it will never be proved, since it is a functional event.

### The Value of Family Histories in Complicated Cases

Even though the family history is the cornerstone of medical intake, its relevance in modern medicine is not fully appreciated. As physicians we look for common threads among family members to estimate the risk for a particular disease process under the auspices of a genetic connection. A family history of cancer predicts an increased risk of cancer for the patient. Similarly, heart disease in the parents suggests a risk for heart disease in the offspring. Same predicts same. Here, the pattern is exactly opposite. With mitochondrial injuries it is the diversity of disease processes within the individual and among the family members that suggests the pattern. This was illustrated with phenotype analysis in Family 1. As modern mitochondrial medicine has become more prominent, patterns such as this become increasingly apparent.[17]

## PEDIATRIC CASES OF THIAMINE RESPONSIVE DYSAUTONOMIAS

To appreciate fully the patterns that emerge among a seeming diversity of clinical symptoms and the underlying relationships to thiamine, the case studies that follow have been grouped by the most conspicuous and easily identifiable symptoms. In each of the case series the key symptoms and laboratory patterns are similar among patients, but the totality or constellation of symptoms presenting in each is always slightly and sometimes hugely different.

### Failure to Thrive in Thiamine-Deficient Infants

The enormous energetic demands required for infant and child development are necessarily influenced by diminished mitochondrial capacity, elicited by thiamine deficiency. In what manner the comorbid symptoms emerge are largely irrelevant inasmuch as they are often unique to the patient and the totality of his/her genetic, epigenetic, and environmental circumstances. Nevertheless, there are patterns that emerge when aggregate patient histories are compiled, such as respiratory difficulties, especially during sleep, dysphagia, and gastrointestinal dysmotility syndromes.

## Case Example 5.1 Three-Month-Old Girl With Suspected Chromosomal Abnormality

This 3-month-old infant was anomalous in appearance and a chromosomal defect was considered to be likely. Chromosome analysis proved to be normal. Red cell TKA was 47.75 mU/L/min (normal 42.1–86.1) and the TPPE was 24.9%. This was a clear indication of TPP deficiency, and for this reason she was treated with thiamine hydrochloride in a dose of 150 mg per day in divided doses.

One month later the parents noticed increased alertness. The TKA was 54.89 mU/L/min and TPPE had decreased to 10.8%. A high potency multivitamin was started and 1 year later there had been a slow, steady improvement. The TKA was 129 mU/L/min and the TPPE was zero. Urinary creatine increased from 3.6 to 13.6 mg/kg body weight per 24 h as creatinine increased from 10 to 19.1 mg/kg/24 h. This suggested that there was an overall increase in metabolism, although there may have been a continued problem in absorbing creatine into muscle cells or storing it as phosphocreatine.

She continued to demonstrate severe temper tantrums and showed signs of learning disability, but became normal in appearance. She went through high school and participated in the marching band. As she grew, the mother would increase the dose of thiamine without medical advice when symptoms suggested deterioration. She died at the age of 27 years from toxic shock syndrome following an infection. The dose that she was receiving before she died was as high as 7 g a day without any evidence of toxicity. There is no way of knowing what she would have been like without any treatment.

## Case Example 5.2 Eighteen-Month-Old Boy, Failure to Thrive, Hypophagia, Apnea, Vomiting

An 18-month-old Caucasian male infant was examined because of failure to thrive, hypophagia, nocturnal breathing difficulty, and vomiting. The birth weight was 4.1 kg. There was no history of maternal mellituria (gestational diabetes). He sat at 6 months, was beginning to walk, and saying a few words. At the age of 6 weeks he began to have "raspy" breathing and repeated vomiting. There was unusual pallor, respiratory congestion, and irritability. At the age of 8 months he had pneumonia, and at 11 months tracheobronchitis.

At 13 months, serous otitis caused his hospital admission for placement of aeration tubes, but infection precluded surgery, which was then postponed until he was 15 months old. On hospital admission for this procedure his night breathing was severely compromised and he was described as gasping for air, snoring loudly, and breathing as though he had croup. After discharge, his mother observed nocturnal breathing problems of major proportions. Loud snoring

*Continued*

## Case Example 5.2 Eighteen-Month-Old Boy, Failure to Thrive, Hypophagia, Apnea, Vomiting—cont'd

would be suddenly interrupted by awakening, frequently with a scream, only to repeat the cycle. Sleep was restless, would last for 17–18h, and was supplemented by frequent naps during the afternoon.

Vomiting of "coffee-ground" material was observed and he was fatigued, irritable, and hypophagic. He drank sweetened fruit juices sporadically, which resulted in frequent choking, and he had excessive oral mucus, a cough, and excessive sweating. On examination he was hyperirritable, pale, and well under the third percentile in weight and height. Loose folds of skin and poor subcutaneous fat suggested chronic dehydration, and inspiratory stridor was heard occasionally during sleep.

The heart rate was 176 per minute with marked sinus arrhythmia and the blood pressure was 120/0 with a 20mm fluctuation at systole in the phases of respiration. Deep patellar tendon reflexes were unpredictable, varying from unobtainable to 1+. Electrocardiography revealed left and right ventricular hypertrophy, although chest roentgenography did not reveal any observed cardiac enlargement.

Red cell TKA was 91.38 mU/L/min and TPPE 6.93%. Serum folic acid was 20.0 ng/mL and vitamin B12 1100 pg/mL. Monitoring of arterial oxygen saturation by night using ear oximetry revealed that oxygen saturation was as low as 72% at night and invariably lower than those of a similar-aged normal child monitored simultaneously. The blood hemoglobin was 6.8 gm/100 mL and the serum iron concentration 2 mcg/100 mL with a normal iron-binding capacity. There was moderate enlargement of the adenoids and adenoidectomy was followed by troublesome persistent laryngospasm.

Snoring cycles continued in spite of surgery and after informed consent by the parent, thiamine tetrahydrofurfuryl disulfide (TTFD), 150 mg per day, and a multivitamin preparation began. When seen 1 month later the child had gained weight and nocturnal snoring and personality were improved. Sleep was no longer disturbed and there was no undue sweating.

### *Points of Consideration*

This chronically ill child suffered from sleep apnea,[18] a relatively common problem in adults. Studies in the sleep laboratory have shown that there is a mixture of airway obstruction and central disturbance, which combines to present a potentially dangerous situation. Nocturnal hypoxia appears to be a physiological phenomenon but the dangerous degree of hypoxia in patients with sleep apnea appears to fail in stimulating reticular activity. Adenoidectomy did not abolish snoring or his sleep restlessness, and TTFD was used empirically, hoping to catalyze an increased uptake of oxygen in both red cells and the brain. This child improved spectacularly, but the clinical observations could not be sustained by laboratory tests, though his ultimate recovery was a surprise to all observers.

# Slowed Growth in Thiamine-Deficient Children

### Case Example 5.3 Prematurity, Dysautonomia, and Developmental Delay

A 5-year-old girl had been born prematurely with a birth weight of 0.5 kg. Respiratory distress, irregular heart rate, jaundice, apnea, and failure to gain weight were initial problems, and there was chronic, intractable diarrhea and recurrent sleep apnea for the first 6 months of life. There was slight developmental delay and she had a continued history of colds, earaches, asthma, recurrent pneumonia, fatigue, croup, night terrors, excessive nocturnal sweating, and tachycardia. She was well under the third percentile in height and weight. Red cell TKA was 85.7 mU and TPPE 19.9%. After 6 months of treatment with thiamine hydrochloride (THCL) and a high-potency multivitamin, urinary creatine decreased and creatinine increased. General health and personality improved.

This kind of case in children has always been a problem of management, and many are treated with continuous antibiotic therapy. Frequently, there are no laboratory studies to suggest an immune defect. The red cell TKA was a clue, possibly to persistent low-grade hypoxia or subnormal oxidation.

# Anorexia and Thiamine Deficiency

Anorexia is both a symptom of, and a contributing factor to, thiamine deficiency. Whether the propensity not to eat originates from a willful decision for dietary purposes, as in the case of anorexia nervosa, or represents appetite loss indicative of mitochondrial damage (see Chapter 4, orexin/hypocretin pathways), both share a final common pathway of thiamine deficiency. The following cases illustrate this point.

### Case Example 5.4 Fifteen-Year-Old Girl With Anorexia Nervosa

A 15-year-old girl presented with anorexia nervosa. In the first 3 months of vitamin therapy, the urinary creatine increased from 1.96 to 22.3 mg/kg/24 h and creatinine decreased from 24.2 to 15 mg/kg/24 h, reflecting a creatine/creatinine ratio (C/CR) of 1.5. At this time, TKA was 74.8 mU and TPPE 16.7%. She was treated with TTFD and in 2 weeks the C/CR decreased to 0.17. The TKA decreased to 57.8 mU and TPPE to 0. These observations suggested that there was a surge of metabolic activity, but there continued to be defective processing of creatine. There was unequivocal improvement in the clinical condition.

## Case Example 5.5 Fifteen-Year-Old Male, Anorexia, Fatigue, Epigastric Pain

A 15-year-old Caucasian male was examined because of anorexia, fatigue, epigastric pain, and weight loss, which became worse after participation in football practice. Taking food was followed by nausea and increased fatigue, forcing him to bed early, often without anything to eat. He had constant rhinorrhea, cough, and hoarseness and was nervous and irritable, exhibiting constant "knuckle cracking," loss of impulse control, and restlessness during sleep. An episode of "flu" with fever, rhinorrhea, cough, nausea, sore throat, and anorexia was followed by severe fatigue, nausea, and frequent temporal headaches. A month later he experienced increased fatigue, cramping abdominal pain, and nausea after running, and he began to lose weight. Similar symptoms occurred on awakening in the morning and he began to miss school. After a weight loss of 15 lb he was admitted to a hospital. Examination reportedly showed an enlargement of axillary lymph nodes and that "a blood test suggested liver damage."

Nutritional history revealed that he practically subsisted on cookies and potato chips, and he was described as a "constant nibbler." He consumed 2 gallons of milk and 1 gallon of carbonated beverage a week. On examination he was found to be well built and muscular. Heart rate was 60 per minute with a grade I systolic murmur audible at the cardiac apex. Femoral pulse was easily audible by auscultation over the inguinal ligament and blood pressure was 130 systolic, with a phase change at 50 and a diastolic disappearance at 20 mm Hg. Both systolic and diastolic components were labile.

Laboratory studies were normal, including red cell TKA and TPPE. Glucose tolerance revealed a fasting blood glucose of 74 mg/100 mL, 72 at 1 h, 80 at 2 h, 66 at 3 h, and 66 mg/100 mL at 4 h. This "flat" curve was shown to be artifactual, because when the tolerance was repeated, blood sugars were measured every 10 min. An adequate increase in blood sugar occurred, and it had returned to the fasting concentration within half an hour. This suggested an accelerated insulin response to glucose. He was treated only with a multivitamin and given diet instruction. One month later he still complained of some fatigue, but nausea, abdominal pain, and headache had disappeared. Examination was normal and blood pressure was 120/60 with no lability. Contact was made by telephone 6 months later, and he had remained well and had indulged in normal sport activity.

## *Points of Consideration*

This young man represents a very common symptomology in American adolescents, which arises from an inordinate consumption of high-calorie "junk" food or empty calories. The stress of athletic activity precipitated symptoms, and the response to proper nutrition, together with an adequate vitamin supplement, strongly suggested that symptoms were caused by nutritional inadequacy. Perhaps the glucose tolerance represented a maladaptive response, which had itself been induced by the high-caloric carbohydrate diet. We know from more recent research that dietary sugars provoke type 2 diabetes and are associated with thiamine malabsorption and increased excretion.[10]

## Cyclic Vomiting

Cyclic vomiting syndrome (CVS) is a poorly understood and underrecognized dysautonomia characterized by recurrent episodes of severe nausea and vomiting that alternate with periods of no symptoms. It was originally believed to affect only pediatric populations but is now recognized to develop and persist across the life span.[19] Comorbid symptoms often include headache, dizziness, fever, sensitivity to light, and diarrhea. At least a quarter of CVS patients have coexisting symptoms of neuromuscular disease.[20] Increasingly, CVS is being recognized among the constellation of mitochondrial diseases,[21] with an apparent matrilineal inheritance pattern.[22] It can emerge in infancy but also later in life in response to a stressor, an illness, or an environmental or pharmaceutical toxicant.[23] Indeed, adult patients report stereotypical stress patterns that trigger episodes.[24] This has been observed in children as well.[25] Autonomic abnormalities have been identified consistent with increased sympathetic activity with a diminished parasympathetic response.[3] The autonomic instability affects vagal modulation of the heart and manifests symptomatically with heart rate variability and postural intolerance.[26]

Among the more effective treatments emerging today include nutrient supplementation with L-carnitine and CoQ10 aimed at correcting mitochondrial deficiencies or injuries.[27] Despite the recognition of nutrient needs in mitochondriopathies such as CVS, to our knowledge thiamine remains overlooked. Decades ago and prior to the current understanding of mitochondrial diseases, Dr. Lonsdale identified thiamine as a critical component of mitochondrial functioning and its deficiency capable of evoking what we now identify as cyclic vomiting. CVS was a relatively common presentation of autonomic disturbance in Dr. Lonsdale's practice. The clinical cases that follow illustrate thiamine responsiveness in pediatric cases of cyclic vomiting.

### Case Example 5.6 Cyclic Vomiting With Complex Regional Pain and Sleep Irregularities

A 5-year-old Caucasian male was examined because of recurrent vomiting. The birth history and development were normal. There was an episode of severe dehydration at the age of 2 years, and he was in a hospital for 9 days. At age 3 years he began to complain frequently of aches and pains in the legs, would cry a great deal, and frequently refused to walk. Swelling of the feet and ankles prevented him from wearing shoes, and a serpiginous rash led to a diagnosis of rheumatic fever elsewhere. He had received injections of penicillin for the next 6 months.

*Continued*

## Case Example 5.6 Cyclic Vomiting With Complex Regional Pain and Sleep Irregularities—cont'd

The swelling improved, but he continued to complain of pain in the left knee. Active streptococcal infection was never confirmed. Subsequently, he began to experience recurrent episodes of vomiting, which created a repetitive pattern. He would awaken in the morning feeling ill, would ask for a drink, but would immediately vomit. Repeated vomiting continued for the next 12 h. Body temperature would rise to 102–104°F, and occasionally there would be an episode of becoming "rigid and stiff for a few minutes." He resented being touched and would scream. The attack would end with "exhaustion."

The family physician had prescribed prednisone because of the painful knee, but he had discontinued it because of nocturnal symptoms attributed to the drug. The child had experienced night terrors, talking of violence in his sleep, and on one occasion crying out that he was unable to move because he was pinned down by a wild animal. At least one myoclonic seizure had occurred before the onset of a vomiting episode. Personality was normal by day and nocturnal symptoms decreased after prednisone was withdrawn, although spontaneous jerking of the leg was noted during sleep, a phenomenon that the child's mother also experienced. Although the child snored, there was no apnea. There was a history of frequent awakening from sleep and recurrent fever of unknown cause in infancy. Tachycardia had been noted with vomiting attacks, and his appetite was capricious and unpredictable.

Examination revealed an intelligent boy with no unusual physical findings other than extreme variability in knee jerks and very sensitive dermographia. Family history disclosed that a brother had had two seizure-like episodes during early childhood and there were a number of diabetic relatives on both sides of the family. One maternal aunt had disturbed ideation and was under psychiatric care, as was the maternal grandmother. The electroencephalogram revealed overall high amplitude and poor regulation but no paroxysmal discharges. Glucose tolerance showed a fasting blood glucose of 70 mg/100 mL, 117 mg/100 mL at 10 min, 106 mg/100 mL at 1 h, 59 mg/100 mL at 3 h, and 78 mg/100 mL at 4 h. Lactic acid dehydrogenase was 280 mU/mL (normal 100–225) and serum glutamic oxaloacetic transaminase (SGOT) 57 mU/mL (normal 17–40). Thiamine hydrochloride 150 mg per day was begun. Although he experienced one or two mild episodes of vomiting within the subsequent month, he was asymptomatic 6 months later.

### Points of Consideration

The dysautonomic element of cyclic vomiting in this case is represented by tachycardia, cephalalgia, fever, and vomiting. Jumping leg syndrome, night terrors, infancy sleep disturbance, and an incident that may have been sleep paralysis all suggest that sleep rhythms in this child were abnormal. The episodes of stiffness and epicritical pain recall perplexing clinical characteristics of "stiff man syndrome" that is related to brain stem dysfunction.[28]

## Case Example 5.7 Infection Triggered Cyclic Vomiting Beginning at 9 Months

A Caucasian girl aged 6 years was examined because of episodes of severe intractable vomiting beginning at the age of 9 months and recurring from two to eight times a year. Each attack occurred in three stages. The attack was precipitated by an upper respiratory infection. This was followed in 2 or 3 days by vomiting and abdominal cramps lasting 4 or 5 days, and frequently resulting in dehydration requiring intravenous fluids. The third stage was characterized by a rapid change to a sense of well-being, cessation of vomiting, a ravenous or voracious appetite, and repeated epistaxis, usually accompanied by pallor and edema of the face and eyelids.

There were associated headaches, tachycardia, and sweating. There were no other unusual physical findings. Routine urinalysis revealed 3+acetone, no sugar, and no albumin. An epinephrine stress test showed a fasting blood glucose of 75 mg/100 mL, 125 mg/100 mL in 0.5 h, and 78 mg/100 mL at 2 h. An intravenous glucose tolerance showed a fasting concentration of 78 mg/100 mL, 40 mg/100 mL after 0.5 h, 70 mg/100 mL at 1 h, 80 mg/100 mL at 2 h, and 76 mg/100 mL at 4 h. This study was repeated with more frequent analyses. The fasting concentration was 87 mg/100 mL, 190 mg/100 mL at 10 min, 150 mg/100 mL at 20 min, 138 mg/100 mL at 30 min, 108 mg/100 mL at 40 min, 91 mg/100 mL at 50 min, and 87 mg/100 mL at 1 h.

An attempt to prevent attacks was made by the administration of thiamine hydrochloride, 150 mg per day, but over the next 10 months there were four further episodes, two of which required hospital admission. One occurred following chickenpox, the other three after colds. Each was associated with extremely irritable behavior. Nocturnal enuresis began after the most recent episode began. There was constant general sweating. On examination, she was pale and conjunctivae suffused. Body weight had increased by 5.5 kg in 10 months. Heart rate was 100 per minute and sinus arrhythmia marked. Blood pressure was 100/50 with systolic lability. Pupils reacted poorly to light and there was striking dermographia.

Thiamine hydrochloride was increased to 300 mg per day and a multivitamin added. One month later a typical episode started with an upper respiratory infection, followed by diarrhea, abdominal cramping, irritability, headache, tachycardia, and vomiting. On examination, she was pale and looked ill. Cardiac rate was 128 and the blood pressure 114/80 with systolic lability. Serum vitamin B12 was 1170 pg/mL (normal 160–900), and folate was greater than 30 ng/mL (normal 4–18). Urinary creatine, creatinine, and uric acid were measured.

Initially, a total of 622 mg of creatine per 24 h and 451 mg of creatinine yielded a creatine/creatinine ratio of 1.3. Total creatinine excretion was 14.1 mg/kg/24 h and uric acid excretion 17.6 mg/kg/24 h. As the vomiting subsided, she experienced one brief epistaxis. After informed consent, she was prescribed TTFD, 150 mg per day, and was seen again in 3 months. Although she had some nasal congestion and a few episodes of epistaxis accompanied by facial edema, there had been no further episodes of vomiting. Examination was normal and the blood pressure was 90/50 with no lability. Urinary creatine had dropped to 193 mg/24 h and creatinine increased to 608 mg/24 h, yielding a ratio of 0.32. Total creatinine excretion had risen to 18.7 mg/kg/24 h and uric acid had fallen to 10.5 mg/kg/24 h. After 2 years of continuous therapy there were no further episodes of vomiting and she remained well.

## Points of Consideration

There are a number of questions raised by the course of this child's recurrent illness and her response to a disulfide derivative of thiamine, but not to a water-soluble salt of thiamine. A distinct personality change occurred at the onset of any one of her individual attacks. Acute irritability and facial pallor invariably heralded an episode of intractable and prolonged vomiting. Individual attacks terminated with voracious appetite accompanied by repeated epistaxis. Perhaps the most important clue to her intermittent disease was well-marked creatinuria. The ratio of creatine to creatinine in the urine was much closer to normal after the use of TTFD. This suggests that there was a genetic abnormality in the absorption of thiamine since TTFD does not require the thiamine transporter system. Although the mechanism was unknown at the time, we now know that alterations in solute carrier (SLC) transporter proteins occur somewhat more broadly than suspected and impair thiamine uptake, necessitating continuous thiamine replacement. Not described here, but when there are thiamine transporter issues there may also be biotin transporter problems, necessitating biotin replacement as well.[29]

### Case Example 5.8 Vomiting and Epistaxis
A 13-year-old girl was referred for an episode of vomiting, followed by a voracious appetite and repeated epistaxis during recovery. The red cell TKA increased from 64.9 to 86.3 mU and TPPE decreased from 19.9% to 3.0% in 8 months of continuous treatment with thiamine hydrochloride at 100 mg a day. Urinary creatine decreased while creatinine increased. The C/CR decreased from 0.55 to 0.11. At the age of 17 years this girl had remained well and had experienced no further episodes of vomiting.

### Case Example 5.9 Cyclic Vomiting in a 10-Year-Old Girl
Another patient, a girl of 10 years, had repeated episodes of symptoms, which might be classified as cyclic vomiting. Three or four times a year she would have an attack of pernicious vomiting that would last several days and which invariably caused her admission to a hospital. On recovery she would develop a voracious appetite for several days, during which she would experience repeated spontaneous epistaxis. Like the other cases presented, urine creatine to creatinine ratio during an attack was greater than 1.0 (Fig. 5.2) and TFFD was started in a dose of 150 mg per day. She had no further attacks, and the ratio of creatine to creatinine and their urinary concentrations, plus that of uric acid, are shown. Again, the evidence is mostly circumstantial. No one could say that the urine changes were proof that the supplement had been responsible, but the complete absence of further episodes of vomiting was dramatic and appeared to be authentic.

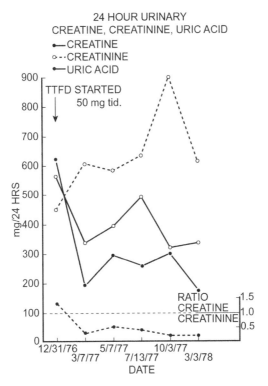

**Figure 5.2** Urinary creatine, creatinine, uric acid, and creatine/creatinine ratios per 24 h in a 10-year-old girl (Case Example 5.9) treated with thiamine tetrahydrofurfuryl disulfide (TTFD) for cyclic vomiting.

## Night Terrors, Sleepwalking, Hyperactivity, and Attentional Deficits

Sleep disorders such as night terrors and sleepwalking are common symptoms of dysautonomic function and are often comorbid with daytime hyperactivity and attentional deficits. With night terrors, the child partially awakens and screams inconsolably with little recognition of what is happening. The episodes are not associated with nightmares per se, but rather with a sympathetic discharge that initiates a state of heightened arousal consistent with a "fear" response. Coincident autonomically driven symptoms include tachycardia, sweating, hyperventilation, and pupillary dilatation. Nocturnal sympathetic discharge may also lead to somnambulism or sleepwalking. The disturbed sleep cycles may be associated with daytime hyperactivity and attention deficit. Daytime hyperactivity and attention deficits may also be attributable to other cases, including high-calorie malnutrition, which as we have shown leads to thiamine and other nutrient deficiencies. Invariably, however, these symptoms arise frequently in pediatrics. A closer look reveals a telling constellation of autonomic symptoms, many remediable by fueling the mitochondria.

### Case Example 5.10 Night Terrors, Piloerection, Enuresis, and Hypothermia

A 5-year-old boy had night terrors. His mother had pregnancy toxemia, and at birth the child had respiratory distress and jaundice, requiring phototherapy, indicating oxidative stress.[30] Severe vomiting and diarrhea caused dehydration that required hospital admission. The night terrors had been observed by the mother who had noted cyanosis, piloerection, shallow respiration, enuresis, hypothermia, and widely dilated pupils unresponsive to light. Red cell TKA was 69.8 mU and TPPE 27.2%. He was treated with thiamine and clinical improvement correlated with decreased urinary creatinine and a decrease in the C/CR.

### Case Example 5.11 Childhood Hyperactivity and Night Terrors

Symptoms in an 8-year-old boy included hyperactivity and night terrors. Red cell TKA was 97.3 and TPPE 19.5%. After 4 months with thiamine supplementation there was a marked improvement in personality and an elimination of night terrors. Red cell TKA was 88.2 mU and TPPE 1.5%. There was a marked increase in both urinary creatine and creatinine. The C/CR remained much the same.

### Case Example 5.12 Night Terrors, Sleep Walking, Hyperactivity, and Reading Difficulties

A 7-year-old Caucasian male child was referred for investigation of night terrors. He was the second of three children, with a normal birth history. Neonatal and early development were normal, with the exception that he did not talk in sentences until after the age of 2 years. He was in second grade and obtaining average grades, but was receiving remedial reading. At the age of 10 months he was hyperactive and this increased with age until it became necessary to attempt to modify it with medication. Night terrors and somnambulism began at the age of 6½ years and had recurred weekly, usually with profuse sweating and frequently with urinary incontinence, with no recollection of the event. Sleep was restless. He snored and would awaken two or three times a night even when no terrors occurred. Fever had been detected after a night terror and occurred occasionally with right hemicranial cephalalgia.

He was indulged liberally with candy and soft drinks. Nasal congestion and mouth breathing persisted in spite of removal of tonsils and adenoids, and he

## Case Example 5.12 Night Terrors, Sleep Walking, Hyperactivity, and Reading Difficulties—cont'd

experienced epistaxis, polydipsia, and frequent micturition. A school psychologist reported short attention span, poor perceptual multiskills, impulsiveness, and poor memory, although testing was in the high range of normal intelligence. Examination revealed transient dermographia and labile patellar reflexes with occasional double or "hung-up" responses.

Blood pressure was 114/20. Laboratory studies showed increased serum concentrations of SGOT and lactate dehydrogenase (LDH). Alkaline phosphatase was 200 mU/mL (normal adult 30–85) and cholesterol 125 mg/100 mL (normal 150–300). There was a family history of migraine headaches in the mother and paternal grandmother, and diabetes was present on both sides of the family. The child was treated with a supplement of 150 mg per day of thiamine hydrochloride and instructed in a high protein, low-carbohydrate diet. He was examined again 2 months later. There had been no further night terrors and he was less hyperactive. Examination was normal.

### *Points of Consideration*

The clues to this child's problem were present in his sleep pattern, which included restlessness, snoring, and night terrors. Other functional disturbance was reflected in headaches, overactivity, and mild learning disability—all of which disappeared quickly after appropriate dietary principles were followed, together with a supplement of thiamine. The laboratory studies were nonspecific but abnormal. Acute cephalalgia had been described in children because of abnormal sympathetic activity following trauma.[31] There was no history of trauma in this case and its disappearance after vitamin administration suggested dysautonomic etiology. The changes in the deep patellar reflexes, transient white dermographia, and increased pulse pressure are all characteristic of early beriberi.

## Recurrent Febrile Lymphadenopathy

Recurrent fevers with swollen cervical glands are common. Most are caused by viral or bacterial infection and almost inevitably treated by antibiotic therapy. The two boys whose case histories are recorded next had their recurrent episodes of febrile lymphadenopathy prevented by the administration of megadose thiamine. We can only try to explain the mechanism by suggesting that their recurrent episodes were initiated by periodic pseudohypoxia in the hypothalamic–autonomic–endocrine axis, initiating a false defensive action.

## Case Example 5.13 Two Boys With Recurrent Fevers

Two Caucasian boys both aged 6 years came to Dr. Lonsdale's attention. Over a period of 2–3 years, each had had repeated episodes of sore throat, fever as high as 104°F, and swollen cervical lymph glands. Both, as expected, had been treated with antibiotics. Because both of these boys had been indulged with ad libitum candy and sweet drinks, they were tested by erythrocyte transketolase. This was abnormal in one of the boys, indicating thiamine deficiency. It was normal in the other, but a urine test revealed the presence of a substance that was purported at that time to inhibit the action of thiamine triphosphate. This test had been reported to be diagnostic for Leigh's disease but was never proved and the research was abandoned for lack of funds.[32] Dr. Lonsdale had found this test to be positive on many occasions in patients that he suspected of being thiamine deficient and could not possibly be interpreted as examples of Leigh's disease. Both of the children were treated with 150 mg of thiamine hydrochloride a day and the febrile episodes disappeared.

## Case Example 5.14 Seven-Year-Old Girl With Recurrent Fever and Cervical Lymphadenopathy

A Caucasian girl aged 7¾ had a history of recurrent cervical lymphadenopathy and fever for 5 months. The first episode was followed several weeks later by malaise and fatigue, repeated vomiting of coffee-ground material, fever to 104°F, and chronic fatigue. She was brought for examination because of yet another episode of fever and cervical lymphadenopathy.

She had a history of restlessness during sleep, sleep talking, and somnambulism. Breathing during sleep was rapid and shallow, and she snored loudly. She was ingesting a significant amount of carbohydrate foods by preference. She complained of frequent fleeting abdominal pain, bloating, and abdominal distension. Examination revealed a pleasant child with flushed cheeks, circumoral pallor, and prominent filiform papillae on the tongue.

The heart was overactive and the rate was 150 per minute. Blood pressure was 110/70 with lability and the femoral pulse audible by auscultation over the inguinal ligament. Deep tendon knee reflexes were erratic. Roentgenography showed an increased adenoidal mass and audiogram demonstrated a mild conductive hearing loss. A few beta-hemolytic streptococci were cultured from the throat for which she had received a course of oral penicillin.

Thiamine hydrochloride 150 mg per day was given orally. Snoring, sleep restlessness, shallow respiration, and nasal congestion disappeared. General well-being increased. On examination she looked well. The heart rate was 128, blood pressure 100/60 without lability, and the audible femoral pulse and dermographia had disappeared. Adenoidectomy was performed. Laboratory tests before and after thiamine supplementation are shown in Table 5.1.

## Points of Consideration

This was a demonstration of abnormal TPP homeostasis, possibly with genetic overtones. The decrease in the elevated TPPE correlated with clinical improvement. The baseline activity of TKA was still below the normal range after treatment although with insignificant increase. The reason for a fall in serum vitamin B12 and an increase in folate represented in the table is unknown. Lymphadenopathy, vomiting, fever, fatigue, abdominal pain, meteorism, constipation, tachycardia, labile blood pressure, and audible femoral pulse are all characteristics of beriberi, and there is reason to believe that this was the reason that her symptoms were responsive to thiamine supplementation.

Diet may not have been the sole cause because, although there was a demonstrably abnormal TPPE, the abnormally low TKA did not change significantly after thiamine supplementation. Blass and Gibson reported genetic changes in transketolase.[33] This case is presented as a possible example of an abnormal host response to stress from infection. The clinical appearance of flushed cheeks, circumoral pallor, and "strawberry tongue" is time honored as characteristic of streptococcal infection that may have represented the attacking stressor. The flushed cheeks, circumoral pallor, and prominent filiform papillae on the tongue, without any evidence of infection, are, in our experience, common in children with this kind of history and without streptococcal infection. Perhaps insufficient attention is given to the symptoms in terms of the organization and nature of the host response and its deviations. The use of vitamins may well be an advantage, irrespective of the etiology of the stressor.

Table 5.1 Baseline and Postthiamine Treatment Vitamin Concentrations in a 7-Year-Old Girl With Recurrent Fevers (Case Example 5.14)

| | First Treatment | Second Treatment | Reference Range |
|---|---|---|---|
| Serum vitamin B12 | 1220 pg/mL | 1050 pg/mL | 160–900 pg/mL |
| Folate | 14.8 ng/mL | >30 ng/mL | 4–18 nv/mL |
| Transketolase | 36.07 mU | 39.05 mU | 42.1–86.1 mU |
| TPP percent uptake | 34.38% | 0% | 0%–17.4% |

*TPP*, thiamine pyrophosphate.

### Case Example 5.15 Nineteen-Month-Old Boy With Repeat Fevers of Unknown Etiology

A 19-month-old Caucasian boy had repeated fevers of unknown cause. Birth history and development were normal. At the age of 2 weeks he had his first episode of nocturnal wheezing with sweating and tachycardia. At the age of 2 months he began to have episodes when he would be found to be hot to the touch at night, interpreted elsewhere as "ear infections." At the age of 11 months he had awakened from a nap with a fever of 106°F. He was admitted to hospital, but no cause was found. Similar recurrent febrile episodes of this nature followed accompanied by hyperactivity, irritability, nocturnal restlessness, starting out of sleep, night terrors, and sweating. Nonspecific leg pain, headaches, and breath holding to cyanosis occurred by day, particularly when he was febrile. Anorexia was indulged by providing ad libitum candy, ice cream, and soft drinks.

Family history revealed a number of individuals who had been affected by a combination of diabetes and cancer, as well as several reported to have pernicious anemia. On examination, height and weight were in the 25th and 97th percentile, respectively. He was hyperactive and irritable. Deep tendon reflexes were overactive. The automated blood profile was normal, except for a slight elevation of LDH. Dietary advice was given and the child began thiamine hydrochloride 150 mg per day. He was examined again 2 months later. He had had no fever, was restful during sleep, less nervous, and more compliant. Profuse sweating and tachycardia had disappeared. Appetite had improved and his mother volunteered that this was the best health that he had enjoyed in a year.

### *Points of Consideration*

This child's symptoms were from deviant brain function. Most physicians would blame maternal anxiety and management, particularly since the mother had undergone surgery during the pregnancy. However, although stress would play a part, all the symptoms could not be attributed to this alone because dietary correction appeared to result in their complete disappearance. Also the family history suggested that there were genetic factors. In three family members there was a combination of cancer and diabetes. Both diabetes and cancer have been linked with autonomic dysfunction.[34,35] We would like to introduce the concept here that it is the combination of genetics, environmental stress, and poor nutrition that variably causes an interplay that must always be considered in the etiology of disease. This will be discussed in more detail in the next chapter. The patients with thiamine-dependent febrile lymphadenopathy mentioned earlier are discussed in more detail in Chapter 4 and were also reported in the medical literature.[36]

## Hypoxias: Reye's Syndrome, Sudden Infant Death Syndrome, and Other Disorders of Altered Hemostasis

Cellular respiration is contingent upon inhaled oxygen and the presence of dietary vitamins and minerals. Thiamine is key among the nutrients required for oxygenation both because of its role in oxidative metabolism but also because it increases oxyhemoglobin concentrations, enabling the delivery of oxygen to the brain.[37] Thiamine deficiency thus evokes a state of molecular oxygen deficiency,[13] a hypoxic state that is absent obstruction but equally dangerous, because the very ability to use oxygen is impaired. The cascade of molecular reactions that ensue is discussed more fully in Chapter 3. Here, let us look at cases where thiamine deficiency induced critical deficits in blood oxygenation.

### Case Example 5.16 Comatose 18-Month-Old Girl With Reye's Syndrome

An 18-month-old Caucasian girl was admitted to hospital in a coma. Four days before she had begun a 48-h episode of repeated vomiting. During the subsequent night she was restless, vomited several times in her sleep, and experienced a grand mal seizure in the morning. She became unconscious and was admitted to a community hospital. Increases in concentrations of SGOT and LDH were noted, and the blood ammonia was 1000 mcg/dL. A diagnosis of Reye's syndrome was made and she was referred to Cleveland Clinic for further care.

Coma was assessed at stage three, and there was Kussmaul respiration with grunting, tightly clenched jaw, and random movements of extremities. There was minimal response to pain and pupils reacted sluggishly to light. Coma deepened rapidly and she became unresponsive to pain. Chest roentgenogram revealed a right mid-lobe infiltrate. Blood ammonia was 856 mcg/dL. An arteriovenous fistula was placed in the left arm and a ventriculostomy tube inserted for monitoring intracerebral pressure. A neurologist performed a two-volume exchange transfusion, without any observed change in the clinical condition. Curare was administered and an automatic respirator set up. On the following day, blood ammonia was 50 mcg/dL and partial thromboplastin time 74 s (control 37 s). The SGOT was 400 mU/mL, LDH 500 mU/mL, and creatine phosphokinase 600 mU/mL. A second exchange transfusion was performed, during which repeated seizures were observed, involving the right arm and face, vertical nystagmus, and blinking. Decadron, 10 mg, and 6 units of insulin were administered. The electroencephalogram (EEG) showed absence of alpha rhythm and high-voltage diffuse slow wave activity. Corneal, gag, and pupillary reflexes were present. There was a downbeat nystagmus; mouthing and flailing limb movements occurred. Intraventricular pressure was 40–45 mm Hg.

*Continued*

### Case Example 5.16 Comatose 18-Month-Old Girl With Reye's Syndrome—cont'd

On the following day her clinical condition was interpreted by a neurologist to be "at the brain stem level." Pupils became fixed and dilated and a decerebrate posturing was seen, although spontaneous respirations occurred independent of the respirator. She was judged to be in a terminal state and the respirator was withdrawn. She began to hyperventilate spontaneously. Serum cholesterol was 152 mg/dL and triglycerides 180 mg/dL.

One week after admission there was no change in her condition. She was deeply comatose and all treatment, other than normal life support, was withdrawn. After informed consent by the parents, TTFD in a dose of 100 mg was given by nasogastric tube every 4 h and she received 150 mg by intravenous injection—a total of 750 mg per 24 h. After 24 h of treatment the lip vermilion was bright red, compared with previous duskiness, and there was flushing of the cheeks. Two days later there was some response to pain and, after 3 days of treatment, there was spontaneous movement of the limbs and diminished hypertonicity. Pupils responded to light and she had a cough reflex. There was some bruxism and lip smacking. The intratracheal tube was removed.

After 1 week, intravenous TTFD was discontinued and the oral dose decreased to 300 mg a day. After 9 days from the beginning of treatment there was a widespread exanthema of small superficial bullous lesions containing clear fluid. The TTFD was withdrawn, the lesions gradually disappeared, and TTFD was then resumed in a dose of 150 mg a day. On the 15th day the patient was in a state of so-called *coma vigilum*. Eye contact could be established and she responded to sounds, but was not conscious. Subsequently, she began to take Jello from a spoon and showed primitive crying responses. The right pupil was seen to be larger than the left. Head control increased, although general muscular hypotonicity remained. On the 21st day she was able to chew and could support her own weight with help. Serum cholesterol had risen to 363 mg/dL and the triglycerides decreased to 134 mg/dL. Gross motor function on the Denver scale was 7 months and a personal social scale of 10 months. She began to walk with her hand held and self-feeding and speech gradually improved. She was discharged from hospital 1 month after TTFD was begun. Medication was continued in the same dose and 3 months later she was clinically well, though muscular tone was diminished. Serum cholesterol was 221 mg/dL and triglycerides 169 mg/dL.

In subsequent follow-up, muscular tone gradually improved, but never became normal. At the age of 8 years she began to experience a seizure disorder, each seizure lasting about 30 s and more likely to occur after she had been reprimanded. She had repeated kindergarten and was in first grade, able to read and do arithmetic. The EEG revealed slow spike and wave complexes.

## Points of Consideration

This child was treated in 1975, and this explains why the conventional treatment of exchange transfusion and use of insulin and glucose are reported. These methods have now been abandoned. Although the disease is now mostly preventable because it is known to be caused by aspirin given to bring the temperature down, it still occurs for unknown reasons and there is still no metabolic treatment for this devastating disease. Better methods of life support are now used and the mortality is consequently less. It is also well recognized that Reye's syndrome can spontaneously improve, sometimes even in very severe cases. This makes any treatment modality very hard to assess, as is the case with any disease capable of remitting spontaneously. However, it would be lacking common sense if we fail to apply a noninvasive, absolutely safe measure if there are clues that it has a beneficial effect, irrespective of hardcore proof, especially in a disease as devastating as this. No claim is made here that this child's life was saved, but the change from a seemingly hopeless state to one of relative normality was impressive, and the effectiveness of TTFD should be explored further. It was not used by us in other cases of Reye's syndrome for a variety of reasons, including skepticism and lack of opportunity.

Since thiamine and perhaps even more TTFD both appear to have a therapeutic effect in conditions where energy metabolism is endangered, it seemed logical to attempt to use TTFD in this case, where "terminal care only" had been ordered. It would be very easy to give the medication to every other case in a series of patients, all of whom would otherwise receive the present care given in this disease.

It is tempting to suggest that the mechanism in Reye's syndrome involves a breakdown in cell membrane physiology, and that systematic research into vitamin and mineral replacement might yield a method of relatively easy medical therapy.

### Case Example 5.17 Reye's-Like Syndrome in a 10-Year-Old Boy

A 10-year-old boy was seen who had experienced more than 30 episodes of a condition that was remarkably like the course of Reye's syndrome, but with repeated spontaneous recovery. Studies elsewhere had not produced any concept of what this recurrent disease represented. After our studies were completed using TTFD, this was discontinued and he subsequently died during one of these episodes. Unfortunately, a totally inadequate autopsy was performed, so that no answer was ever obtained. A brother of this child had died from a similar condition, and another sibling had experienced rheumatoid arthritis,

*Continued*

## Case Example 5.17 Reye's-Like Syndrome in a 10-Year-Old Boy—cont'd

which remitted spontaneously. Two such episodes were studied, one over a period of 3 days and another over a 9-day period. One of these (Fig. 5.3) revealed a falling urinary concentration of creatine and rising creatinine. The recovery was spontaneous and totally untreated. During the second episode (Fig. 5.4) he received a supplement of 150 mg TTFD a day in divided doses. The same phenomenon was observed; the creatine and uric acid fell, and creatinine remained relatively steady. Since this child's disease was capable of spontaneous recovery, it becomes virtually impossible to ascertain whether TTFD had any therapeutic effect. Nevertheless, the experiment revealed the sequential difference in the metabolites and this may well be of significance in demonstrating a dynamic change in the disease.

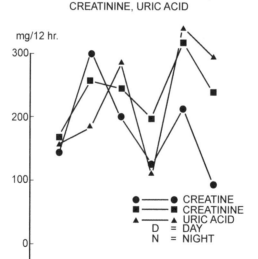

Figure 5.3 Twelve-hour day and night urinary creatine, creatinine, and uric acid concentrations in a 10-year-old boy (Case Example 5.17) during an illness resembling Reye's syndrome that resolved spontaneously.

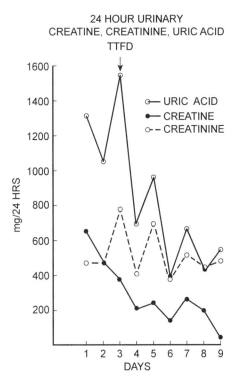

**Figure 5.4** Twelve-hour day and night urinary creatine, creatinine, and uric acid concentrations from the same patient (Case Example 5.17) in a subsequent episode of illness resembling Reye's syndrome but with thiamine tetrahydrofurfuryl disulfide (TTFD) at 150 mg/day.

## Case Example 5.18 Recurrent Episodes of Diaphoresis, Cyanosis, and Sudden Infant Death Syndrome-Like Episodes in a 2-Year-Old Boy

A 2-year-old Caucasian male child was referred because of episodes of pallor, diaphoresis, and cyanosis. Birth history and neonatal and early development were normal. Mucous rhinorrhea from the fifth day of life was attributed to "milk allergy." At 9 months he developed a series of ear infections and tympanic aeration tubes were placed. At 11 months of age he had repeated episodes of diarrhea. At 15 months a nocturnal episode of crying was followed by a seizure, and labile blood pressure and increases in urinary catecholamines were reported elsewhere as the only abnormalities. Diarrhea ceased at 18 months and urinary catecholamines were reported to be only equivocally increased. At the age of 20 months he was found in his crib early one morning pale and lethargic, with cyanotic lips

*Continued*

**Case Example 5.18 Recurrent Episodes of Diaphoresis, Cyanosis, and Sudden Infant Death Syndrome-Like Episodes in a 2-Year-Old Boy—cont'd**

and nails, and he recovered spontaneously. At the age of 22 months, similar episodes began to occur regularly, usually when awakening from an afternoon nap. Pallor, lethargy, diaphoresis, and cyanosis were repeatedly observed. Urinary catecholamine increases and labile blood pressure were reported, and there was frequently bronchial wheezing and tachycardia. Following sedation for electroencephalography he became pale, lethargic, and exhibited patchy cyanotic mottling of the skin. Extreme activity was accompanied by an enormous appetite, estimated to be greater than his older brother, aged 5 years. Family history revealed one case each of diabetes in the paternal and maternal family, respectively. On examination the child was in the 75th percentile for height and weight and looked well. Blood pressure was 100/80, and there was cardiac sinus arrhythmia. Urinary amino and keto acid profiles were normal. Fasting serum pyruvate was 2.0 mg/100 mL 4 h after epinephrine. Glucose tolerance was normal.

Thiamine hydrochloride was begun empirically in a dose of 150 mg per day. He was asymptomatic 3 months later. Weight had increased by 0.7 kg and height by 3.1 cm, revealing a slight acceleration on the growth grid. It is notable that only concentrations of vanillylmandelic acid correlated with clinical improvement. Changes in other urinary amino acids were not consistent. Symptoms were similar to those seen in threatened sudden infant death syndrome, but occurred at a later than usual age. Symptoms recurred subsequently when attempts were made to discontinue thiamine. The relationship between catecholamine concentrations and thiamine deficiency is reported in animal studies.[38]

*Points of Consideration*

This was a case of functional dysautonomia. Remission in all symptoms occurred while he was receiving the vitamin supplement, suggesting that he was dependent upon it during a period of accelerated growth. It is uncertain whether the child's problem can be classified strictly as "nutritional" since there may well be underlying genetic factors that were not understood. Most of the episodes described were related to the state of sleep.

## Variations in Presentation

In the following section we present additional cases of dysautonomic symptoms, often with widely different clinical presentations that were amenable to thiamine therapy.

## Case Example 5.19 Metabolic Instability and Severe Vomiting and Diarrhea in a 22-Month-Old Girl

A 22-month-old girl, the younger sister of a cerebrally handicapped child, was found to have a persistently increased urinary C/CR ratio of 1.5. When she developed severe diarrhea and vomiting, followed by seizure, it was viewed in terms of possible metabolic abnormality. Red cell TKA was 65.9 mU/L/min and TPPE 18.2%. She was treated with large doses of thiamine hydrochloride.

When seen again 2 months later the C/CR had decreased to 0.48. Red cell TKA was 42.09 mU and TPPE 0. Since she was then well, the vitamin supplement was discontinued. She was seen again 4 months later and C/CR had increased to 1.2. It is suggested that this represented an unstable state, which created susceptibility to sudden onset of disease. It was strongly suspected that an inherited factor, such as a defect in cell membrane function, was present in the two children, and that it had affected the older sister more severely. This also suggests that the C/CR cannot be used as an unequivocal test of a disease state and would obviously depend upon the state of nutrition as well as the degree of environmental stress.

## Case Example 5.20 Two-and-a-Half-Year-Old With Poor Visual Acuity, Hyperactivity, and Multinutrient Deficiencies

A 2½-year-old child was examined by an ophthalmologist regarding poor visual acuity. The lenses in both eyes were dislocated and the child was referred for metabolic evaluation. Hyperactivity and poor attention span suggested that the active underlying condition might be homocystinuria[39] but urine was negative by the nitroprusside test, and no homocysteine could be identified by chromatography. Amino acid analysis of urine revealed that there was some increase in histidine. An oral dose of L-methionine (100 mg/kg of body weight) was given to the child, and plasma and urine amino acid analysis performed sequentially over 24 h. Plasma methionine increased moderately and had returned to normal within 24 h, indicating no obstruction in normal methionine metabolism.

Urine revealed the presence of the mixed disulfides of cysteine and homocysteine, also interpreted as a normal response. The child was then referred to Dr. Gaull for further study, and he was unable to detect any abnormally hypoactive state of any of the enzymes in transmethylation and transsulfuration, which have been reported previously in cases of homocystinuria.[40]

Serum folate was greater than 30 ng/mL and B12 was 1450 pg/mL. Red cell TKA was 29.7 mU/L/min (normal 42.1–86.1 mU/L/min) and TPPE 32.3% (normal 0%–17.4%). The TKA and TPPE clearly indicated that the child's red cells were deficient in the cofactor TPP, and it is tempting to speculate that the raised serum levels of folate and B12 were secondary to the slow rate of oxidative metabolism

*Continued*

## Case Example 5.20 Two-and-a-Half-Year-Old With Poor Visual Acuity, Hyperactivity, and Multinutrient Deficiencies—cont'd

that might be predicted under these circumstances resulting in a partial deficiency of ATP. The interesting suggestion has been raised that homocystinuria might be brought about by an abnormal state of oxidative metabolism in chromosomal disease.[41] It is not unreasonable to use an analogy: defective mechanisms in an automobile. Oxidative metabolism would represent the engine, whereas the energy-consuming processes of transmethylation would represent transmission. These important biochemical relationships are understood by the biochemist, but seldom used by clinicians. The situation might be summarized as follows:

1. Serum concentration of folate can apparently be increased when cells show evidence of "active" folate deficiency as indicated by polymorphonuclear hypersegmentation. This suggests that the biologic deficiency is brought about by accumulation of methylated folate. The active form of the vitamin is formed when the labile methyl group is transferred to methionine.
2. Deficiency of dietary protein might result in lack of sufficient concentration of methionine to receive the labile methyl group, thus causing accumulation of methylated folate and possibly B12.
3. Defective synthesis of S-adenosyl methionine may give rise to accumulation of methylated folate, which is overproduced because of failure in the negative feedback loop regulating activity of the methylene tetrahydrofolate reductase. This might occur because of a genetic defect of methionine-activating enzyme, or by inability for some reason to use ATP in converting methionine to S-adenosyl methionine.
4. Transmethylation is a complicated vital mechanism performing energy transmission and is dependent upon oxidative metabolism, and hence an adequate provision of ATP. The integration of folate and B12 in remethylation of methionine is a vital part of the internal balance that must be maintained for this function to proceed normally.
5. For the reasons enumerated, the process depends upon proper nutrition since many of the ingredients are essential nutrients.

## Case Example 5.21 Functional Dysautonomia in a 6-Year-Old Boy

A 6-year-old boy had functional dysautonomia and abnormal labs. After beginning THCL, the urinary creatine increased from 0.4 to 8.3 mg/kg/24 h, while creatinine increased from 2.4 to 22.8 mg/kg/24 h in 1 month. The C/CR increased

## Case Example 5.21 Functional Dysautonomia in a 6-Year-Old Boy—cont'd

from 0.17 to 0.36. In the following 2 months, urinary creatine decreased to 4.1 and creatinine only to 18.1 mg/kg/24 h. Thus there was a symmetrical increase in both urinary creatine and creatinine, followed by a relative decrease in creatine. It is suggested that this would be consistent with a period of "paradox" when metabolism increased, but there remained a temporary abnormality in processing creatine. As this mechanism improved, so the C/CR decreased.

## Case Example 5.22 Life-Threatening Croup in a 6-Year-Old Boy

A 6-year-old boy had severe life-threatening croup and his three siblings had an identical history. Similar attacks had been occurring five or six times a year since the age of 1 year and during the winter months only. Each began between 2:00 a.m. and 4:00 a.m., and they were characterized by difficulty in respiration, tachycardia, barking cough, typical croup, and sometimes accompanied by repeated vomiting. His poor appetite had caused great maternal anxiety, resulting in attempts to feed him. He had frequent temper tantrums, slept restlessly, and frequently talked in his sleep. Previous history revealed that he had an illness at the age of 4 years characterized by rash and low-grade fever for 2 weeks, which terminated by desquamation of hands and feet. On examination there was intercostal retraction, inspiratory wheezing, and stridor. The epiglottis was inflamed and petechial hemorrhages were seen on the face.

Rapid resolution followed symptomatic therapy and he was examined again 2 weeks later. He was pale and rough ichthyosiform skin below the knees was noted. Knee reflexes were difficult to obtain without reinforcement. Red cell TKA was 46.49 mU/L/min and TPPE 23.6%. Decreased concentrations of creatine and increased concentrations of creatinine were observed. In the next 2 months he experienced two further attacks of nocturnal croup. Blood pressure was 100/0 and much "overflow" movement of a choreiform nature was seen. After 1 month's trial with thiamine hydrochloride his general health was improved. He had a normal appetite, was sleeping restfully, and had no more croup. The supplement was continued and 1 year later he had remained completely well with no further episodes of croup.

Thiamine supplement was discontinued and another episode of croup occurred 3 weeks later, requiring admission to hospital. Red cell TKA was 47.1 mU and TPPE 18.3% before thiamine was restored. Interestingly, the main change in C/CR was by day, for this was initially 0.9 and 0.08 1 year later, although there was an increase from 0.35 to 0.49 in the night C/CR in the same time period. The night C/CR may have been a clue to attacks of croup that had occurred invariably at night, as is so common in croup. The blood pressure recorded in this child is typical of beriberi vasomotor changes and a diastolic pressure of zero was a common finding in many of the children examined by Dr. Lonsdale.

### Case Example 5.23 Pyridoxine and Thiamine in Infantile Myoclonus

A 6-month-old boy had infantile myoclonus. His EEG showed hypsarrhythmia. He was treated only with pyridoxine (vitamin B6), 150 mg per day. He quickly became seizure free and 2 months later the EEG was normal. However, he had four or five green-colored liquid stools a day, suggesting the green-colored stools of infancy beriberi discussed in Chapter 1, and had begun to refuse feedings. Thiamine was started in a dose of 150 mg per day and pyridoxine continued. Diarrhea ceased and appetite returned. A few months later, both vitamins were discontinued and he remained well. Urinary C/CR was not recorded.

There appeared to be a synergistic therapeutic effect when large doses of thiamine and pyridoxine were given together, each covering possible functional abnormalities in the patient when administered singly. In some cases, infantile myoclonus may be vitamin dependent without there being any clue other than a response to clinical trial. A tryptophan load in this child had not revealed any increase in urinary xanthurenic acid, a test that is often positive in deficiency of pyridoxine.

## Seizures

## Pyridoxine, Thiamine, and Brain Inflammation

In recent years, the role of pyridoxine in brain inflammation[42–44] has been more clearly elucidated. The chemistry is complicated but deserves mention as the relationship between thiamine and pyridoxine is critically important to brain health and not routinely recognized. Not only is pyridoxine (pyridoxal 5′-phosphate) a necessary cofactor in over 140 enzymes required for the synthesis, degradation, and interconversion of amino acids that are necessary for neurotransmitter synthesis, but it plays an essential role in mitochondrial energetics and is critical for both the folate and methionine cycles.[45] See Figs. 5.5 and 5.6.

Errors in tryptophan catabolism result in altered neurotransmitter balance, but also lead to cell death or apoptosis in vital brain regions via a range of mechanisms that intersect at the mitochondria. When all is functioning well, excess tryptophan is degraded resulting in the by-products nicotinic acid and nicotinamide adenine dinucleotide ($NAD^+$), a niacin product. The NAD–NADH reaction occurs throughout the citric acid cycle and the electron transport chain. Loss of niacin metabolism from this pathway can lead to significant disease processes, most recognizably in pellagra.

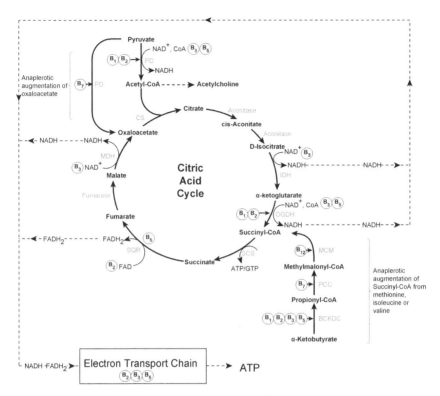

**Figure 5.5** *B vitamins in mitochondrial functioning.*[45] The role of B vitamins in mitochondrial energy production. The citric acid cycle (tricarboxylic/Krebs cycle) is a series of chemical reactions that generate energy in the form of ATP in the mitochondria of eukaryotes. Carbohydrates, fats, and proteins are first converted to acetyl-CoA, most often via pyruvate, and then undergo eight enzymatic reactions that result in the production of NADH and FADH2, which transfer the energy generated by the citric acid cycle to the electron transport chain. This in turn leads to the synthesis of ATP, the energy currency of cells. B vitamins contribute (as shown) to this process as cofactors/enzymes such as FAD (B2), NAD (B3), and as a component of CoA (B5) or coenzyme Q10 (B5). The intermediate compounds of the cycle are also sequestered as substrates for the synthesis of other compounds, including amino acids and fatty acids, and several subsequently have to be replenished by anaplerotic synthesis, taking place outside of the cycle. The most prevalent examples are the augmentation of succinyl-CoA from α-ketobutyrate generated from methionine within the methionine cycle (see Fig. 5.2), and synthesis of oxaloacetate direct from pyruvate. *BCKDC*, branched-chain α-ketoacid dehydrogenase complex; *CS*, citrate synthase; *CoA*, coenzyme A; *FAD/FADH2*, flavin adenine dinucleotide (oxidized/reduced); *IDH*, isocitrate dehydrogenase; *NAD*, nicotinamide adenine dinucleotide (+/H = oxidized/reduced); *MDH*, malate dehydrogenase; *MCM*, methylmalonyl-CoA mutase; *OGDH*, α-ketoglutarate dehydrogenase; *PCC*, propionyl-CoA carboxylase; *PC*, pyruvate carboxylase; *PD*, pyruvate dehydrogenase; *SCS*, succinyl-CoA synthetase; *SQR*, succinate-coenzyme Q reductase.

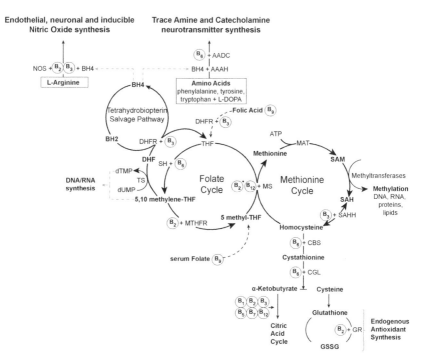

**Figure 5.6** *Pyridoxine in folate and methionine cycles.*[45] The interlinked folate and methionine cycles. Dietary folate enters the folate cycle and rotates through several enzymatic modifications that generate the one-carbon units required for the synthesis of DNA/RNA and the methyl groups required to regenerate methionine from homocysteine. The "methionine cycle" provides the methyl groups required for all genomic and nongenomic methylation reactions in the form of S-adenosyl methionine (SAM). These two enzymatic cycles are essential to cellular function, including via interactions with other pathways. As an example of the latter, the resalvaging from dihydrobiopterin of tetrahydrobiopterin, an essential cofactor in trace amine and catecholamine neurotransmitter synthesis and nitric oxide production, is rate limited by provision of the enzyme dihydrofolate reductase produced by the folate cycle. * FAD (vitamin B2) is a cofactor for methionine synthase reductase in the recycling of the vitamin B12 cofactor for methionine synthase. *AADC*, Aromatic L-amino acid decarboxylase; *AAAH*, aromatic amino acid hydroxylases; *ATP*, adenosine triphosphate; *BH2*, dihydrobiopterin; *BH4*, tetrahydrobiopterin; *CBS*, cystathionine beta synthase; *CGL*, cystathionine gamma-lyase; *DHFR*, dihydrofolate reductase; *dTMP*, thymidine monophosphate; *dUMP*, deoxyuridine monophosphate; *GR*, glutathione reductase; *GSSG*, glutathione disulfide; *MAT*, methionine adenosyltransferase; *MS*, methionine synthase; *MTHFR*, methyltetrahydrofolate reductase; *NOS*, nitric oxide synthase; *SAH*, S-adenosylhomocysteine; *SAHH*, S-adenosylhomocysteine hydrolase; *SAM*, S-adenosyl methionine; *SH*, serine hydroxymethyltransferase; *THF*, tetrahydrofolate; *TS*, thymidylate synthase.

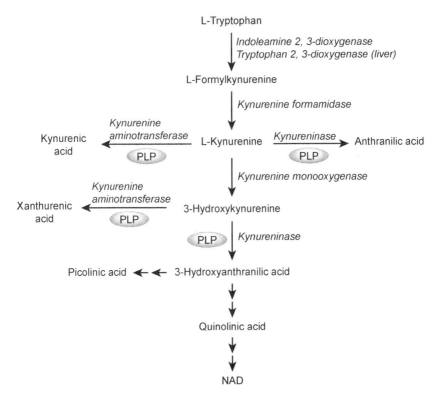

**Figure 5.7** Pyridoxine in tryptophan degradation.[48] *NAD*, nicotinamide adenine dinucleotide; *PLP*, pyridoxal phosphate (active form of vitamin B6).

Pyridoxine deficiency disturbs tryptophan catabolism producing several metabolites that are neurotoxic, including one called quinolinic acid. Quinolinic acid is a potent and self-perpetuating neurotoxin when unopposed in the brain.[46] It generates excess ROS and hyperstimulates *N*-methyl-D-aspartate (NMDA) glutamate receptors, elevating glutamate synthesis significantly,[47] which then induces apoptosis via cytotoxicity, while simultaneously inhibiting brain astrocytes' ability to clean up the excess glutamate. Once that cycle becomes initiated, quinolinic acid potentiates its own release and that of other neurotoxins, ensuring continued brain inflammation and damage. Fig. 5.7 illustrates the role of pyridoxine in quinolinic acid balance.

With the appropriate vitamin B6 concentrations, quinolinic acid is not the final product of tryptophan catabolism, $NAD^+$, and any damage initiated by quinolinic acid as a natural by-product within this pathway is offset by two neuroprotective factors, kynurenine and picolinic acid. Vitamin B6 is critical for the kynurenine aminotransferase and kynurinase enzymes; enzymes that lead to neuroprotective compounds, kynurenine or picolinic acid. Kynurenine blocks the cytotoxic effects of quinolinic acid by blocking the NMDA receptor, making it unavailable to quinolinic acid, while picolinic acid is the primary metal chelator in the brain. Alone, pyridoxine deficiency can evoke seizures. However, its role in NAD conversion, which begins with the pyruvate to acetyl-CoA and repeats throughout the citric acid cycle, suggests a relationship with thiamine. The fact that thiamine coadministered with pyridoxine in pyridoxine-dependent seizures, in the Case Example 5.23 presented here as well as in others, further supports the relationship.[49]

## Reassessing Complicated Cases

All of these cases represent relatively common pediatric problems where treatment is mostly unsatisfactory by the use of medication. Many of them were referred to Cleveland Clinic as a referral center and were not treated on any form of protocol. Each one presented as a problem of clinical management. TKA is a useful test, but only if the TPPE is used as well. To our knowledge the only advanced laboratories that are doing this test perform only the TKA. TPPE has been described as "nonspecific" and is not used. Dr. Lonsdale's experience doing thousands of these tests strongly indicates that the TKA can be normal when the TPPE is grossly abnormal. The clinical response, the upgrading of TKA, and the decrease in the TPPE all represent a very objective analysis of the clinical situation.

## THIAMINE-RESPONSIVE DYSAUTONOMIAS IN ADULTS

Dr. Lonsdale practiced as a pediatrician at Cleveland Clinic between 1962 and 1982 when most of the children described here were researched. In 1982, he entered private practice specializing in nutrient therapy and began to see adult patients as well as children. This work is notable in that it illustrates the greater degrees of complexity of symptom expression in older patients. With time and as life stressors present, autonomic and mitochondrial adaptions become progressively more exaggerated but more easily indicative of beriberi.

## Cardiac Irregularity and Associated Symptoms

### Case Example 5.24 Progressive Autonomic Instability in a 36-Year-Old Woman

A 36-year-old woman complained of cardiac irregularity. She had "whooping cough" at the age of 4 years and at 5 years an illness characterized by a morbilliform rash on the upper trunk and face, associated with high fever and photophobia. At the age of 12 years she experienced inappropriate emotional responses, recurrent diplopia, constant lacrimation with sneezing, and photophobia. Subsequently, she began to have increased academic difficulties in school. At the age of 26 years her first pregnancy terminated prematurely. The second pregnancy was followed by a bleeding duodenal ulcer and the third by thrombophlebitis.

Following dental local anesthesia with epinephrine she had respiratory distress, irregular heart rate, and hypertension for several hours. Repeated episodes of cardiac palpitations, fatigue, heat and cold intolerance, anorexia, and weight loss followed. There was an episode of hemoptysis and respiratory distress and on another occasion she awakened at night with palpitations and asthma. Cardiac irregularity was treated with digitalis. A series of dental abscesses were accompanied by postural hypotension, anorexia, lassitude, weakness, and recurrent cardiac arrhythmia.

Other symptoms included ichthyosiform patches of skin on the elbows and knees, epigastric pain, constipation, dysphagia, hoarseness or aphonia, insomnia, and unwarranted fear. On the current admission to hospital, examination revealed a pale, haggard woman with obvious weight loss, cold cyanotic extremities, pitting edema of the feet, and calf tenderness.

Blood pressure varied from 194/50 to 144/88 and the pulse rate increased from 100 supine to 150 when standing. A heart murmur was caused by MVP.[16] A 24-h urine revealed an increase in the total keto acid content and 196 mg of 1-methyl histidine per gram of creatinine (normal less than 108). After beginning a multivitamin supplement she experienced tachycardia, followed by bradycardia and cardiac irregularity. After commencing a supplement of thiamine hydrochloride she had temporary insomnia but there followed a rapid improvement in general well-being and resolution of symptoms. Fig. 5.8 shows the pedigree of this family. There was an unusual incidence of sudden death in family members by unknown mechanism.[50]

### *Points of Consideration*

The clinical characteristics are consistent with a diagnosis of an incomplete form of familial dysautonomia[51,52]. A marked improvement occurred in the patient after the diet was supplemented with moderate doses of thiamine and a multivitamin. MVP is now known to occur in association with autonomic dysfunction.[16]

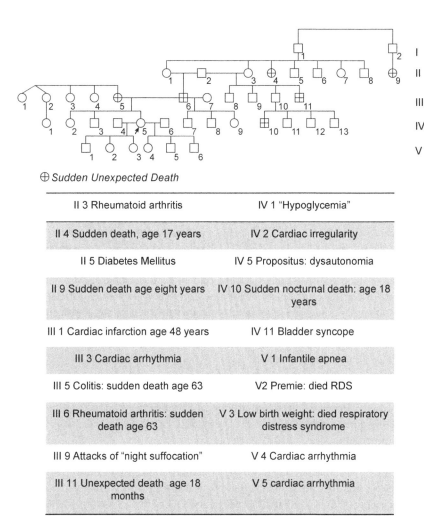

Figure 5.8 Pedigree for family with history of sudden and unexplained deaths (Case Example 5.24).

## Case Example 5.25 Twenty-Six-Year-Old Female Post-Gardasil With Thiamine Deficiency, Postural Orthostatic Tachycardia Syndrome, Hashimoto's, and Other Dysautonomias

A 26-year-old female, 9 years post-Gardasil, suffering from postural orthostatic tachycardia syndrome (POTS), chronic fatigue syndrome, swelling/edema, gut dysmotility problems, severe food allergies, and thyroid issues, reached out to Dr. Lonsdale. Prior to the vaccination, she was an extremely healthy 18-year-old, at college on a cross-country running scholarship.

### Case Example 5.25 Twenty-Six-Year-Old Female Post-Gardasil With Thiamine Deficiency, Postural Orthostatic Tachycardia Syndrome, Hashimoto's, and Other Dysautonomias—cont'd

Following the second dose of the vaccination she experienced extreme fatigue and swelling, developed chronic Epstein–Barr virus, plus additional recurring viruses, and Hashimoto's thyroiditis. Before reaching out to Dr. Lonsdale she had been bedridden for 3 years. Her symptoms included brain fog, extreme swelling and fatigue, heart palpitations, fluctuations in blood pressure, anxiety, *Bartonella*, and food allergies. Conventional labs showed mostly normal ranges, with the exception of low vitamin D and B12 and aberrant fatty acid metabolism.

Tranketolase testing showed extremely severe thiamine deficiency. In addition to the wide range of supplements, she was already taking vitamins C and B, magnesium, and minerals; she worked up to five Allithiamine (TTFD; 250 mg thiamine) daily.

After approximately 8 weeks of TTFD treatment she had a marked decrease in swelling, an improvement in energy levels, and a reduction in brain fog. Her lab values improved significantly. The thiamine appeared to help her other supplements to work better. Notably, if she decreases or stops taking the thiamine she has a resurgence in symptoms.

Although she has improved significantly, the patient rates her recovery at about 85%, and she continues to struggle with POTS, food allergies, and anxiety. Recent genetic testing showed several mutations in the thiamine SLC transport genes.

### *Points of Consideration*

The details of this case were reported to Dr. Lonsdale by email. The mother had done her own research following 4 years of futile treatment and she had come to the conclusion that her daughter had beriberi. She was able to obtain an erythrocyte transketolase study that proved thiamine deficiency, suggesting that the POTS from which her daughter suffered was masking as beriberi. It can only be suggested that this remarkable association represented the vaccination as a nonspecific stressor imposed on marginal thiamine deficiency, thus precipitating clinically expressed thiamine deficiency.

## Fatigue as the Presenting Complaint

### Case Example 5.26 Severe Fatigue in a 77-Year-Old Woman

A 77-year-old woman complaining of severe fatigue that caused her to fall asleep while driving. Also, with morning dizziness and constipation, sought evaluation by Dr. Lonsdale and his colleagues. Additional symptoms included increased eye pressure in one eye, a longstanding need for triiodothyronine supplementation,

*Continued*

### Case Example 5.26 Severe Fatigue in a 77-Year-Old Woman—cont'd

and osteoporosis. Testing revealed normal TKA but abnormal TPPE (18%), indicating a mild thiamine deficiency. She was treated with a multivitamin, 3 g of ascorbic acid (bowel tolerance), 300 mg of magnesium/potassium/aspartate, 250 mg of calcium with 166 mg magnesium in a combination tablet taken at bedtime, 5 mg of phytonadione (vitamin K1), 200 mg of lipoic acid, and 150 mg of TTFD.

After 2 months of treatment the patient reported increased energy with some symptom abatement, but testing revealed declining TKA and increasing TPPE values. After 3 months of treatment her lab values continued to worsen and IV nutrients were administered. Subsequently, TPPE values decreased to 3%.

### Case Example 5.27 Fifty-Six-Year Old Male With Fatigue, Severe Muscle Cramps, and Occasional Hypogastric Pain With Exercise

A 56-year-old male with a 15-year history of easily pulled muscles and severe carpopedal spasms with exercise was seen at Dr. Lonsdale's clinic. Clinical intake revealed longstanding dietary indiscretions involving sweets and simple carbohydrates. Testing indicated an abnormal TPPE. Multinutrient supplementation including TTFD and magnesium/potassium/aspartate was given. Two months later, although there was improvement in the TPPE values, his symptoms remained troubling. Nutrients were given by serial IVs, at which point his symptoms dissipated and the lab values normalized. Upon cessation of the IV treatments, symptoms returned and TKA values began to increase, although TPPE remained normal.

### Case Example 5.28 Seventy-Two-Year-Old Woman With Repeat Flu-Like Symptoms Following Exertion

Like clockwork this patient experienced typical flu-like symptoms including fever, chills, nausea, and fatigue every 2 weeks after square dancing. Each episode would last approximately 4 days. She would recover, only to reexperience the same symptoms after her dancing activity. Testing indicated thiamine deficiency and hemoconcentration. After treatment with IV vitamins that included thiamine, these repetitive episodes ceased and she was able to resume square dancing. The hemoconcentration returned to normal levels. It was concluded that thiamine deficiency had produced pseudo-hypoxia that affected oxygen sensors in brain stem. The physical activity initiated the equivalent of mountain sickness.

## FAMILIAL DYSAUTONOMIA AND EPIGENETICS

Though the focus of this chapter has been functional dysautonomias where thiamine and mitochondrial dysfunction are implicated, emerging evidence suggests that inherited dysautonomias may also be affected by nutrient availability. Specifically, the mechanisms involved in propagating the mutation involved in familial dysautonomia corresponds to the presence and absence of nutrient cofactors in coincidence with stressors that directly influence mitochondrial respiratory capacity. In light of these discoveries, a review of familial dysautonomia and the molecular mechanisms uncovered in recent years is warranted.

### Familial Dysautonomia

Familial dysautonomia is an autosomal recessive mutation that affects individuals of Ashkenazic Jewish heritage with an incidence of 1 in 3700.[53] The primary lesion in this disease is caused by a point mutation in the IKBKAP (inhibitor of kappa light polypeptide gene enhancer in B-cells) gene that affects the splicing of IKAP, also called elongator proteins (ELP).[54] The splicing error results in the errant development and survival of afferent sensory neurons.[55] Familial dysautonomia presents in infancy and is considered a high-mortality rate disease, likely caused by an unusual susceptibility to infection as well as sudden death. Since first described by Conrad Milton Riley and Richard Lawrence Day in 1949, the symptoms have been well described in the literature. A review of the symptoms suggests concordance with the functional dysautonomias, differing only by magnitude of severity and scope of pathology. The symptoms of familial dysautonomia include the following:
- A failure of general body growth despite normal growth hormone.
- Difficulty in feeding, choking, and defective swallowing coupled with a failure to thrive.
- Severe prostrating episodes of vomiting, possibly explained by failure in the brain stem and reticular system, although other brain mechanisms could also be involved.
- Anorexia.
- The absence of fungiform papillae and taste buds on the tongue. This is considered to be related to the trophic failure of autonomic denervation.
- Excessive sweating, especially on the head during sleep.

- A failure to produce tears. This is also a cholinergic function and supports the lesion being related to the central control of the system rather than to the synthesis of the peripheral neurotransmitter.
- Vasomotor instability with frequent but transient morbilliform rash when eating or excited; a phenomenon seen in many otherwise normal but "nervous" people.
- Indifference to pain.
- Absence of deep tendon reflexes.
- Inappropriate emotional responses (in older children).
- A high prevalence of scoliosis.

The symptoms of familial dysautonomia are also similar to those of the mitochondrial disease, Leigh's subacute necrotizing encephalomyelopathy, for example, a disease in which the pathology is clearly delineated in brain stem and upper cord but of mitochondrial origins. Although mitochondrial involvement has not yet been directly implicated in familial dysautonomia, the interplay between nDNA and mtDNA warrants this consideration and new research supports this possibility.

## Molecular Components of Familial Dysautonomia

Recall from Chapter 3 that the majority of the ~1500 proteins required for proper mitochondrial functioning are transcribed from nuclear genes and translated in the cell cytosol before being transported into the mitochondria[56]; a contingent reciprocity when one considers that transcription and translation processes are themselves ATP dependent. When we explore IKBKAP, the gene encoding the IKAP/ELP proteins[57] responsible for familial dysautonomia, we find that the IKAP/ELP proteins play a critical role in cellular response to stress, particularly nutrient stressors, but also temperature and chemical stressors. This is in addition to their role in transcription/chromatin remodeling, teleomere silencing, DNA damage response signals, and cell division.[58] In other words, the IKAP/ELP proteins contribute significantly to what researchers call the mitochondrial regulome, acting as "environmental" sensors that respond to and affect epigenetic modifications. Though the mechanisms remain to be elucidated fully, in the HeLa cell line, at least, the ELP protein complex influences mitochondrial signal transduction directly.[59] Similarly, researchers have identified both enzymatic[60] and nonenzymatic[61] mitochondrial processes regulated by the ELP protein complex, mostly via its role in lysine acetylation processes.

Most notably for our purposes, the IKAP/ELP nutrition/starvation stressor-sensing capability extends the possibility that, at least evolutionarily, the splicing error was in response to dietary constraints; one that may yet be modified by overriding those conditions. Indeed, some research suggests this is the case. Specifically, the soy isoflavones genistein and daidzein (phytoestrogens), in addition to tocotrienol (vitamin E), the flavinoid epigallocatechin gallate (EGCG; an antioxidant found in green tea[62]), and the plant cytokinin kinetin (a component of coconut milk[63]), all favorably modulate IKBKAP splicing in familial dysautonomia-derived cells. That is, these compounds, alone or together, increase the proportional number of wild-type to mutated proteins.[64] The combination of EGCG plus genistein restored the ratio of wild-type to mutated proteins equivalent to those in normal cells.

While not directly related to thiamine, the notion that compounds found in consumed foods regulate the transcriptional activity of proteins involved in nutrient sensing with direct and indirect ties to mitochondrial function suggests the inherent modifiability of processes that we heretofore considered hardwired. It is not such a big jump to think that there may be other nutrient compounds capable of supporting healthy development and/or functionally overriding genetic errors.

## CONCLUSION

Many physicians are under the impression that the only use of vitamins is when there is either dietary deficiency or a genetic effect exclusive to the ability of the vitamin to bind to its enzyme. Zbinden reported 696 published papers in which thiamine therapy had been attempted in more than 230 different diseases with varying degrees of success.[65] This information, important to the health of millions, was abandoned until relatively recently when vitamins have reemerged in the medical press for their true therapeutic value. Because so many different diagnosed conditions sometimes responded to the administration of thiamine as a single entity, it offended the medical model for disease as it presently exists. Since healing is a function of the body itself, all it requires is energy and it seems that a new model for disease is required. We have shown that thiamine deficiency or anything that affects thiamine homeostasis reduces the synthesis of energy, most prominently affecting the hypothalamic autonomic endocrine axis and the heart. High-calorie carbohydrate malnutrition is in the forefront of etiology.

## REFERENCES

1. Clark VL, Kruse JA. Clinical methods: the history, physical, and laboratory examinations. *JAMA* 1990;**264**(21):2808–9.
2. Di Leo R, Musumeci O, de Gregorio C, Recupero A, Grimaldi P, Messina C, Coglitore S, Vita G, Toscano A. Evidence of cardiovascular autonomic impairment in mitochondrial disorders. *J Neurol* 2007;**254**(11):1498–503.
3. Axelrod FB, Chelimsky GG, Weese-Mayer DE. Pediatric autonomic disorders. *Pediatrics* 2006;**118**(1):309–21.
4. Parsons T, Weiner L, Engelstad K, Linker A, Battista V, Wei Y, Hirano M, DiMauro S, Darryl C, Kaufmann P. Autonomic symptoms in carriers of the m. 3243A>G mitochondrial DNA mutation. *Arch Neurol* 2010;**67**(8):976–9.
5. Williams RD, Mason HL, Power MH, Wilder RM. Induced thiamine (vitamin B1) deficiency in man: relation of depletion of thiamine to development of biochemical defect and of polyneuropathy. *Arch Intern Med* 1943;**71**(1):38–53.
6. Shimazono N, Katsura E. *Review of Japanese literature on beriberi and thiamine*. 1965.
7. McCandless DW, Schenker S. Encephalopathy of thiamine deficiency: studies of intracerebral mechanisms. *J Clin Invest* 1968;**47**(10):2268.
8. Fattal-Valevski A. Thiamine (vitamin B1). *J Evid Based Complement Altern Med* 2011;**16**(1):12–20.
9. Irwin JB. *The natural way to a trouble-free pregnancy: the toxemia/thiamine connection*. Aslan Publishing; 2008.
10. Pácal L, Tomandl J, Svojanovský J, Krusová D, Štěpánková S, Řehořová J, Olšovský J, Bělobrádková J, Tanhäuserová V, Tomandlová M, Mužík J. Role of thiamine status and genetic variability in transketolase and other pentose phosphate cycle enzymes in the progression of diabetic nephropathy. *Nephrol Dial Transpl* 2011;**26**(4):1229–36.
11. Martin PR, Singleton CK, Hiller-Sturmhofel S. The role of thiamine deficiency in alcoholic brain disease. *Alcohol Res Health* 2003;**27**(2):134–42.
12. Naviaux RK. Metabolic features of the cell danger response. *Mitochondrion* 2014;**16**:7–17.
13. Sweet RL, Zastre JA. HIF1-α-Mediated gene expression induced by vitamin B. *Int J Vitam Nutr Res* 2013;**83**(3):188–97.
14. Higashimoto T, Baldwin EE, Gold JI, Boles RG. Reflex sympathetic dystrophy: complex regional pain syndrome type I in children with mitochondrial disease and maternal inheritance. *Arch Dis Child* 2008;**93**.
15. Styres KS. The phenomenon of dysautonomia and mitral valve prolapse. *J Am Acad Nurse Pract* 1994;**6**(1):11–5.
16. Coghlan HC, Phares P, Cowley M, Copley D, James TN. Dysautonomia in mitral valve prolapse. *Am J Med* 1979;**67**(2):236–44.
17. Taylor RW, Turnbull DM. Mitochondrial DNA mutations in human disease. *Nat Rev Genet* 2005;**6**(5):389–402.
18. Guilleminault C, Eldridge FL, Dement WC. Insomnia with sleep apnea: a new syndrome. *Science* 1973;**181**(4102):856–8.
19. Pareek N, Fleisher DR, Abell T. Cyclic vomiting syndrome: What a gastroenterologist needs to know. *Am J Gastroenterol* 2007;**102**(12):2832–40.
20. Boles RG, Powers AL, Adams K. Cyclic vomiting syndrome plus. *J Child Neurol* 2006;**21**(3):182–9.
21. Boles RG, Williams JC. Mitochondrial disease and cyclic vomiting syndrome. *Dig Dis Sci* 1999;**44**(Suppl. 8):103S–7S.
22. Boles RG, Adams K, Li BUK. Maternal inheritance in cyclic vomiting syndrome. *Am J Med Genet Part A* 2005;**133**(1):71–7.

23. Abell TL, Adams KA, Boles RG, Bousvaros A, Chong SKF, Fleisher DR, Hasler WL, Hyman PE, Issenman RM, Li BUK, Linder SL. Cyclic vomiting syndrome in adults. *Neurogastroenterol Motil* 2008;**20**(4):269–84.
24. Fleisher DR, Gornowicz B, Adams K, Burch R, Feldman EJ. Cyclic Vomiting Syndrome in 41 adults: the illness, the patients, and problems of management. *BMC Med* 2005;**3**(1):1.
25. Kaul A, Kaul KK. Cyclic vomiting syndrome: a functional disorder. *Pediatr Gastroenterol Hepatol Nutr* 2015;**18**(4):224–9.
26. To J, Issenman RM, Kamath MV. Evaluation of neurocardiac signals in pediatric patients with cyclic vomiting syndrome through power spectral analysis of heart rate variability. *J Pediatr* 1999;**135**(3):363–6.
27. Boles RG. High degree of efficacy in the treatment of cyclic vomiting syndrome with combined co-enzyme Q10, L-carnitine and amitriptyline, a case series. *BMC Neurol* 2011;**11**(1):1.
28. Gordon EE, Januszko DM, Kaufman L. A critical survey of stiff-man syndrome. *Am J Med* 1967;**42**(4):582–99.
29. Ygberg S, Naess K, Eriksson M, Stranneheim H, Lesko N, Barbaro M, Wibom R, Wang C, Wedell A, Wickström R. Biotin and thiamine responsive basal ganglia disease–A vital differential diagnosis in infants with severe encephalopathy. *Eur J Paediatr Neurol* 2016;**20**(3):457–61.
30. Dahiya K, Tiwari AD, Shankar V, Kharb S, Dhankhar R. Antioxidant status in neonatal jaundice before and after phototherapy. *Indian J Clin Biochem* 2006;**21**(1):157–60.
31. Vijayan N, Dreyfus PM. Posttraumatic dysautonomic cephalalgia: clinical observations and treatment. *Arch Neurol* 1975;**32**(10):649–52.
32. Cooper JR, Itokawa Y, Pincus JH. Thiamine-triphosphate deficiency in subacute necrotizing encephalomyelopathy. *Science* 1969;**164**(3875):74–5.
33. Blass JP, Gibson GE. Abnormality of a thiamine-requiring enzyme in patients with Wernicke-Korsakoff syndrome. *N Engl J Med* 1977;**297**(25):1367–70.
34. Bennett T, Evans D, Hampton JR, Hosking DJ. Abnormal cardiovascular reflexes in subjects with autonomic neuropathy. *J Physiol* 1975;**246**(2):47P.
35. IVY HK. Renal sodium loss and bronchogenic carcinoma: associated autonomic neuropathy. *Arch Intern Med* 1961;**108**(1):47–55.
36. Lonsdale D. Recurrent febrile lymphadenopathy treated with large doses of vitamin B1: report of two cases. *Dev Pharmacol Ther* 1979;**1**(4):254–64.
37. Ishimaru T, Yata T, Hatanaka-Ikeno S. Hemodynamic response of the frontal cortex elicited by intravenous thiamine propyldisulphide administration. *Chem Senses* 2004;**29**(3):247–51.
38. Cannon WB. "Voodoo" death. *Psychosom Med* 1957;**19**(3):182–90.
39. Carson NA, Cusworth DC, Dent CE, Field CMB, Neill DW, Westall RG. Homocystinuria: a new inborn error of metabolism associated with mental deficiency. *Arch Dis Child* 1963;**38**(201):425.
40. Gaull GE. Clinical importance of enzymatic diagnosis: the homocystinurias. *J Pediatr Ophthalmol Strabismus* 1973;**10**(4):247–51.
41. Lejeune J. On the mechanism of mental deficiency in chromosomal diseases. *Hereditas* 1977;**86**(1):9–14.
42. Lehmann M, Regland BOR, Blennow K, Gottfries CG. Vitamin B12-B6-folate treatment improves blood–brain barrier function in patients with hyperhomocysteinaemia and mild cognitive impairment. *Dement Geriatr Cogn Disord* 2003;**16**(3):145–50.
43. Zysset-Burri DC, Bellac CL, Leib SL, Wittwer M. Vitamin B6 reduces hippocampal apoptosis in experimental pneumococcal meningitis. *BMC Infect Dis* 2013;**13**(1):1.

44. Stockler S, Plecko B, Gospe SM, Coulter-Mackie M, Connolly M, van Karnebeek C, Mercimek-Mahmutoglu S, Hartmann H, Scharer G, Struijs E, Tein I. Pyridoxine dependent epilepsy and antiquitin deficiency: clinical and molecular characteristics and recommendations for diagnosis, treatment and follow-up. *Mol Genet Metab* 2011;**104**(1):48–60.
45. Kennedy DO. B vitamins and the brain: mechanisms, dose and efficacy—a review. *Nutrients* 2016;**8**(2).
46. Zinger A, Barcia C, Herrero MT, Guillemin GJ. The involvement of neuroinflammation and kynurenine pathway in Parkinson's disease. *Parkinson's Dis* 2011;**2011**.
47. Baumeister FA, Shin YS, Egger J, Gsell W. Glutamate in pyridoxine-dependent epilepsy: neurotoxic glutamate concentration in the cerebrospinal fluid and its normalization by pyridoxine. *Pediatrics* 1994;**94**(3):318–21.
48. Paul L, Ueland PM, Selhub J. Mechanistic perspective on the relationship between pyridoxal 5′-phosphate and inflammation. *Nutr Rev* 2013;**71**(4):239–44.
49. Alfadhel M, Sirrs S, Waters PJ, Szeitz A, Struys E, Coulter-Mackie M, Stockler-Ipsiroglu S. Variability of phenotype in two sisters with pyridoxine dependent epilepsy. *Can J Neurol Sci* 2012;**39**(04):516–9.
50. Lown B, Verrier RL, Rabinowitz SH. Neural and psychologic mechanisms and the problem of sudden cardiac death. *Am J Cardiol* 1977;**39**(6):890–902.
51. Pearson J, Axelrod F, Dancis J. Current concepts of dysautonomia: neuropathological defects. *Ann NY Acad Sci* 1974;**228**(1):288–300.
52. Riley CM, Moore RH. Familial dysautonomia differentiated from related disorders. Case reports and discussions of current concepts. *Pediatrics* 1966;**37**(3):435–46.
53. Dietrich P, Yue J, Shuyu E, Dragatsis I. Deletion of exon 20 of the Familial Dysautonomia gene Ikbkap in mice causes developmental delay, cardiovascular defects, and early embryonic lethality. *PLoS One* 2011;**6**(10):e27015.
54. Rubin BY, Anderson SL. The molecular basis of familial dysautonomia: overview, new discoveries and implications for directed therapies. *Neuromolecular Med* 2008;**10**(3):148–56.
55. Norcliffe-Kaufmann L, Slaugenhaupt SA, Kaufmann H. Familial dysautonomia: history, genotype, phenotype and translational research. *Prog Neurobiol* 2016. http://dx.doi.org/10.1016/j.pneurobio.2016.06.003.
56. Stewart JB, Chinnery PF. The dynamics of mitochondrial DNA heteroplasmy: implications for human health and disease. *Nat Rev Genet* 2015;**16**(9):530–42.
57. Anderson SL, Coli R, Daly IW, Kichula EA, Rork MJ, Volpi SA, Ekstein J, Rubin BY. Familial dysautonomia is caused by mutations of the IKAP gene. *Am J Human Genet* 2001;**68**(3):753–8.
58. Tigano M, Ruotolo R, Dallabona C, Fontanesi F, Barrientos A, Donnini C, Ottonello S. Elongator-dependent modification of cytoplasmic tRNALysUUU is required for mitochondrial function under stress conditions. *Nucleic Acids Res* 2015:gkv765.
59. Barton D, Braet F, Marc J, Overall R, Gardiner J. ELP3 localises to mitochondria and actin-rich domains at edges of HeLa cells. *Neurosci Lett* 2009;**455**(1):60–4.
60. Stilger KL, Sullivan WJ. Elongator protein 3 (Elp3) lysine acetyltransferase is a tail-anchored mitochondrial protein in *Toxoplasma gondii*. *J Biol Chem* 2013;**288**(35):25318–29.
61. Wagner GR, Payne RM. Widespread and enzyme-independent Nε-acetylation and Nε-succinylation of proteins in the chemical conditions of the mitochondrial matrix. *J Biol Chem* 2013;**288**(40):29036–45.
62. Du GJ, Zhang Z, Wen XD, Yu C, Calway T, Yuan CS, Wang CZ. Epigallocatechin Gallate (EGCG) is the most effective cancer chemopreventive polyphenol in green tea. *Nutrients* 2012;**4**(11):1679–91.

63. Ge L, Yong JWH, Goh NK, Chia LS, Tan SN, Ong ES. Identification of kinetin and kinetin riboside in coconut (*Cocos nucifera* L.) water using a combined approach of liquid chromatography–tandem mass spectrometry, high performance liquid chromatography and capillary electrophoresis. *J Chromatogr B* 2005;**829**(1):26–34.
64. Anderson SL, Liu B, Qiu J, Sturm AJ, Schwartz JA, Peters AJ, Sullivan KA, Rubin BY. Nutraceutical-mediated restoration of wild-type levels of IKBKAP-encoded IKAP protein in familial dysautonomia-derived cells. *Mol Nutr Food Res* 2012;**56**(4):570–9.
65. Zbinden G. Therapeutic use of vitamin B1 in diseases other than beriberi. *Ann NY Acad Sci* 1962;**98**(2):550–61.

# CHAPTER 6
# High-Calorie Malnutrition and Its Impact on Health

## Contents

| | |
|---|---|
| High-Calorie Malnutrition: a Different Kind of Mitochondrial Stress | 215 |
| From the Obvious to Not so Obvious Signs of High-Calorie Malnutrition | 216 |
|    Obesity, Type 2 Diabetes, and Cardiovascular Disease | 216 |
|    High-Calorie Malnutrition, Warburg, and Cancer: Adaptive Mechanisms in Energy Homeostasis | 218 |
|    Autism Spectrum Disorders, Sugar, and Thiamine | 220 |
|       *Transketolase Activity* | *221* |
|       *Thiamine Pyrophosphate Effect* | *222* |
|       *Points of Consideration* | *222* |
|    Thiamine in Sudden Infant Death Syndrome | 222 |
|       *Points of Consideration* | *233* |
|    Thiamine in Hypoxia and Ragged Red Fibers | 235 |
|    Thiamine in Menstrual and Reproductive Disorders | 237 |
|    Thiamine in Neurodegenerative Disorders | 239 |
|    Thiamine in Obstetrics | 240 |
| High-Calorie Malnutrition and Thiamine: Clinical Cases | 241 |
|    Eosinophilic Esophagitis | 241 |
|    Disorders of the Skin: Urticaria, Angioedema, and Dermatitis | 243 |
|       *Points of Consideration* | *245* |
|    Repeat Infections, Immunity, and Autoimmunity in Dysautonomic Patients | 246 |
|       *Points of Consideration* | *248* |
|       *Points of Consideration* | *250* |
| Conclusion | 253 |
| References | 254 |

Previous chapters have considered the function of the normal autonomic system and have reviewed some of the literature that described the clinical pattern of autonomic dysfunction. No proof exists at the present time as to whether autonomic dysfunction is the forerunner of a given disease entity or merely an associated phenomenon. We have seen that it appears, however, in many seemingly totally unrelated disease states and it would seem to be rational to attempt to elucidate this further. It is interesting history that Selye started his investigations because of a very simple and rather obvious fact. As a medical student he noticed and was impressed by the fact that a series of individuals with various diseases, who were presented to his class, all looked alike. In short, they all looked "sick or ill."

Much like Newton, who questioned the reason for the falling apple, Selye asked himself why this appearance should be similar and what the mechanism behind it could be. Humanity has occasionally made giant steps in understanding by taking such simple and direct common observations and examining them, rather than merely accepting them as unexplained facts of life. Much like Selye did, we too must look for the commonalities. We must look for the patterns that underlie the taxonomic distinctions and ask the very basic question—what causes this? When we track the myriad disturbed molecular pathways that correspond with each disease process back to their origins we find ourselves at the mitochondria. Mitochondria, by way of their control over cellular metabolism, sit at the nexus of all disease, sometimes initiating and other times simply adapting and responding to a diseased environment. In either case, mitochondria control regulatory functions that determine whether and how cells live or die.[1,2] They are the drivers of the metabolic response to cell danger[3,4] and therefore represent both the beginning and end points of disease. Inasmuch as the autonomic system regulates higher-order responses to cell danger signals, it is not unreasonable to suspect that autonomic perturbations across disparate disease processes are markers of mitochondrial distress. Therefore in asking the most basic question—why, across diseases, do all patients look "sick or ill?"—we see the most obvious of answers: disturbed mitochondrial function. It is this sameness of illness behaviors amid the kaleidoscope of disparate symptoms that leads us to where we are now, standing at a crossroads where we have a choice between placing yet another taxonomic notch in the ever-increasing disease pegboard or moving beyond the taxonomy altogether to look for commonalities among the distinctions.

In the previous chapters we outlined the extensive nutrient requirements involved in mitochondrial function, the autonomic chaos that ensued when oxidative metabolism becomes disrupted, and clinical cases that highlighted both. Here we would like to delve more deeply into one of the more common but infrequently recognized culprits in disordered oxidative metabolism: high-calorie malnutrition. Despite decades of evidence,[5] whenever dietary indiscretion is implicated as the harbinger of ill health, it is inevitably dismissed as being somehow "unscientific" and a form of quackery that only "those whacky alternative medicine folks practice."[6,7] As a result, it is not until all other treatments have been exhausted that patients and their doctors consider the possibility of dietary remediation and nutrient therapy. Even then it is considered a "Hail Mary" of sorts, a half-hearted and final attempt to salvage an unsalvageable situation. When it works and the patient improves, the very real mechanisms by which nutrients influence enzyme activity are summarily disregarded in favor of a placebo effect or some other cognitively dissonant magical thinking. As we have contended throughout this book, we believe the approach should be exactly opposite. Dietary correction and nutrient therapies, particularly those targeting the mitochondria, ought to be considered first and medications ought to be used much more sparingly.

## HIGH-CALORIE MALNUTRITION: A DIFFERENT KIND OF MITOCHONDRIAL STRESS

A common theme across the case studies presented thus far is the presence of high-calorie malnutrition. In contrast to the malnutrition induced by an absolute food shortage, where there is a concordant absence of both calories and micro nutrients, with high-calorie malnutrition excessive calories correspond to diminished noncaloric nutrients, while simultaneously overloading mitochondrial capacity to process the carbons into ATP and remove the foodstuff-related toxicants ingested daily. High-calorie malnutrition comes with the added stressors of excess sugars; trans fats; and the chemicals used to grow, process, and preserve modern foods. This type of malnutrition therefore provides three hits to the body: gross metabolic overload, coupled with excessive demands for detoxification, in the absence of nutrient substrates to perform these tasks. The net result is metabolic inefficiency and inflexibility,[8] making the individual ever more susceptible to illness in the face of additional stressors.

At the most fundamental level there is insufficient energy to maintain basic functions, mount an immune response, and clear toxicants.[9,10] This may explain why dysautonomic symptoms emerge and/or exacerbate with minor illness or in conjunction with medication and vaccine reactions.[11] To the extent resources are reallocated, energy availability becomes inconsistent and that inconsistency then nets the autonomic chaos that characterizes dysautonomia. How and where that energy deficit presents is unique to the individual, but that it presents should not be considered unique. We would expect no less chaos from energy disruptions in our electricity grid, but somehow expect the human energy grid to maintain homeostasis in the face of limited resources and abundant stressors. This is illogical at best.

Subsistence on calorie-rich, nutrient-poor foodstuffs therefore overrides mitochondrial capacity for oxidative metabolism, forcing protective cascades that ultimately become deleterious to health and survival.[12] Oxidative stress represents a key component of modern disease[13] and the ensuing damage leaves no tissue unscathed. In the brain and heart, metabolic homeostasis is absolutely critical and why we see thiamine deficiency expressed so explicitly in those systems, particularly as the disease processes progress in severity and chronicity. We must remember, however, that even though the disruptions in the brain and heart energetics are acutely obvious, they remain components of a larger and multilayered process of energetic compensations.

At the molecular level, where thiamine and other nutrients regulate energy capacity, the oxidative insufficiency resembles anoxic/ischemic insults.[14] The absence of nutrients[15] alone, but especially in combination with chronic toxicant exposure, initiates homeostatic cascades such as hypoxia inducible factor expression[16,17] that become manifest as biochemical lesions wherever the combination of genetics and epigenetics sees fit. Admittedly, we can derail mitochondrial functioning by a multitude of other mechanisms. Many, if not all, pharmaceuticals, for example, damage mitochondria.[18] No matter where the insults originate, however, the final common pathway is reduced oxidative capacity[19] and unless and until oxidative capacity is restored, any therapeutic approach that fails to address that function should be considered ancillary at best.

## FROM THE OBVIOUS TO NOT SO OBVIOUS SIGNS OF HIGH-CALORIE MALNUTRITION

### Obesity, Type 2 Diabetes, and Cardiovascular Disease

Obesity rates are one among the most troubling trends of modernity, considered responsible for a long litany of disease processes from type 2 diabetes to cardiovascular disease and myriad other metabolic disturbances. On its face, obesity is a simple math problem: too many calories in and not enough out. When we dig a little deeper, however, we see that while this basic arithmetic accounts for a percentage of cases, it does not account for all cases. Similarly, weight as an absolute marker for disease prospect is misleading at best. Indeed, additional weight confers a protective measure against all-cause mortality,[20] suggesting that fat storage by itself is not the mechanism of illness per se. Indeed, it may be a protective mechanism.[21,22] Similarly, normal weight[23] and even skinny individuals make up 21% of the type 2 diabetes population,[24] suggesting that weight is not the sole contributing factor to type 2 diabetes. Rather, the determining factor is metabolic health,[25] or more specifically, metabolic flexibility.[26]

Metabolic flexibility refers to the combination of factors, environmental and intrinsic, that allow an individual to adapt to perturbations in energy availability. Arguably, metabolic inflexibility necessarily underpins the dysautonomias, particularly when paired with high-calorie malnutrition, whether manifestly expressed in body weight or not. Thus to the extent that excessive, nonnutrient, high-chemical foodstuffs limit molecular oxygen and force compensatory mechanisms such as anaerobic metabolism, diseases typically associated with weight alone would more appropriately be addressed as signs of metabolic inflexibility with the expectation of upstream autonomic compensations. Autonomic compensations are all too frequently considered separate disease processes, such as comorbid fatigue,[27] neuropathies,[28,29] hormonal disruptions,[30] cognitive deficits,[31,32] and mood lability.[33] From this perspective, weight is no longer the issue. It is no longer a discrete taxonomic notch on our diagnostic pegboard. Instead, the nutrient status that allows the mitochondria to respire and process macronutrients becomes more important because that is what determines metabolic health and flexibility. With this simple shift in perspective we begin to see Selye's sameness of "illness behaviors" amid the constellation of disparate symptoms. More importantly, we initiate the very real possibility of illness resolution, not just symptom management.

With type 2 diabetes specifically, thiamine and other nutrient deficiencies are prevalent.[34] One study found 72% and 64% of type 1 and type 2 diabetics, respectively, were thiamine deficient.[35] The constant state of hyperglycemia triggers an accumulation of triosephosphates because of a faulty thiamine-dependent clearance pathway.[36] Triosephosphates disposal requires a thiamine-sufficient transketolase in the pentose phosphate pathway. Thiamine deficiency also limits the entry of glucose and fats into the system because of its position in the pyruvate pathway,[37,38] the HACL1 enzyme,[39] and the absolute requirement of thiamine in cellular respiration—molecular oxygen consumption.[40] In other words, excess sugars and processed food substances, absent appropriate nutrients hamper mitochondrial processing, limiting energy output.[41] This simultaneously derails detoxification efforts,[42] inducing reactive oxygen species (ROS),[43] and inflammatory pathways[44] and aberrant immune function.[45] Notably, extreme stress such as trauma or critical illness induces a state of hyperglycemia,[46] one that demands additional thiamine to compensate.[47] In the case of obesity, the increased storage of fat[48] and the insulin-resistant cascades[49] may be merely incidental, even protective, to mitochondrial starvation and hypoxia. Interestingly, single nucleotide polymorphisms in the thiamine transporter

SLC1943 confer protection against diabetic vascular damage,[50] presumably by increasing thiamine uptake even in the face of sustained hyperglycemia.

With cardiovascular disease, dyslipidemia, and hypertension, similar processes evolve. Indeed, dyslipidemia is directly associated with sugar intake and not the intake of fats as is so often proscribed.[51] Excessive sugars elevate triglycerides,[52] increase white adiposity, and, most importantly, lead to the nonalcoholic fatty liver disease (NAFLD),[53] putatively responsible for perturbations in insulin usage[54] that underpin type 2 diabetes and is linked to mitochondrial disturbances.[55] Excessive sugar ingestion by itself is deleterious to metabolism, but in the absence of other nutrients, and/or in combination with genetic and epigenetic variables that limit the absorption and utilization of nutrients, leads to significant morbidity and mortality. Although researchers and clinicians have been sounding this alarm for decades, the role of dietary sugars in disease is a point missed by most of modern medicine. Attempts to correct hyperglycemia all too often rely largely on pharmaceutical and surgical interventions such as metformin and gastric bypass. Both treatments increase thiamine deficiency, exacerbating the already disturbed metabolic state.[34,56,57] Metformin, the number one drug prescribed to control hyperglycemia in type 2 diabetics, overrides thiamine uptake[58] while simultaneously reducing the typical exercise-induced insulin sensitivity,[59] exercise capacity,[60] and units of ATP by as much as 48%.[61] This is in addition to depleting vitamin B12,[62] cQ10,[61] and initiating cascades that induce fatty liver,[63] the putative cause of insulin resistance.[64] Similarly, a common consequence of gastric bypass surgery is Wernicke's encephalopathy,[65] caused by the blockage of intestinal lumen that absorbs dietary thiamine. A more prudent approach may be to rectify nutrient status and eliminate dietary sugars.

## High-Calorie Malnutrition, Warburg, and Cancer: Adaptive Mechanisms in Energy Homeostasis

One of the unsolved problems in cancer is the unusual use of glucose in cancer cells. In oncology, the Warburg effect is the observation that most cancer cells predominantly produce energy by a high rate of glycolysis followed by lactic acid fermentation in the cytosol rather than by a comparatively low rate of glycolysis followed by oxidation of pyruvate in mitochondria.[66,67] Although Warburg postulated that this was the cause of cancer, mutations in oncogenes and tumor suppressor genes are thought today to be responsible for malignant transformation, though there yet remains much debate.[68]

As we have reported throughout this text, thiamine deficiency is increasingly recognized in severely ill patients. The prevalence of thiamine deficiency among cancer patients is unknown. However, recent study suggested it may be very common. Among 217 patients with various types of cancer, deficiency was found in no less than 55.3%. Risk factors included significant weight loss and undergoing active cancer treatment. Almost all patients were normal in weight and a few had vitamin B12 or folate deficiency as well. Measurement of serum thiamine concentration preceded psychiatric consultation in only 10.6% of cases. The conclusion of these authors was that thiamine deficiency is highly prevalent among inpatients with cancer and in the absence of other vitamin deficiencies. Interestingly, evaluation of thiamine deficiency was most commonly not initiated by oncologists,[69] suggesting the recognition of thiamine deficiency has yet to reach the clinicians whose patients may benefit the most.

What role high-calorie malnutrition, or specifically dietary sugar consumption, plays in the pathogenesis of cancer has come into focus over recent decades. Epidemiologically, type 2 diabetes is associated with a higher incidence of all cancers and 41% increase in mortality.[70] Type 2 diabetes represents one of the many effects of high-calorie malnutrition. Chronically high intake of dietary sugars initiates changes in liver mitochondria that results in accumulation of both peripheral adipocytes and the NAFLD responsible for the insulin dysregulation and persistent hyperglycemia.

From a molecular perspective, hyperglycemia has long been recognized for its role in the glycolytic switch integral to the cancer phenotype.[67] Hyperglycemia deranges mitochondrial morphology, increases ROS production, and promotes mitochondrial DNA mutations.[71] In an effort to compensate and reduce the damage, mitochondrial respiration is reduced (the hypoxic cascades initiated) and mitochondrial dynamics are adjusted (fission/fusion). Concomitantly, we get increased production of lactate, which feeds anaerobic respiration and tumorigenesis,[70] but we also have a notable increase in aerobic glycolysis, suggesting an adaptation to states of both normoxia and hypoxia.[66] All of this occurs in the presence of a microenvironment where hyperglycemia is forced upon the cells and must cause an adaptive response. Tumorigenesis appears to be the mechanism of choice, where the excess sugars can be sequestered and metabolized independently of mitochondrial and normal cellular function.

In an elegant study using a 3D cell culture model with breast cancer cells, researchers found that glucose in the microenvironment of cells would induce or inhibit oncogenesis. The forced metabolism of excessive glucose was the oncogenic event that initiated the cancer pathways and the inhibition of glucose uptake reversed the oncogenic pathways.[72] Although mitochondrial ATP production was not impaired in this model, there was a reciprocal relationship between ATP and several oncogenic proteins upregulated by persistent glucose.

Returning to the role of thiamine in mitochondrial oxidative function, it has not yet become clear how cancer cells regulate cellular homeostasis of cofactors adaptively. Putatively, however, we know that thiamine must be involved given its requirement in both cytosolic and mitochondrial glucose metabolism. We also know that thiamine deficiency is common in cancer, as are alterations in thiamine transporter functioning.[73] One review discusses the current knowledge in the alterations in thiamine availability, homeostasis, and exploitation of thiamine-dependent pathways by cancer cells.[74] It appears that thiamine supplementation follows an unexpected dose–response curve. Low and moderate doses of thiamine increase tumor activity, whereas supraphysiological doses inhibit or reverse tumor growth.[74] Dr. Lonsdale has long observed that when thiamine deficiency is chronic and/or severe, high doses of the vitamin are required to reengage enzyme activity. Whether this is the case here or not remains to be investigated, but it does present an intriguing possibility and a novel opportunity for treatment. Similarly, it is difficult not to speculate whether widespread sugar consumption, perhaps by its induction of thiamine deficiency, is causative in oncogenesis.

## Autism Spectrum Disorders, Sugar, and Thiamine

Dr. Lonsdale's interest in thiamine arose from his study of a 6-year-old child with intermittent episodes of cerebellar ataxia that proved to be the first case of thiamine dependency.[75] Many cases of emotional disease in children were referred to him, and it soon became obvious that it was dietary excess of simple carbohydrates and dietary mayhem rather than abnormal parental control that was a decisive factor. Erythrocyte transketolase activity (ETKA) and thiamine pyrophosphate effect (TPPE)[76] became a tool by which he was able to prove thiamine deficiency. It soon became obvious that there could be many ways in which thiamine deficiency could be clinically projected and that there was no particular phenotype. When the epidemic of autism began, Dr. Lonsdale found that many of these children did in fact have abnormal ETKA.

Because of these findings, Dr. Lonsdale performed a pilot study to see how many autistic children would respond to thiamine tetrahydrofurfuryl disulfide (TTFD).[77] Although this was an uncontrolled study, parents filled in forms that had been developed by the Autism Research Institute in San Diego. These forms, read by computer analysis, had been tested for years and were found to be remarkably accurate in predicting outcome in autistic children. The study showed that 8 out of 10 had definite symptomatic responses, strongly suggesting that this disease had a mitochondrial etiology that has since been supported.[78] Subsequently, the case histories of a mother and two children were reported.[79]

The mother was a recovered alcoholic. She and her two children, both of whom had symptoms typical of autism spectrum disorder (ASD), had dysautonomia diagnosed from symptoms. All had intermittently abnormal erythrocyte transketolase studies and both children had unusual concentrations of urinary arsenic. They all had symptomatic improvement with diet restriction and supplementary vitamin therapy, including thiamine, but quickly relapsed after ingestion of sugar, milk, or wheat. The stress of a heavy metal burden superimposed on existing genetic or epigenetic risk factors, coupled with sugar consumption, may be important in the etiology of ASD when in combination. Both of these children appeared to be totally incapable of staying away from sugar, even though their symptoms relapsed extremely quickly after such ingestion.

It has recently been shown that sugar and alcohol both have a relationship with the distribution and potential etiology of autism in the United States. An analysis of breast milk showed that its concentration of vitamin B was less than that in bovine milk. Binge drinking in pregnancy was found to be widespread and was found also to relate to the incidence of autism. The author suggested that the rising intake of sugar throughout the population had a direct relationship with vitamin B deficiency in the breast milk.[80] The incidence of brain disease from thiamine deficiency caused by alcoholism has long been known.

Dr. Lonsdale surveyed the records of 157 children with ASD. There were 128 boys (81.5%) and 29 girls (18.5%). Because this information was gleaned from practice records rather than a study, he found that only 91 of these patients had the ETKA and TPPE performed as part of their laboratory investigation.

## *Transketolase Activity*

This is the baseline activity of the transketolase and 82 (90%) children were found to have this in the normal range. Only two of them (2%) were below the normal range and seven (8%) above the normal range.

*Thiamine Pyrophosphate Effect*
Of 91 tests, the TPPE was over the acceptable range of 18% in 19 (21%), while only 6 (7%) showed no acceleration in the TPPE. Of a total of 91 records, the TPPE was between 1% and 18% in 66 (72%) of these ASD children.

*Points of Consideration*
Over many years of practice, Dr. Lonsdale found repeatedly that the transketolase activity (TKA) was in the normal range when the TPPE was clearly well above the acceptable limit of 18% acceleration. He came to the conclusion that the only strictly normal TPPE would be zero, indicating that the transketolase enzyme was fully saturated with thiamine as its cofactor. The normal range of the TPPE was derived originally from people who were ostensibly healthy, meaning that they had no symptoms that indicated loss of health. It might well be that a gradually increasing acceleration of the TPPE is on a sliding scale from zero to a percentage acceleration that is commensurate with symptoms in a given individual. If that is true, the 66 ASD children with a TPPE between 1% and 18% might be classified with ASD where mitochondrial dysfunction is from causes other than thiamine deficiency[78] but where a minor degree of deficiency plays a part. The best proof of this would be by including thiamine in a cocktail of nutrient supplementation and repeating the transketolase test at a later date after symptomatic improvement. Basal TKA below the normal range may indicate an unusually severe degree of thiamine deficiency or a genetically determined handicap in thiamine homeostasis.[81] A TKA above the normal range reportedly was able to distinguish between vitamin B12 and folate deficiency pernicious anemia,[82] and might suggest that mitochondrial dysfunction in autism has variable biochemical lesions where genetic susceptibility is at risk, coupled with some form of stress such as a vaccination and high-calorie malnutrition.

## Thiamine in Sudden Infant Death Syndrome

The syndrome of sudden infant death remains incompletely solved. Its existence has been recognized in all parts of the world, and the failure to find an obvious cause of death at autopsy has remained a puzzling feature. This in itself has suggested that an unbalanced pathophysiologic state is responsible. There are almost as many theories to explain the syndrome as there are investigators.[83] At a series of workshops, planned by the National Institute of Child Health and Human Development, infection and immunity, behavioral considerations, neurophysiologic factors, epidemiology, and pathology were discussed without reaching a definite conclusion as to etiology,[84] although some studies have pointed increasingly toward the autonomic system as the origin of the process that leads to sudden death.[85–89] The question arises as to how the infant at risk is identified and how such deaths can be prevented. There are some important statistics that have been recognized from a collection of public health data.

- Peak incidences between 1 and 4 months of age[90]
- Greater incidence in males than females[90]
- Greater incidence with low socioeconomic status[91]
- Low birth weight[92]
- Cold weather months predilection with peak incidence in late winter and early spring[93]
- Death between midnight and 6:00 a.m.[94]

The results of a great deal of work have been reported on the clinical presentation and pathology to be able to point increasingly to the relation between brain stem, reticular activating system, and cardiopulmonary function that implicates the mechanism within the autonomic system. Steinschneider[85] was one of the first investigators to report on studies during sleep in infancy, and he described some of the characteristics of the infant at risk for sudden death. His studies revealed alterations in frequency, variability, and character of respirations during sleep, and a decrease in the responsiveness of the respiratory centers to alterations in $CO_2$ concentration. In five cases he reported the infants at risk had frequent episodes of sleep apnea, some associated with cyanosis and severe enough in some instances to require resuscitation. Two of the five infants subsequently died.

Other investigators have also related the syndrome to poor autonomic control, and their findings suggested a brain stem disorder.[86] Naeye[95] described a 38-year-old patient whose death was attributed to the respiratory center associated with abnormalities in the pulmonary vascular bed. Clinical features included general muscular weakness, tachycardia, and cardiomegaly with pulmonary hypertension. Laboratory studies revealed a blood sugar of 198 mg/dL, increased $CO_2$, hypochloremia, hyperkalemia, and elevation of spinal fluid pressure. Death followed recurrent hematemesis and irreversible laryngospasm. The brain was reported to be unremarkable on gross examination, but many areas showed vascular congestion and neuronal degeneration. Hemodynamic features of this case were related to chronic arterial oxygen desaturation and explained the pulmonary hypertension, hypertrophy of pulmonary arterial smooth muscle, and dilatation of the pulmonary arterial bed related to polycythemia. It is particularly important to draw attention to the fact that Asian influenza virus was recovered from the lungs of this patient if "stress" factors are to be considered, and "there was some resemblance to lesions in certain metabolic and nutritional disorders such as Wernicke's encephalopathy, but other evidence of such disturbances was lacking." No nutritional history was recorded.

The same investigator reported similar pulmonary arterial abnormalities in sudden infant death syndrome (SIDS) and related them to chronic recurrent hypoxemia in these infants.[96] Known chronic hypoxemia in infancy causes the retention of a large proportion of the brown fat cells that are normally replaced by white fat cells after birth. Such infants also have an abnormal retention of extramedullary hematopoiesis, abnormalities that were found in many victims of SIDS.[97]

It may be possible to substitute "pseudohypoxia" for hypoxemia. This would then remove the stigma of failure to detect adequate oxygenation of arterial blood flowing to the brain. It would embrace a need to look at all possible aspects of oxidative metabolism, including the necessary vitamin and mineral catalysts and the ability of cells to utilize oxygen adequately. Evidence has suggested a very distinct possibility that defective phosphorylation may be one of the common denominators in the pathophysiology.[98]

Davis et al.[99] reported high concentrations of thiamine in infants dying of crib death and suggested that this represents accumulation of an inactive form of the vitamin (personal communication). Our own experience[100,101] has suggested that this may lead to a therapeutic approach in some of the infants with threatened SIDS. Similar thinking led another investigator to suggest aberrant thiamine neurochemistry as a possible cause in some patients dying of SIDS.[102] An article refuted thiamine deficiency as an important factor, citing negative red cell TKA as the criterion.[103] The authors reported normal TPPE; but of perhaps greater importance, this study tells nothing about the state of thiamine triphosphate in the brain, and it may be this component that fits better into the hypothesis. Thiamine triphosphate deficiency was reported in the phrenic nerve of a SIDS victim.[104]

Our experience suggests that an infant at risk for SIDS can be identified with one or more symptoms of autonomic dysfunction, including varying severity of apnea, choking, vomiting, gasping, extreme pallor, muscular hypotonia, bradycardia, tachycardia, excessive pharyngeal mucus, or defective body temperature control; in other words, comorbid symptoms of dysautonomic function. The history from parents has been confirmed in some cases by admission of the infant to the hospital and cardiorespiratory monitoring around the clock. In one instance a 3-month-old female infant had a history of gasping, vomiting, pallor, muscular weakness, and tachycardia. Urine from a symptomatic infant was examined for urinary monoamines by a physician of Dr. Lonsdale's acquaintance on admission at the age of 5 months. No treatment was given, but the patient remained attached to a nighttime cardiorespiratory monitor unit until it was considered that she had matured beyond the period of considered risk.

Table 6.1 shows the changes in urinary biogenic amines that occurred spontaneously in a period of only 2 months. Note the increase in dihydroxyphenylalanine (DOPA), decrease in dopamine, reduced concentrations of serotonin, and 5-hydroxyindoleacetic acid and normal concentration of 5-hydroxytryptophan. The conversion of DOPA to dopamine and 5-hydroxytryptophan to serotonin are catalyzed by the pyridoxine-dependent enzyme, L-aromatic amino acid decarboxylase, and these results suggested a temporary obstruction in this enzyme system. Similar changes were described in familial dysautonomia.[105] It is not yet possible to state that sudden infant death can be caused by unbalanced or unilateral action of the autonomic system.

Table 6.1 Urinary Biogenic Amines From a Female Infant With Threatened Sudden Infant Death Syndrome at 3 Months, When Symptomatic, and Again at 5 Months, When Asymptomatic

| Controls | ng/mg | Creatinine | 3 Months | 5 Months |
|---|---|---|---|---|
| DOPA | 236.5 | +/−106.1 | 2,370 | 219.2 |
| Dopamine | 1,199 | +/−46.6 | 415 | 950.5 |
| Norepinephrine | 84.4 | +/−32.3 | 81.9 | 43.4 |
| Epinephrine | 47.6 | +/−21.0 | 41.0 | 27.1 |
| HVA | 13,500 | +/−6,500 | 12,500 | 11,090 |
| VMA | 13,500 | +/−14,200 | 1,620 | – |
| Serotonin | 510 | +/−157 | 133.8 | – |
| 5-HTP | 2,138 | +/−1,633 | 3,600 | 2,690 |
| 5-HIAA | 7,220 | +/−3,350 | 3,760 | 10,500 |

*5-HIAA*, 5-hydroxyindoleacetic acid; *5-HTP*, 5-hydroxytryptophan; *DOPA*, dihydroxyphenylalanine; *HVA*, homovanillic acid; *VMA*, vanillylmandelic acid.

Dr. Lonsdale has presented the evidence that some SIDS deaths, if not all, are related to abnormal thiamine metabolism.[89] Not only from his own clinical experience, Dr. David Read, a physiologist at the University of Sydney, had found evidence that thiamine metabolism was involved in the etiology of SIDS.[102,107] This concept was supported by the finding of abnormal brain stem auditory evoked potentials, suggesting an electrochemical etiology.[108]

Supporting the hypothesis of impaired oxidative metabolism, researchers have shown significantly diminished orexin immunoreactivity in postmortem analysis of SIDS infants compared to non-SIDS infants.[109] SIDS infants exhibited a 21% reduction in orexin immunoreactivity in the hypothalamus compared to non-SIDS infants, but also a 50% reduction in the pontine nuclei. Notably, the researchers found no correlations between reduced orexin and the more conventional correlates of SIDS, such as sleep position or exposure to cigarette smoke. The reduced orexin provides an interesting clue to SIDS suggesting a molecular approach not often considered; one that corresponds with thiamine-deficient dysautonomic function.

Recall from Chapter 3 that the orexin/hypocretin nuclei are located in the hypothalamus and fire to maintain wakefulness.[110] They have vast innervation tracts throughout the brain, directly influencing autonomic function,[111] including synapses in the brain stem pons—the nuclei responsible for maintaining motor control of respiration.[112] Recall also that the orexin neurons are ATP sensors, glucose sensors, and thermosensors. When ATP is low, the orexin neurons cease firing.[110] When extracellular glucose concentrations are high, orexin neurons cease firing[113] and when temperature is elevated, orexin neurons cease firing.[114] Reduced ATP[115] and elevated extracellular glucose are direct correlates with thiamine insufficiency and fever is a common stressor in infancy. When these signals are sensed by the orexin neurons, arousal and sympathetic tones are impaired. In an infant, where brain stem coordinated activity is not well developed, this can be deadly.

Notably, if we look at family histories where sudden deaths are disproportionally represented, we see clear evidence of functional dysautonomia, which when taken in total should point us toward disturbed bioenergetics. To illustrate this point, eight cases and associated family histories are presented. In five of the families, there were six infants brought for examination to determine whether they were at risk for SIDS. In each case there had been at least one infant in the family who had been found dead in the crib. Although the criteria for accepting such an event as an example of SIDS are poorly defined, a sudden unexplained infancy death is always a dramatic event, and in each of the cases reported here the history was that of finding a previously healthy infant dead in the crib. Each was 7 months of age or less, with the exception of a few for whom the age was unknown. None had been under immediate treatment for any symptoms preceding the discovery.

### Case Example 6.1 Sudden Death in a 2-Month-Old Female
A 2-month-old female infant was delivered by cesarean section at full term because of pregnancy toxemia and hypertension. The mother had smoked one pack of cigarettes a day throughout pregnancy. The infant had been asymptomatic and physical examination was normal except for clinically judged poor neck tone. A home-going infant apnea alarm was prescribed and 3 days later the apnea alarm sounded twice at night. The infant was found breathing normally on each occasion. The electrodes were attached appropriately and the monitor was functioning normally. The pedigree is shown in Fig. 6.1.

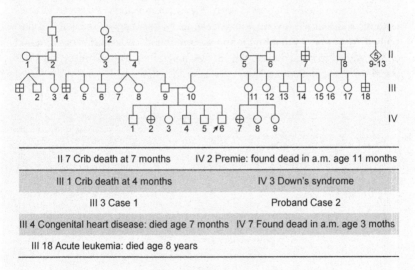

| | |
|---|---|
| II 7 Crib death at 7 months | IV 2 Premie: found dead in a.m. age 11 months |
| III 1 Crib death at 4 months | IV 3 Down's syndrome |
| III 3 Case 1 | Proband Case 2 |
| III 4 Congenital heart disease: died age 7 months | IV 7 Found dead in a.m. age 3 moths |
| III 18 Acute leukemia: died age 8 years | |

**Figure 6.1** Family history for Case Examples 6.1 and 6.2.

## Case Example 6.2 Three-Week-Old Male

A 3-week-old male infant, related to the infant in Case Example 6.1 (Fig. 6.1), was delivered at the 36th week of pregnancy by cesarean section because of hemorrhage from placenta previa. The Apgar score was two at 5 min and six at 10 min. He required resuscitation and 11 days of intensive care, including continuous oxygen for 7 days. Physical exam was normal, with the exception of clinically judged poor neck tone and limb tone. A home-going infant apnea alarm was prescribed. During the following week the apnea alarm sounded four times and on each occasion the infant was found apneic. Physical stimulation restored normal respiration. At age 3 months he had four or five explosive, green colored, watery stools, and developed fever, cough, and bronchial wheezing, for which he had been admitted to another hospital. After hospital discharge, the bradycardia alarm sounded repeatedly during a 24-hour period, and the mother had confirmed the heart rate of less than 80 bpm by palpitation of the carotid pulse. She reported that the fingernails and lips were bluish in color during this 24-h period. This case was lost to follow-up.

## Case Example 6.3 Two-Week-Old Female at Risk for SIDS

A 2-week-old asymptomatic female infant was brought for examination because of SIDS risk. The mother had smoked half a pack of cigarettes a day through pregnancy. She had lost two previous infants from sudden death, each one by a different father. There was a family history of eight male maternal relatives with unknown slowly progressive neuromuscular disorder (Fig. 6.2). The two infancy deaths were also males. The mother reported that she had observed tachypnea and periodic short apneas in the infant during sleep. Physical examination revealed mild acrocyanosis and clinically judged poor neck tone. An infant apnea monitor was prescribed. At the age of 2 months the apnea alarm sounded and the infant was found apneic. After physical stimulation she gasped and resumed normal respiration. This was the only event reported. This case was lost to follow-up.

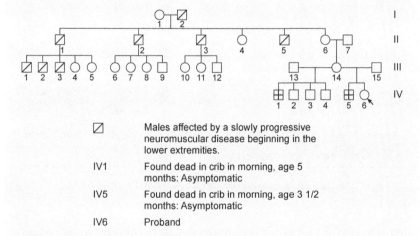

Figure 6.2 Family history of 2-week-old female at risk for sudden infant death syndrome (Case Example 6.3).

## Case Example 6.4 Four-Week-Old Female With Family History of SIDS

A 4-week-old female with a family history of autopsy supported SIDS (Fig. 6.3) was delivered at full term by cesarean section. During pregnancy the mother smoked half a pack of cigarettes a day. She had passed some renal calculi. The infant reportedly had choked occasionally during sleep and appeared to be unduly sensitive to noise, demonstrating frequent sleep starting. Physical examination was normal, with the exception of clinically judged poor neck tone and some diffuse mottling of the skin. At the age of 3 months, the infant apnea alarm sounded three or four times in a 10-day period and one apnea to cyanosis had been observed while she was awake. This case was lost to follow-up.

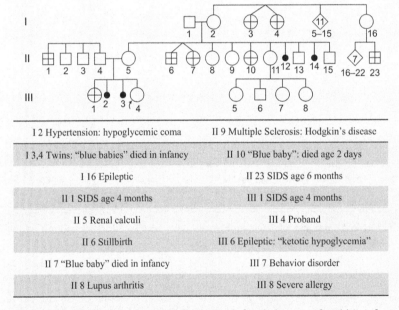

| | |
|---|---|
| I 2 Hypertension: hypoglycemic coma | II 9 Multiple Sclerosis: Hodgkin's disease |
| I 3,4 Twins: "blue babies" died in infancy | II 10 "Blue baby": died age 2 days |
| I 16 Epileptic | II 23 SIDS age 6 months |
| II 1 SIDS age 4 months | III 1 SIDS age 4 months |
| II 5 Renal calculi | III 4 Proband |
| II 6 Stillbirth | III 6 Epileptic: "ketotic hypoglycemia" |
| II 7 "Blue baby" died in infancy | III 7 Behavior disorder |
| II 8 Lupus arthritis | III 8 Severe allergy |

Figure 6.3 Pedigree of 4-week-old female with family history of sudden infant death syndrome (SIDS) (Case Example 6.4).

## Case Example 6.5 Five-Week-Old Male With Family History of SIDS

A 5-week-old asymptomatic male infant was brought for examination because of a family history of two sudden infancy deaths (Fig. 6.4). The mother had been diagnosed elsewhere with sleep apnea. Delivery was by cesarean section. Physical examination was normal, but neck tone was judged to be poor in the flexors. An

*Continued*

## Case Example 6.5 Five-Week-Old Male With Family History of SIDS—Cont'd

infant alarm was prescribed, though the father was opposed. At the age of 2 months, the apnea alarm sounded and the infant was found apneic and limp. Physical stimulation restored normal respiration. The incident convinced the father of the wisdom of using the monitor, since he believed that the event might have been lethal. This case was also lost to follow-up.

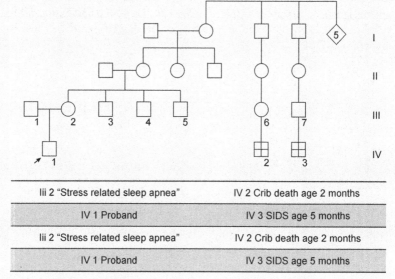

| Iii 2 "Stress related sleep apnea" | IV 2 Crib death age 2 months |
|---|---|
| IV 1 Proband | IV 3 SIDS age 5 months |
| Iii 2 "Stress related sleep apnea" | IV 2 Crib death age 2 months |
| IV 1 Proband | IV 3 SIDS age 5 months |

Figure 6.4 Pedigree of 5-week-old male with family history of sudden infant death syndrome (SIDS) (Case Example 6.5).

## Case Example 6.6 One-Month-Old Infant With Family History of Sudden Death

A 1-month-old infant was brought for examination because of familial unexplained infancy death. The mother had gestational diabetes mellitus and there was a family history of this condition (Fig. 6.5). The infant had been noted to wheeze occasionally during feeding and experienced unusual nasal congestion and irritability. Physical examination was normal. An apnea alarm was prescribed but no events were reported.

## Case Example 6.6 One-Month-Old Infant With Family History of Sudden Death—Cont'd

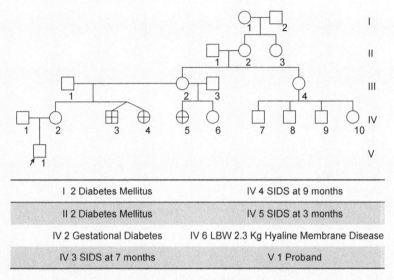

| I 2 Diabetes Mellitus | IV 4 SIDS at 9 months |
|---|---|
| II 2 Diabetes Mellitus | IV 5 SIDS at 3 months |
| IV 2 Gestational Diabetes | IV 6 LBW 2.3 Kg Hyaline Membrane Disease |
| IV 3 SIDS at 7 months | V 1 Proband |

**Figure 6.5** Pedigree of 1-month-old infant with family history of sudden death.

## Case Example 6.7 Eleven-Year-Old Girl With Episode of Cyanosis

The proband, an 11-year-old girl, had a history of headaches, recurrent abdominal pain, unexplained fever, and dizziness. After an upper respiratory infection she experienced a morbilliform rash on the neck and chest, protracted vomiting, difficulty in breathing, choking, and cyanosis, which had been treated in an emergency room with administration of oxygen. In this large family the symbols with crosses in Fig. 6.6 represent nine infants who had been found dead in the crib. In each case the death had been completely unexpected, but details of age and circumstances were not available.

There were many diseases claimed by the mother of the proband. These included hypertension, cancer, diabetes, mental retardation, and cardiomyopathy of unknown cause. There was a surprising incidence of sudden infantile deaths in the first year of life. In each case, the child had been found dead in the crib in the morning, without any adequate explanation. In the proband analysis below (Fig. 6.7), cases of sudden death are marked with a cross. The exact ages could not be ascertained in every case.

*Continued*

## Case Example 6.7 Eleven-Year-Old Girl With Episode of Cyanosis—Cont'd

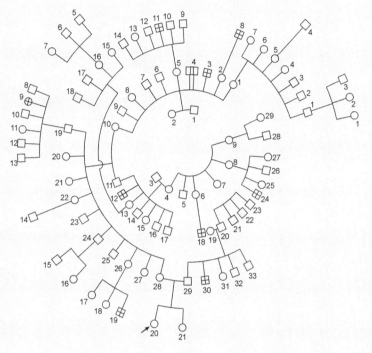

| | |
|---|---|
| II 3 Death at 2 months | III 11 Death in first year |
| II 12 Death at 2 months | III 30 Death in first year |
| II 18 Death at 6 months | IV 9 Death in first year |
| II 24 Death in first year | IV 19 Death in first year |
| III 8 Death at 6 weeks | IV 20 Proband: Dysautonomia |

**Figure 6.6** Proband analysis and pedigree of 11-year-old girl with episodes of cyanosis (Case Example 6.7).

## Case Example 6.8 Sudden Death in Consanguineous Family With History of Dysautonomia

The proband in this family (Fig. 6.7) required extensive resuscitation at birth. Throughout childhood she experienced recurrent fatigue, periorbital edema, unexplained fever, profuse nocturnal sweating, cold intolerance, and extreme irritability. The mother was not aware of her family history until she made

## Case Example 6.8 Sudden Death in Consanguineous Family With History of Dysautonomia—Cont'd

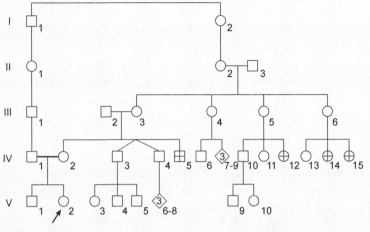

| | |
|---|---|
| III 3 "Heart attack" age 28 | IV 15 Crib death age ? |
| IV 5 Sudden death: postmeasles: age 7 years | V 2 Proband |
| IV 6 CP: hemiplegia: no speech | V 5 Premie: recurrent pneumonia/vomiting |
| IV 12 Crib death at 4 months | V 9 Brain tumor: blind |
| IV 14 Crib death age ? | |

**Figure 6.7** Proband analysis of consanguineous family with history of dysautonomia and sudden death (Case Example 6.8).

enquiries. She found that she was related to her husband and that there were three infants who had typical histories of crib death. Sudden death had occurred in one 7-year-old child recovering from measles and III 3 had been pronounced dead following an apparent heart attack, but had revived spontaneously.

## *Points of Consideration*

This clinical experience is not open to any kind of statistical analysis. But with infinite variability of biological expression, statistics have a limited role at best, and may on occasion be misleading. In these families, there does appear to be a series of patterns and their interpretation may be of utmost importance in our approach to the frustrating problem of SIDS. In the first place, if the death is from abnormal function, it is not likely to leave in its wake any evidence of gross structural damage and we find this to be the case in autopsy studies of SIDS victims.

In five families there were six infants with either minimal or no symptoms, a phenomenon with which every physician who deals with SIDS has become painfully aware. It is impossible to state whether any one of the episodes that came to light through the alarm system would have been lethal. Some would probably not have been discovered at all. However, incidents of greater or lesser severity did occur in five of the six infants who were considered to be at risk from a historical and clinical standpoint.

It has become fairly obvious that pregnancy factors are of utmost importance in predicting risk—perhaps the most notorious of all being smoking, which was recorded as a possible factor in three of these case histories. In four of the six cases, the babies had been delivered by cesarean section, but this may have been a reflection of the mothers' health and therefore has indirect importance. In one case the section was performed because of toxemia, in another for placenta previa, and in the third case the mother had passed renal calculi and had a urinary tract infection.

Within the seven families, there were 26 infants who had died unexpectedly and for whom there was no adequate explanation. Only eight autopsies were known to have been performed and in six cases the death had been attributed to SIDS. In two infants in one family (Fig. 6.1), autopsy had revealed the presence of pneumonia, although neither of these infants had had symptoms recognizable to the mother. Riley and Moore[116] reported sudden pulmonary edema associated with sudden death in a patient with familial dysautonomia, but were unable to decide whether or not it was related to the autonomic dysfunction.

Some evidence of heredity factors appears to emerge from these case histories. In each of two families (Figs. 6.2 and 6.5) there were deaths in infants by two different fathers, respectively, and in one (Fig. 6.2) there was a history of progressive neuromuscular disease. In our present preoccupation with Mendelian inheritance, this might be considered as an entirely different and unrelated disorder. However, in a biochemical sense the deaths in the infants might well have been either mitochondrial or a defect in cholinergic neurotransmission, which could also explain the neuromuscular condition. In Case Example 6.6 (Fig. 6.5) there was a strong family history of diabetes mellitus and the proband's mother was a gestational diabetic. The potential relationship between diabetes and dysautonomia has already been discussed[117] and is now a well-known complication of the disease to be considered in a later chapter. In Case Example 6.5 (Fig. 6.4) the proband's mother was reported to have experienced sleep apnea, and evidence exists that some parents of SIDS victims have reduced ventilatory responsiveness to hypercapnia and reduced compensatory response to added resistive respiratory loads as compared with parents of healthy infants.[118]

A remarkable incidence of disease is demonstrated in the family of Case Example 6.4 (Fig. 6.3) and there were two autopsy-certified SIDS victims. Again, on Mendelian lines this is meaningless, but there may well have been constitutional factors of which we are presently unaware and which yet may make sense out of this kind of family history.

The proband in Case Examples 6.7 (Fig. 6.6) and 6.8 (Fig. 6.7) had symptoms that included unexplained fever, pulmonary abnormalities, irritable personality, excessive sweating, a morbilliform rash on the chest, vomiting, unusual fatigue, abdominal pain, headache, and cold intolerance—all of which have been described in familial and other forms of dysautonomia.[119–121] Centrally mediated abnormal autonomic reflexes have been described in infants who later succumb to SIDS.[85,86]

These brief case histories indicate that sudden death occurs in some families in greater incidence. The two families in whom the probands demonstrated autonomic dysfunction are of interest, since in neither case were the proband's mothers aware of sudden death in family members. In Case Example 6.7 the mother was asked to make enquiries of her relatives and she was very surprised to find such a high incidence of nine infant deaths. In the other case (Case Example 6.8) the mother was ignorant of family history details. She was also surprised to find that her marriage was consanguineous and that there was an incidence of infants dying unexpectedly in the crib. It is by no means clear whether this indicates dominance of constitutional, environmental, or nutritional associations or combinations of all three. However, based upon what we now know about orexin, mitochondria, and thiamine, it is not difficult to imagine involvement.

## Thiamine in Hypoxia and Ragged Red Fibers

Any biochemical phenomenon that prevents the normal consumption of oxygen in cellular metabolism is referred to here as pseudohypoxia. Neuropathy and mild mitochondrial changes as seen in the "ragged red" diseases are induced by thiamine deficiency.[122] A decrease in high-energy phosphates is found in biopsies from painful muscle and the most characteristic morphological finding is ragged red fibers, a finding that can be seen in mitochondrial disorders.[123] The author suggested that this is a consequence of longstanding hypoxia. Two siblings with a mitochondrial myopathy and familial thiamine deficiency with an A3243G mutation of mitochondrial DNA were studied. Thiamine deficiency was present in the siblings and parents and ragged red fibers were noted in muscle biopsies. Thiamine therapy resolved the symptoms.[124] Perhaps this begs the question whether the mutation was acquired from thiamine deficiency or whether it was primarily genetic. It certainly emphasizes the potential relationship between genetics and nutrition.

A boy with Leigh's disease, caused by altered oxidative phosphorylation, developed his symptoms at the age of 2½ years after a minor respiratory infection. Studies revealed partial cytochrome C oxidase deficiency and an abnormal lactate/pyruvate ratio. Although muscle biopsy revealed isolated fiber atrophy, there were no ragged red fibers, raising the question of oxidative dysfunctional specificity or degree of severity in their cause. The authors reported that he had responded clinically to levodopa, creatine, and therapeutic doses of thiamine and lipoic acid.[125] It suggests that oxidative metabolism was marginal at the genetic level and a simple infection acted as a stressor, consuming energy and introducing eventually the clinical effects. Although much progress has been made in defining the biochemical defects and molecular mechanisms of oxidative phosphorylation disorders, there is limited information on effective treatment. A dose-dependent increase in ATP synthesis was reported in lymphocytes from patients undergoing cofactor treatment with therapeutic use of coenzyme Q10.[126] This emphasizes the necessity of trying to define the biochemical lesion.

The presence of "ragged red fibers" in muscle biopsies appears to be an important clue to mitochondrial disease. A 9-year-old boy developed generalized muscle weakness, growth retardation, generalized convulsions, and stroke-like episodes at the age of 5 years (mitochondrial encephalomyopathy, lactic acidosis, and stroke-like episodes, MELAS). A muscle biopsy revealed numerous ragged red fibers with excessive accumulation of lipid droplets of glycogen particles. Scattered fibers had no cytochrome C oxidase. Although the authors claim that high-dose oral thiamine administration together with a high-fat diet induced "remarkable neurological and biochemical improvement," he died from cardiac and renal failure at the age of 9 years.[127] Mitochondrial diseases have great clinical variation. A typical case of myoclonic epilepsy with ragged red fibers showed rapid deterioration with the introduction of sodium valproate that was partly reversed on the introduction of a "mitochondrial cocktail" and withdrawal of the offending drug. The authors stated that phenobarbital, chloramphenicol, and many antiviral agents are mitochondrial poisons and may do more harm than good.[128] MELAS and diabetes coexisted in a patient as well as her brother, both of whom exhibited the A3243G mutation.[129] MELAS is a progressive, multisystem-affected mitochondrial disease with unpredictable presentations and clinical course. It is commonly misdiagnosed as encephalitis, cerebral infarction, or brain neoplasm. The relationship between mutations and phenotypes remains unclear but evidence of maternal inheritance family history and a muscle biopsy showing ragged red fibers represent important clues.[130] Biotin and thiamine-responsive basal ganglia disease is a treatable and underdiagnosed disease where magnetic resonance imaging of the brain can be used in diagnosis.[131]

Two siblings were reported with a mitochondrial myopathy. An A3243G mutation of the mitochondrial DNA was found. Thiamine deficiency was present in the siblings and parents, and ragged red fibers were noted in muscle biopsies from the siblings. Thiamine treatment decreased the serum concentration of lactate and pyruvate in one of the siblings but not the other.[124] The abnormalities seen in the muscles of thiamine-deficient rats, but not in controls, indicated that motor neuropathy and mild mitochondrial changes such as those seen in the "ragged red" diseases are induced by pure thiamine deficiency.[122] Although this animal study was reported in 1975, it appears to be an important observation that certainly needs further research.

## Thiamine in Menstrual and Reproductive Disorders

The menstrual cycle in a healthy woman is a fairly regular 28-day rotation, governed by a biological time clock. Whether this time clock is influenced by outside stimulus is unknown, although it is known that women living in a dormitory tend to synchronize their menstrual cycles. For another example, it might be that the powerful gravitational pull of the moon could be an influence, since the cycle is similarly timed. Virtually nothing is known about the effects of natural environmental rhythms upon humans, but there are many examples in animals and it is not unreasonable to deduce that the unconscious response of the hypothalamus is regulated or influenced by something of this nature.

Women with premenstrual tension syndrome (PMTS) (now called premenstrual dysphoric disorder [PMDD]) develop alarming symptoms before a menstrual cycle and these are conventionally considered as psychogenic in origin. The symptoms vary from severe depression (cholinergic?) to extreme irritability and aggressiveness (adrenergic?). This may be associated with changes in breasts, varying from tenderness to formation of cysts or mastitis. This is endocrine in nature. During the menstrual flow there are often severe cramps and, since the nerve supply to the uterus is known, this must be sympathetic in character. The craving for food, usually chocolate or something sweet, that occurs premenstrually can be viewed as a maladaptive mechanism in the hypothalamus and is similar to the cravings seen in pregnancy.

During the cycle, an array of neurologic or functional symptoms include exquisite fatigue, changes in sleep patterns, postural hypotension, poor cold tolerance, coldness in the extremities, parasthesiae, urinary frequency, urinary tract infection, abdominal pain, vaginal yeast infection, pseudoangina, a sense of suffocation, nasal congestion, cardiac palpitations, excessive sweating, and piloerection (typical of sympathetic dominance). Marked extremes in the appetite may be experienced and there may be diarrhea or constipation. Such individuals are maladapted to their environment and cannot handle the metabolic stresses associated with menstruation.

The key to understanding this syndrome lies in recognizing lack of hypothalamic coordination. The frequency of yeast infection is related to this, since yeast is a predator that is able to detect the biochemical changes that are to its advantage and disadvantageous to the host. Many such women with this syndrome have "hypothalamic tongue" as described previously. It may be associated with "geographic tongue" or an increase in reddened appearance of the filiform papillae. Many women also suffer from temporomandibular joint syndrome.

It is suggested that the mechanism of PMTS is causally related to inefficient oxidative metabolism in hypothalamic control and that this explains the multiplicity of dysautonomic and endocrine symptoms. Since the brain is extremely sensitive to oxygen deprivation, or to put it into a more accurate perspective, oxidative metabolism, it is easy to see how PMTS is caused by a combination of malnutrition and increased internal stress. Treatment with drugs occasionally helps to suppress the symptoms, but only an effective approach with nutritional resources is therapeutic.

Mitral valve prolapse is not uncommon in this syndrome, probably because of the dysautonomia that is part of the syndrome.[132] The associated dysautonomia can be profound. Dr. Lonsdale observed a patient with the syndrome whose pulse rate doubled immediately on standing upright, and she experienced severe postural hypotension. She was virtually crippled and yet she had been discharged from a hospital with the explanation that "nothing was found wrong." As has been repeatedly emphasized, changes in function can be severe without there being any evidence of organic disease, and clinical observation is the easiest and least expensive way of making the diagnosis. A relatively recent and rapidly emerging state of scientific understanding has focused on the generation of free oxygen radicals. The excessive formation of oxygen in this form is considered to be oxidatively destructive in the cell, but perhaps another hypothesis might be added. If the oxygen in this form is not available to the cell in oxidative phosphorylation, the energy efficiency might be proportionately affected, resulting in the loss of cellular function. Increased rate of cellular death might then result in accumulation of organic debris, which stimulates yeast growth, since the ecological objective of yeast is to recycle organic matter.

This syndrome makes it clear that the basic reason for the dysfunction is central in origin and has a definable biochemical cause. Furthermore, many physicians know that it is responsive to applied nutritional therapy, since they have seen clear-cut clinical benefit repeatedly. It is no longer sufficient to offer the patients one of the many tranquilizers available and hormonal treatment appears only to create further problems, since hormones have their own effect in the hypothalamus. If the role of nutrition can be perceived appropriately as the source of both fuel and ignition, it is relatively easy to make the transition in concept and the idea of treating a complicated syndrome by such a simple means appears less bizarre.

## Thiamine in Neurodegenerative Disorders

In the autopsied cerebral cortex of 18 patients with Alzheimer's disease compared with 20 matched controls, the levels of thiamine diphosphate were significantly reduced in all three cortical brain areas examined. The authors suggested that this decrease could be explained by deficiency of ATP that is needed for the synthesis of thiamine diphosphate. Although the magnitude of the thiamine diphosphate reduction was mild, the authors suggested that a chronic subclinical deficiency of this nature could contribute to impaired brain function in Alzheimer's disease and might provide the basis for the modest improvement by thiamine in the cognitive status of some patients with this disease.[133] The dream enactment of rapid eye movement sleep behavior disorder (RBD) is often the first indication of an impending alpha-synuclein disorder such as Parkinson's disease. Because RBD is a prodromal syndrome of Parkinson's disease and related disorders, it represents an opportunity for developing disease-modifying therapy with the cofactor.[134]

Fifty patients with Parkinson's disease were treated with 100 mg of thiamine administered intramuscularly twice a week. This treatment led to significant improvement of motor and nonmotor symptoms. Some patients with a milder phenotype had complete clinical recovery. The clinical improvement was stable over time in all the patients.[135] Alzheimer's disease is the most common form of dementia. Thiamine levels and the activity of thiamine-dependent enzymes are reduced in the brains and peripheral tissues of patients with this disease. Genetic studies have provided the opportunity to determine what proteins link thiamine to Alzheimer's pathology.

Parenteral thiamine has been used successfully in treatment and further studies are needed. Absorption of orally administered thiamine is poor in elderly individuals.[136] This would strongly suggest a clinical trial with TTFD, an open ring form of thiamine that is reduced nonenzymatically at the cell membrane. It does not require thiamine transporters and since it has been shown to cross the blood–brain barrier, it would appear to be the ideal oral agent for clinical trial.[137]

## Thiamine in Obstetrics

The information that follows is extracted from a book by John B. Irwin, MD, FACOG, *The Natural Way to a Trouble-Free Pregnancy*.[138] The US maternal death rate is about 8–11 per 100,000 live births, suggesting 400 maternal deaths a year. Diet has long been suspected to play a large part in the outcome of pregnancy and vitamin supplementation has become standard practice. Even though many billions of dollars have been spent looking for the cause of toxemia, it is still unknown. Its incidence varies from 4% to 6% of all pregnancies and the toxemia-related fetal death rate far exceeds the maternal mortality, amounting to more than 30,000 fetal deaths a year and over 30,000 severely disadvantaged children in the United States. The majority of obstetrical lawsuits concern the adverse effects of toxemia and approximately 25% of American babies are delivered by cesarean section, mostly because of threatening fetal heart patterns. The medical community has long believed that toxemia and pregnancy-induced heart disease have no known cause and no known specific therapy other than removing the fetus, regardless of its prematurity. This book clearly describes how the author became aware of the role of thiamine in preventing or curing toxemia. By using 100 mg of thiamine a day he describes how more than 1000 prenatal patients who were given this protection had trouble-free pregnancies and delivered strong, vigorous infants with no prematurity, no growth retardation, no fetal death, no premature separation of the placenta, and no need for cesarean deliveries because of fetal heart irregularities. Philip C. Dennen, an obstetrician colleague, after hearing this from Dr. Irwin, endorsed the book. He started all pregnant patients on 100 mg of thiamine daily. In several years of practice he had a zero incidence of toxemia or pregnancy-induced hypertension.

This exquisitely simple and harmless method of prevention seems to us to be a "no-brainer." It took a few years for the acceptance of megadose folate supplementation in pregnancy as a prevention for neural tube defects. It is not difficult to extend the principle to the use of thiamine and other water-soluble vitamins in megadose form. It seems that the present dose of prenatal vitamins is far too low, perhaps because the overall quality of high-calorie malnutrition is the mostly acceptable form of food ingestion.

## HIGH-CALORIE MALNUTRITION AND THIAMINE: CLINICAL CASES

Given the diversity of symptoms resolved with thiamine supplementation, it is difficult not to be suspect of this treatment approach. In medicine we tend toward a one medication, one disease approach. How is it possible that any one compound could be beneficial in so many different disease processes? To answer this we have to remind ourselves continuously that the body requires a lot of noncaloric nutrients and when those nutrients are missing, the survival cascades that ensue are severely disturbed. When we look at the absolute bare minimum requirements for mitochondrial functioning, the importance of thiamine emerges because of its position in the pyruvate pathway and is therefore key among them.

As we present additional case studies we invite you to map the mechanisms by which diet influences each layer of homeostatic regulation, from the autonomic system down to mitochondria and back up. Keep in mind, however, that although we focus on thiamine, the mitochondria require at least 22 vitamins and minerals to function and produce ATP, to manage redox cycles and the myriad other processes from steroidogenesis through inflammatory signals, dependent on mitochondrial integrity.

### Eosinophilic Esophagitis

Eosinophilic esophagitis (EoE) is an inflammatory condition of the esophagus, causing dysphagia, food impaction, and chest pain. A minimum of 15 eosinophils per high-power field by esophageal biopsy is necessary for diagnosis. It has become an increasingly important cause of gastrointestinal morbidity in the past two decades,[139] representing the most recent form of food allergy. It is often poorly responsive to therapy and there is no commonly accepted long-term treatment. The usual treatments include dietary restriction, topical corticosteroids, gluten freedom, and an amino acid–based diet. The diagnosis has to be made by endoscopy and it is distinguished from other causes of inflammation by finding eosinophils in the inflammatory area. When we look at the constellation of comorbid symptoms, it becomes clear that EoE is more than just a disorder of esophageal function. It clearly follows a dysautonomic pattern; one that appears directly linked to mitochondrial dysfunction, with direct dietary influence. Consider the following case.

## Case Example 6.9 A 14-Year-Old Boy With Eosinophilic Esophagitis, Dysautonomic Responses, and Slowed Growth

A 14-year-old boy with EoE came to Dr. Lonsdale's attention 6 years after the diagnosis had been made and after repeated examinations and conventional treatments at prestigious institutions failed. His full case history is reported in the literature.[140] Briefly, however, the child presented with a constellation of health issues from infancy onward that extended well beyond what might be expected from inflammation of the esophagus. These included:

- An early history of repeated ear infections and asthma, which the reader should recall is suggestive of inefficient oxidative metabolism[141]
- The association of eosinophils with asthma in some cases[142]
- Hyperalgesia (a dramatic response to any physical pain producing stimulus), emotional instability, unusual fatigue, headaches, dizziness, panic attacks, and increased sensitivity to both sound and light
- An exaggerated nocturnal cough reflex
- Nightmares
- Daytime attentional deficits and hyperactivity
- Obsessive compulsive behavior
- Slowed growth

The diversity of his symptoms was misattributed to psychosomatic reactions until endoscopy was performed when he was 8 years old and the esophagitis was discovered. From that time on he had been examined repeatedly and had received conventional EoE treatments without success at several prestigious institutions. Because of the "psychosomatic" symptoms, Dr. Lonsdale suspected autonomic nervous system dysfunction. The medical history also indicated that he was addicted to sugar, and alcoholism was widespread on both sides of the family, both being related to thiamine metabolism.

Because of this family history of alcoholism his addiction to sugar, and the known relationship of thiamine deficiency with autonomic dysfunction, the thiamine testing ensued, revealing an extremely abnormal erythrocyte transketolase, proving a severe degree of thiamine deficiency or abnormal thiamine metabolism.

He was treated with a series of intravenous infusions of water-soluble vitamins that contained thiamine hydrochloride. Although his symptoms began to improve, the transketolase test became much more abnormal, suggesting that thiamine was not being absorbed into the cells that needed it. TTFD was substituted for the thiamine hydrochloride with the result that the transketolase improved greatly.

Symptoms continued to improve but the most surprising thing that happened was the tremendous growth spurt that occurred throughout a year of treatment. Body weight at the beginning of treatment was 105 lb, placing him in the 25th percentile. After 1 year of treatment his weight had increased to 122 lb

## Case Example 6.9 A 14-Year-Old Boy With Eosinophilic Esophagitis, Dysautonomic Responses, and Slowed Growth—Cont'd

(+17 lb), placing him in the 50th percentile. His stature increased in the same time period from 64.5 to 68.5"(+4"), raising it from the 50th to the 75th percentile.

From these data it was concluded that an addiction to sugar, coupled with the family history of alcoholism and the possibility of a genetically determined transport defect, had resulted in thiamine deficiency dysautonomia. His dramatic increase in height and weight suggested that his failure to thrive before treatment was similar to the failure to thrive associated with familial dysautonomia and the functional dysautonomias we described in Chapter 5. It was hypothesized therefore that the EoE represented unsuppressed esophageal inflammatory response to food allergy, particularly sugar, related to cholinergic failure of the vagus resulting from thiamine deficiency. Recall that the cholinergic neurons require pyruvate dehydrogenase-derived acetyl coenzyme A to synthesize acetylcholine. Thiamine deficiency limits this capacity for providing a mechanism for the esophagitis and the comorbid dysautonomic symptoms. Indeed, given the necessity of acetylcholine in autonomic function, perturbations by any mechanism suggests we should expect comorbid symptoms.

Although this case certainly does not indicate that abnormal thiamine metabolism is the ultimate cause of EoE, it does represent a mechanism to explore, particularly when EoE presents with the constellation of dysautonomic symptoms. Whether this was an unusual example of the disease or not, it certainly draws attention to the part played by the brain and the autonomic nervous system in producing the variegated symptoms and the esophageal inflammation, symptoms that can be linked directly to high-calorie malnutrition and thiamine deficiency.

## Disorders of the Skin: Urticaria, Angioedema, and Dermatitis

Inflammatory disorders affecting the skin when viewed in isolation are often dismissed as simple allergic reactions of some sort and treated in this way. Although dietary triggers are considered,[143] little consideration is given to the mechanisms by which diet can trigger skin reactions, beyond of course mast cell activation and histamine release. However, when viewed in the context of a wholly connected physiological system, we see an abundance of evidence linking many skin disorders to the aberrant biochemistry underlying the dysautonomias[144] with mitochondrial involvement.[145] The following cases illustrate the value of evaluating the total health of the patient when skin conditions are the primary complaint.

## Case Example 6.10 Five-Year-Old Boy With Recurrent Urticarial, Hypertonic Movements

A 5-year-old Caucasian male was seen and examined because of recurrent urticaria. Withdrawal of eggs, chocolate, aspirin, and the use of either antihistamine or steroid had no effect. A search for stool parasites was negative. Nutritional history revealed that he consumed an average of one candy bar and 32 ounces of a popular carbonated beverage every day. He was enuretic, overactive, and constantly thirsty or hungry. He exhibited choreiform and tic-like activity, which occurred throughout the examination. With hands extended he demonstrated the hypotonic positioning frequently seen in children with Sydenham's chorea. Dietary excess of carbohydrate was withdrawn and a high-protein diet offered. Thiamine hydrochloride in a dose of 150 mg per day was started. Urticaria and hyperactivity disappeared, and because of the obvious and marked improvement, the child's 9-year-old sister had her excessive carbohydrate withdrawn. As a result her longstanding insomnia was relieved.

The rapid reversal of symptoms in both children was testimony to their dysfunctional nature. Appearance of giant urticaria was presumably related to unusual release of histamine caused by excessive neurotransmission.[146] The withdrawal of excessive carbohydrate and the addition of thiamine as the rate-limiting factor in processing glucose metabolism resulted in major therapeutic benefit.

## Case Example 6.11 Eleven-and-a-Half-Year-Old Girl With Swollen Fingers, Bruising, Stiffness, Headaches, and Dizziness

An African American female aged 11½ years was first seen with the complaint of swollen fingers. Her birth weight was 3.1 kg and she was described as "severely bruised." Her early development was normal and she was receiving average grades in an appropriate class for her age. Swollen fingers had been chronically and intermittently present for 2 months and she complained of aching and stiffness in the morning that improved as the day wore on. She became relatively easily fatigued and complained of transient pains in various muscles and would occasionally have a headache, accompanied by "dizziness" and "lightheadedness." Her legs ached after running, her moods changed very quickly, and she had sudden flares of temper. Physical examination was normal.

During the next few years she was treated for eczematous dermatitis of unknown etiology, with varying degrees of success. At the age of 16 years she was examined because of increased fatigue, pain in the abdomen, and diarrhea. About 3 months previously she had started to return from school with extreme fatigue, and she would go immediately to bed, sometimes without or after an indifferent supper. The dermatitis had flared particularly on the palms and soles; her fatigue had gradually worsened and she had frequent left temporal and

## Case Example 6.11 Eleven-and-a-Half-Year-Old Girl With Swollen Fingers, Bruising, Stiffness, Headaches, and Dizziness—Cont'd

frontal headaches. Recurrent pain in the right hypochondrium had been intermittently present for 2 or 3 years. More recently she had developed severe diarrhea, abdominal distension, and constant loud audible bowel sounds.

Diet history revealed that her daily intake of "empty calories" was large, including at least one pack of potato chips, 16 ounces of carbonated beverages, 16 ounces of chocolate milk, four to six cups of tea containing one to two full teaspoons of sugar, one to two cups of black coffee, and ad libitum cookies. In a week she consumed at least half a gallon of ice cream and six chocolate bars. Sleep was restless and accompanied by night sweating, and her menses were heavy and accompanied by cramping and nausea. She had occasional stabbing chest pains.

On examination there was striking conjunctival suffusion, and her tongue was shiny and smooth, except for prominent filiform papillae. The blood pressure was 110/60 and there was absence of knee reflexes, which could be elicited only after reinforcement. The palms and soles were covered with rough, dry, scaling dermatitis. Without further investigation, she was referred to a dietician for proper dietary instruction and she began a supplement of 150 mg/day of thiamine hydrochloride. Two months later her appetite was normal and headaches, joint pain, abdominal pain, and fatigue had disappeared. Her weight had increased by 3.3 kg. She looked well and the conjunctival suffusion had disappeared. She still had an absence of knee jerks without reinforcement, normal ankle jerks, and her blood pressure was 116/50. The dermatitis had improved.

### *Points of Consideration*

The early symptoms of swollen fingers and gelling were those generally considered to occur in early arthritis. The later symptoms could easily have been those of chronic infection or early connective tissue disorder. These symptoms slowly improved when appropriate diet was begun. The underlying principles are not new. They are as old as modern nutrition itself, and the relationship between common symptoms in adolescence and ingestion of large amounts of high-calorie food is related in many cases. Symptoms such as these must raise the question of the incidence of marginal malnutrition in an industrialized and affluent society. It is quite easy to accept some of the present personality characteristics of children and adolescents as normal since they are so widespread. It must be pointed out, however, that malnutrition abuse is also widespread and little or no medical attention has been paid to it as a potential source of disease. The symptoms of functional dysautonomia are readily discerned.

## Repeat Infections, Immunity, and Autoimmunity in Dysautonomic Patients

It has long been noted that patients with familial dysautonomia succumb more frequently to and suffer more severely with common infections.[147] Similarly, common infections present difficult physiological stressors for individuals with primary mitochondrial diseases.[148] Repeat infections, however, are not often considered a sign of the more functional dysautonomias, especially in pediatrics where infections are viewed as a normal part of childhood. From a purely logical standpoint, infection is a stressor that must be dealt with to maintain survival. In cases where energy capacity is limited to begin with, mounting the appropriate energy-dependent defenses is difficult and likely to trigger dysautonomic symptoms in individuals so predisposed.

At the most fundamental level, mounting an inflammatory or immune response is a highly energy-dependent activity that necessitates a host of tissue-level metabolic shifts that include:
- A local depletion of nutrients
- Increased oxygen consumption
- The increased generation of ROS[149]

To the degree that the metabolic demands can be met and compensated for determines the severity and chronicity of tissue-level changes. Sensing and signaling those shifts in metabolism fall to the mitochondria.[3] When the stressor is significant and/or metabolic capacity is underpowered, hypoxic cascades are initiated, both of which are influenced by thiamine and other nutrients.

### Case Example 6.12 Nine-and-a-Half-Year-Old Boy With Severe Herpangina Infection and Four-and-a-Half-Year-Old Sister With Repeat Infections

A Caucasian boy aged 9½ years was examined for an unusually severe herpangina infection. Since infancy he had been seen repeatedly for unexplained fevers, colds, vomiting, myringitis, and "habit cough." Episodes were usually accompanied by extreme irritability and anorexia, and they were invariably assumed to be viral in nature, since no bacterial cause could be demonstrated. The onset of herpangina was marked by fever, earache, irritable personality, and anorexia. Bright red hyperemia of the palms of the hands frequently alternated with their being pale and cold. After a short course of oral penicillin, a multivitamin preparation was started. He was seen 3 months later, and his weight had increased by 1.8 kg and his height by 5 cm. His general health, activity, and personality were much improved. With modern knowledge this child can be seen as an excellent example of oxidative stress, resulting in hyperreflexia of the limbic system.

## Case Example 6.12 Nine-and-a-Half-Year-Old Boy With Severe Herpangina Infection and Four-and-a-Half-Year-Old Sister With Repeat Infections—Cont'd

The 4½-year-old sister of Case Example 6.12 was first seen for routine pediatric care at the age of 1 week. Throughout the next few years her history was similar to that of her brother. Unexplained fever, cough, pharyngitis, diarrhea, and croup had been treated as viral infections. She had an unusually severe episode of cough, croup, and fever of 2 days' duration treated symptomatically, but she returned 2 weeks later because of persistence of fever and cough. There was an intermittent pruritic rash and she complained of feeling cold and shivery. She developed pains behind the knees and in the elbows, a fever of 103°F, anorexia, and abdominal pain. Her palms and soles were pruritic. On examination she was pale and acutely ill. *Alae nasi* dilatation was seen occasionally, and her respirations were 40 per minute. Palms and soles were erythematous and edematous. She had lost 0.9 kg body weight in 2 weeks. Radial pulse was labile, thready, and 160 per minute. She had pronounced sinus arrhythmia and a blood pressure of 140/80. Urticarial lesions were randomly situated on the trunk, her course was acutely febrile, and laboratory studies showed mild, persistent acetonuria without glycosuria. Serum fibrinogen was 1050 mg/100 mL and glycoproteins 229 mg/100 mL (normal 110–155 mg/100 mL). The sedimentation rate was increased and C-reactive protein 6+positive. Cold agglutinins were present to a titer of 1:128 and electrocardiographic examination revealed nonspecific myocardial changes. Chest roentgenogram revealed consolidation of the anteromedial segment of the left lower lobe, and a diffuse interstitial infiltrate in the right lower lobe.

A presumptive diagnosis of *Mycoplasma pneumoniae* was made. A multivitamin was begun, and the patient was discharged from the hospital afebrile and asymptomatic 1 week after admission. Two weeks later there were no unusual physical signs. Blood pressure was 120/40. Serum fibrinogen concentration was 320 mg/100 mL and glycoproteins 123 mg/100 mL. Her sedimentation rate was normal and her weight had increased by 0.7 kg. Two months later examination revealed increased heart activity. The radial pulse was full with marked sinus arrhythmia and the blood pressure was 114/0. The femoral pulse was audible by auscultation. The multivitamin had been discontinued. Three weeks later the child's appetite abruptly decreased and she became irritable, started to yawn repeatedly, and developed a fever of 102°F. She complained of neck and head pain, abdominal pain, and unusual thirst. On examination, the radial pulse was full and 124 per minute. The cardiac impulse was forceful and visible, and the femoral pulse audible by auscultation. The blood pressure was 130 systolic with a distinct phase change at 60 mm Hg and was still clearly audible at zero. The TKA was 66.69 mU/L/min and TPPE 22.1%. Thiamine hydrochloride 150 mg/day was begun. Two weeks later the patient's weight had increased and the cardiac rate was 88 per minute. The pulse was less bounding and heart activity had diminished. Blood pressure was 116/60/30. Three months later her weight had

*Continued*

### Case Example 6.12 Nine-and-a-Half-Year-Old Boy With Severe Herpangina Infection and Four-and-a-Half-Year-Old Sister With Repeat Infections—Cont'd

increased by 1 kg and she was asymptomatic. She had experienced one episode of "24-h flu," another of nocturnal vomiting, and some brief episodes of croup. Her general health had remained otherwise good, and she had experienced less fatigue and her appetite was improved. Pulse rate was 80 per minute and cardiac activity within normal limits.

### *Points of Consideration*

The similarity in the history of these siblings is more impressive than their separate courses. The father was a biochemist who expected near perfection of his children, and he had been rigid in enforcing discipline, school performance, and general compliance. This had caused severe family tensions. Repeated episodes of phenomena interpreted as viral or bacterial in etiology may have been caused by abnormal host response. The symptoms of cough, fever, vomiting, diarrhea, abdominal pain, and croup are perceived as derailed sympathetic stress responses, and unequivocal evidence of thiamine pyrophosphate deficiency was obtained by TPPE in the red cells of one of the children. Both children had been allowed ad libitum intake of carbohydrate, which was contributory. Erythroderma of palms and soles and myocardial changes have been reported in mucocutaneous lymph node syndrome.[150] Although the presumptive diagnosis of *Mycoplasma* was made on the basis of positive cold agglutination, perhaps the symptomatology represented an altered host response, which in turn was identified with a temporary defect in energy metabolism required to meet the stress of the infection. Oxidative stress was clearly at the root of the symptoms and may well have been initiated by the compulsive attitude of the father.

### Case Example 6.13 Eight-Year-Old Girl With Rheumatoid Arthritis

An 8-year-old Caucasian girl was first examined for juvenile rheumatoid arthritis, a diagnosis made elsewhere. She had been born prematurely with a birth weight of 1.6 kg. Early development was normal and she was receiving high scholastic grades. Six months previously her right knee became swollen and stiff. Fluid was aspirated and she received an intraarticular injection of corticosteroid. Laboratory tests showed no systemic effects and culture of the synovial fluid was sterile. Three months later the same knee became swollen and the joint was reported to be warm to the touch and

## Case Example 6.13 Eight-Year-Old Girl With Rheumatoid Arthritis—Cont'd

tender. Laboratory tests were again reportedly negative. Appropriate doses of acetylsalicylic acid were started, which she was unable to tolerate because of nausea.

Other symptoms reported were constantly cold hands, recurrent abdominal pain with nausea, easy fatigue, and pallor. Stiffness in the joint was more marked in the morning. Her sleep requirement was noticeably increased compared with her two siblings, and she was described as persistently irritable and bad tempered.

On examination she was normal for height and weight and looked pale. Filiform papillae on the tongue were prominent. The heart rate was 140 bpm and blood pressure 120/66 mm Hg. Both legs were mildly cyanotic and the feet cold to the touch. Dermographic stimulation produced obvious blanching, which was more marked on the right leg. The right knee was swollen with some patellar tap elicited and the circumference of the left thigh was measurably greater than that of the right.

A qualified dietician reported that her nutrient intake was adequate and she was counseled. Two weeks later she developed some swelling in the left knee. Examination revealed facial flush with circumoral pallor, overactive heart, audible femoral pulse by auscultation, unpredictable deep patellar knee reflexes varying from nonreactive to double in nature, and mild cyanosis of the feet and hands together with well-marked hippus of the pupils. Laboratory studies (Table 6.2) revealed an abnormal TPPE in red cell TKA, elevation of serum B12, and moderately increased ratio of creatine to creatinine in urine (Table 6.3).

After informed consent of both the child and her parents, TTFD, 150 mg per day, and a comprehensive high-potency multivitamin were started. Two months later it was reported that there was no change in her knees but that her disposition was improved. Body weight had increased by 1 kg. Recurrent cyanosis and coldness of the feet were still present. The right knee was swollen and there was about 5 degrees of flexion deformity. No patellar tap could be elicited.

Three months later she reported the disappearance of pain and stiffness and her activity included running and riding a bicycle. After 7 months she reported full physical activity without pain or stiffness and great improvement in personality. She looked well. There was a mild livid mottling of the skin in the legs. Blood pressure was 100/60 mm Hg and heart rate was normal. Thigh circumference was greater on the left, but no deformity or swelling was detectable in either knee. Red cell TKA had increased and TPPE had fallen to 1.8%. The dose of TTFD was decreased to 100 mg per day.

In the next few months it was revealed that there had been some stresses within the family, although their nature was not discussed, and 8 months after decreasing the dose of TTFD there was found to be some synovial effusion and swelling in the left knee. Urinary ratio of creatine to creatinine had again increased. The dose of TTFD was increased to 200 mg/day. Four months later TTFD was replaced by thiamine hydrochloride, 300 mg per day. General health was good and she was asymptomatic. At the age of 12 years when last examined she was completely well and free from symptoms.

## Points of Consideration

The graph (Fig. 6.8) shows the consistent fall in the urinary ratio of creatine to creatinine and Table 6.2 shows the changes in laboratory studies that were performed repeatedly. There was a temporary rise in the creatine to creatinine ratio in October 1979, which was coincident with a recurrence of symptoms.

There are a number of questions that arise from this case. In spite of normal conventional laboratory studies, could this child really have rheumatoid arthritis? Each physician who had examined her had stated this to be the diagnosis. A diagnosis of reflex sympathetic dystrophy was suggested by the obvious vascular changes that were observed. In spite of the lack of history of trauma, this seemed to be appropriate. Can this condition be a precursor to the fixed pathological changes of fully developed rheumatoid arthritis?

Was the irritability and poor disposition in this child directly related to the state of sympathetic dominance, or was it secondary? Are we justified in assuming that the undisputed personality changes seen in this condition are merely because the child does not feel well? Can the blood pressure and the overactive heart be equated with sympathetic dominance, or are they the nonspecific effects of an illness as we usually have assumed? The serial changes in TPPE were slow and this suggested that it was a biochemical phenomenon, which was adjusting, for it certainly was not a simple dietary insufficiency. The urinary studies are virtually valueless taken by themselves, but the changes that occurred serially do seem to conform to the clinical changes that were observed and may be a very simple way of monitoring the metabolic response, suggesting improved transport of creatine across the plasma membrane or its trapping as phosphocreatine within the cell.

The changes seen in folate and B12 may be purely random or related to the administration of vitamins. We have already seen, however, that these values can be related to metabolic changes that are poorly understood and are by no means a simple reflection of dietary intake.

Finally, it must be recognized that this treatment was possible in this child because the parents themselves had sought a nutritional approach and were disenchanted with the treatment that had been offered previously. They were told that they had a choice at all times of changing to the care of a rheumatologist. Much more study is required in ascertaining whether such an approach is valid for other similar cases. It also seems quite important to take into consideration the fact that family stresses may have played a part in causing a temporary exacerbation of symptoms. The course of the condition is consistent with the viewpoint that the initial stages of the child's disease was functional in nature, and that her ability to cope with it depended on whether she could muster sufficient cellular energy to meet the threat.

**Table 6.2** Lab Values for Case Example 6.13: Eight-Year-Old Girl With Rheumatoid Arthritis

| Test | April 1978 | October 1978 | February 1979 | May 1979 | October 1979 | May 1980 | September 1980 |
|---|---|---|---|---|---|---|---|
| Day creatine | 85 | 56 | 41 | 62 | 85 | 11 | 50 |
| Creatinine | 187 | 266 | 305 | 296 | 206 | 319 | 320 |
| Creatine/Creatinine (C/Cr) ratio | 0.45 | 0.21 | 0.13 | 0.2 | 0.41 | 0.03 | 0.16 |
| Uric acid | 163 | 218 | 247 | 209 | 210 | 218 | 265 |
| Night creatine | 79 | 48 | 37 | 43 | 125 | 25 | 38 |
| Creatinine | 281 | 272 | 285 | 242 | 400 | 325 | 429 |
| C/Cr ratio | 0.28 | 0.18 | 0.12 | 0.18 | 0.31 | 0.08 | 0.09 |
| Uric acid | 173 | 170 | 165 | 120 | 275 | 175 | 192 |
| Total creatine | 164 | 104 | 78 | 105 | 210 | 36 | 88 |
| Creatinine | 468 | 538 | 590 | 538 | 606 | 644 | 749 |
| C/Cr ratio | 0.35 | 0.19 | 0.13 | 0.19 | 0.35 | 0.05 | 0.12 |
| Uric acid | 336 | 388 | 412 | 329 | 485 | 393 | 457 |

**Table 6.3** Transketolase Activity (TKA), Thiamine Pyrophosphate Effect (TPPE), Folate, and Vitamin B12 Values for Case Example 6.13

| Test | Value | | | | |
|---|---|---|---|---|---|
| | April 1978 | October 1978 | February 1979 | May 1979 | September 1980 |
| TKA (42.1–86.1 mU/L/min) | 58.2 | 67.8 | 83.9 | 114.2 | 99.3 |
| TPPE (0%–18%) | 22.7 | 19.9 | 2.2 | 10.5 | 8.8 |
| Folate (4.18 ng/mL) | 7.8 | 1.6 | 14.8 | 22.0 | 22.0 |
| B12 (170–700 pg/mL)[a] | 1450.0 | 1150.0 | 1810.0 | 940.0 | 1790.0 |

[a]Cobalamin analogs removed, erythrocyte transketolase activity (ETKA), TPPE, serum folate and B12 as recorded throughout treatment.

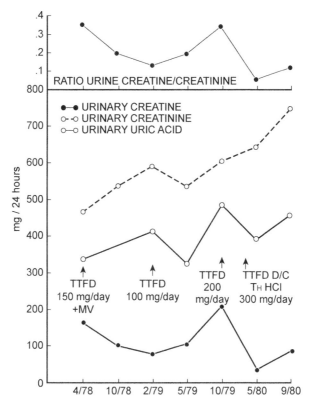

**Figure 6.8** Urinary creatine, creatinine, and uric acid for Case Example 6.13: Eight-year-old girl with rheumatoid arthritis. *D/C*, discontinue; *MV*, multivitamin; *TH HCl*, thiamine hydrochoride; *TTFD*, thiamine tetrahydrofurfuryl disulfide.

Graphs showing 24-h urinary concentrations of creatine, creatinine, and uric acid, and the ratio of creatine to creatinine. Note the sharp rise in creatine and uric acid in Oct. 1979, and their subsequent decrease after increased dose of thiamine tetrahydrofurfuryl disulfide (TTFD). Creatinine gradually increased throughout the entire treatment period, although this would also be influenced by increasing age of the patient.

## CONCLUSION

Vitamins were only synthesized in the early part of the 20th century. It caused a lot of scientific interest at that time. Vitamin enrichment of many foods was initiated, leading to the concept that vitamin deficiency had been conquered. It was natural that the scientific interest would wane, for the idea of them being used for therapy, other than replacing deficiency, was thought to be impossible. The tiny concentrations that were required in the diet were regarded as being absolute in the reaction; that any excess of water-soluble vitamins, for which there is no body storage, would simply have no effect and be excreted. No thought was given to the possibility of decline in enzyme activity from a prolonged cofactor deficiency because such a deficiency was thought to be nonexistent. All the machinery of scientific research became focused on pharmacy and the use of drugs. This was so deeply ingrained in the medical psyche that any clinical research on the subject of vitamin therapy was regarded as being fictitious or "quackery." What truly surprised Dr. Lonsdale was the reaction of his colleagues. In several cases they were able to see the results for themselves. In some of those cases the patients were considered to be beyond medical help.

The explanation by his colleagues for the surprising patient improvement or recovery was always the same, "spontaneous remission." This is a common phrase used by doctors to explain a recovery that has no known explanation. He never had a single question from anybody asking for his reasons for the approach used or his concepts of a potential explanation. A time-honored exercise in medicine has always been the initiation of a conference surrounding obscure cases. Only one of his "spontaneous remissions" was ever conferenced. It involved the case of the two boys with febrile lymphadenopathy described previously who responded to thiamine therapy. It intrigued one of the pediatric residents who presented it to the remainder of the pediatric residents. Not a single question was raised by his audience. To them it "had to be an infection and the idea of a vitamin deficiency being involved was laughable." To be "out of the box" with a new concept has to go through its ordeals of proof.

In a multiple specialty, clinic patients are classified according to the organ system in the body, which is considered to be the seat of the disease. Diseases of the heart go to cardiologists. Diseases of the brain and nervous system go to neurologists or psychiatrists. Diseases in children go primarily to a pediatrician, but if the heart is concerned in the disease it is virtually mandatory for the pediatrician to consult a pediatric cardiologist who then takes over the case as a specialist. It creates a situation that discourages a breakaway from the current "party line" of medical thinking. Nobody ever seems to have the big picture in mind, that each organ is a member of a team that relies on communication with the brain to coordinate action. It is reminiscent of the parable of the blind men and the elephant. Each blind man had a particular part of the elephant and was able to describe that with meticulous accuracy, but none of them could see the whole elephant.

In an earlier chapter we described a middle-aged woman whose case had not been recognized as being full-scale beriberi. She was under the care of a rheumatologist and it was an ear, nose, throat surgeon who knew of Dr. Lonsdale's interests and drew the case to his attention after he had performed the required tracheostomy. Dr. Lonsdale approached the rheumatologist, told her of the simple studies that would prove the diagnosis of beriberi, and asked for the case to be conferenced. The idea of this person having a classic vitamin deficiency disease in modern America was so absurd to this physician that bringing it to conference never materialized. The idea of treating disease with nutrients is not new. It was the method used by Hippocrates in 400 BC. There is still the overriding view that vitamin deficiency can only be replaced by the small doses required to replace that deficiency. It is logical to consider that an enzyme, lacking its essential cofactor(s) for a long enough time, would deteriorate in its action. Perhaps the megadose of the cofactor(s) stimulates the enzyme to recover its function. If that is how this therapy works, it would seem appropriate that the dose of the cofactor(s) would need to be reduced as enzymatic action recovers. These thoughts and the evidence that we have shown should stimulate research.

## REFERENCES

1. Pinkoski M, Waterhouse N, Green D. Mitochondria, apoptosis and autoimmunity. In: *Apoptosis and Its Relevance to Autoimmunity*. vol. 9. Karger Publishers; 2006. p. 55–73.
2. Kroemer G, Dallaporta B, Resche-Rigon M. The mitochondrial death/life regulator in apoptosis and necrosis. *Annu Rev Physiol* 1998;**60**(1):619–42.
3. Naviaux RK. Metabolic features of the cell danger response. *Mitochondrion* 2014;**16**:7–17.

4. Galluzzi L, Kepp O, Kroemer G. Mitochondria: master regulators of danger signalling. *Nat Rev Mol Cell Biol* 2012;**13**(12):780–8.
5. Johnson RJ, Segal MS, Sautin Y, Nakagawa T, Feig DI, Kang DH, Gersch MS, Benner S, Sánchez-Lozada LG. Potential role of sugar (fructose) in the epidemic of hypertension, obesity and the metabolic syndrome, diabetes, kidney disease, and cardiovascular disease. *Am J Clin Nutr* 2007;**86**(4):899–906.
6. Barrett S. The dark side of Linus Pauling's legacy. *Skept Inquirer* 1995;**19**(1):18–20.
7. Gavura S. *A closer look at vitamin injections.* 2013. https://sciencebasedmedicine.org/a-closer-look-at-vitamin-injections/.
8. Muoio DM. Metabolic inflexibility: when mitochondrial indecision leads to metabolic gridlock. *Cell* 2014;**159**(6):1253–62.
9. Reuter S, Gupta SC, Chaturvedi MM, Aggarwal BB. Oxidative stress, inflammation, and cancer: how are they linked? *Free Radic Biol Med* 2010;**49**(11):1603–16.
10. Cloonan SM, Choi AM. Mitochondria: commanders of innate immunity and disease? *Curr Opin Immunol* 2012;**24**(1):32–40.
11. Lonsdale D. Dysautonomia, a heuristic approach to a revised model for etiology of disease. *Evid based Complement Altern Med* 2009;**6**(1):3–10.
12. Ceriello A, Motz E. Is oxidative stress the pathogenic mechanism underlying insulin resistance, diabetes, and cardiovascular disease? The common soil hypothesis revisited. *Arterioscler Thromb Vasc Biol* 2004;**24**(5):816–23.
13. Pham-Huy LA, He H, Pham-Huy C. Free radicals, antioxidants in disease and health. *Int J Biomed Sci* 2008;**4**(2):89–96.
14. Mailloux RJ, Lemire J, Appanna VD. Hepatic response to aluminum toxicity: dyslipidemia and liver diseases. *Exp Cell Res* 2011;**317**(16):2231–8.
15. Sweet RL, Zastre JA. HIF-1-α-Mediated gene expression induced by vitamin B. *Int J Vitam Nutr Res* 2013;**83**(3):188–97.
16. Lin Q, Yun Z. The hypoxia-inducible factor pathway in adipocytes: the role of HIF-2 in adipose inflammation and hypertrophic cardiomyopathy. *Front Endocrinol* 2015;**6**:39.
17. Solaini G, Baracca A, Lenaz G, Sgarbi G. Hypoxia and mitochondrial oxidative metabolism. *Biochim Biophys Acta (BBA)-Bioenergetics* 2010;**1797**(6):1171–7.
18. Wallace KB. Drug-induced mitochondrial neuropathy in children: a conceptual framework for critical windows of development. *J Child Neurol* 2014. 0883073814538510.
19. Ames BN. Low micronutrient intake may accelerate the degenerative diseases of aging through allocation of scarce micronutrients by triage. *Proc Natl Acad Sci USA* 2006;**103**(47):17589–94.
20. Hainer V, Aldhoon-Hainerová I. Obesity paradox does exist. *Diabetes Care* 2013;**36**(Suppl. 2):S276–81.
21. Thompson MM, Manning HC, Ellacott KL. Translocator protein 18 kDa (TSPO) is regulated in white and brown adipose tissue by obesity. *PLoS One* 2013;**8**(11):e79980.
22. Veenman L, Papadopoulos V, Gavish M. Channel-like functions of the 18-kDa translocator protein (TSPO): regulation of apoptosis and steroidogenesis as part of the host-defense response. *Curr Pharm Design* 2007;**13**(23):2385–405.
23. Ruderman N, Chisholm D, Pi-Sunyer X, Schneider S. The metabolically obese, normal-weight individual revisited. *Diabetes* 1998;**47**(5):699–713.
24. Carnethon MR, De Chavez PJD, Biggs ML, Lewis CE, Pankow JS, Bertoni AG, Golden SH, Liu K, Mukamal KJ, Campbell-Jenkins B, Dyer AR. Association of weight status with mortality in adults with incident diabetes. *Jama* 2012;**308**(6):581–90.
25. Hamer M, Stamatakis E. Metabolically healthy obesity and risk of all-cause and cardiovascular disease mortality. *J Clin Endocrinol Metab* 2012;**97**(7):2482–8.
26. Storlien L, Oakes ND, Kelley DE. Metabolic flexibility. *Proc Nutr Soc* 2004;**63**(2):363–8.
27. Vgontzas AN, Papanicolaou DA, Bixler EO, Hopper K, Lotsikas A, Lin HM, Kales A, Chrousos GP. Sleep apnea and daytime sleepiness and fatigue: relation to visceral obesity, insulin resistance, and hypercytokinemia. *J Clin Endocrinol Metab* 2000;**85**(3):1151–8.

28. Miscio G, Guastamacchia G, Brunani A, Priano L, Baudo S, Mauro A. Obesity and peripheral neuropathy risk: a dangerous liaison. *J Peripher Nerv Syst* 2005;**10**(4): 354–8.
29. Valensi P, Paries J, Attali JR, French Group for Research, Study of Diabetic Neuropathy. Cardiac autonomic neuropathy in diabetic patients: influence of diabetes duration, obesity, and microangiopathic complications—the French multicenter study. *Metabolism* 2003;**52**(7):815–20.
30. Pasquali R, Pelusi C, Genghini S, Cacciari M, Gambineri A. Obesity and reproductive disorders in women. *Hum Reprod Update* 2003;**9**(4):359–72.
31. Farr SA, Yamada KA, Butterfield DA, Abdul HM, Xu L, Miller NE, Banks WA, Morley JE. Obesity and hypertriglyceridemia produce cognitive impairment. *Endocrinology* 2008;**149**(5):2628–36.
32. Kanoski SE, Davidson TL. Western diet consumption and cognitive impairment: links to hippocampal dysfunction and obesity. *Physiol Behav* 2011;**103**(1):59–68.
33. McElroy SL, Kotwal R, Malhotra S, Nelson EB, Keck PE, Nemeroff CB. Are mood disorders and obesity related? A review for the mental health professional. *J Clin Psychiatry* 2004;**65**(5):634–51.
34. Via M. The malnutrition of obesity: micronutrient deficiencies that promote diabetes. *ISRN Endocrinol* 2012;**2012**.
35. Thornalley PJ, Babaei-Jadidi R, Al Ali H, Rabbani N, Antonysunil A, Larkin J, Ahmed A, Rayman G, Bodmer CW. High prevalence of low plasma thiamine concentration in diabetes linked to a marker of vascular disease. *Diabetologia* 2007;**50**(10):2164–70.
36. Thornalley PJ. The potential role of thiamine (vitamin B1) in diabetic complications. *Curr Diabetes Rev* 2005;**1**(3):287–98.
37. Kaufman RE. Influence of thiamine on blood sugar levels in diabetic patients. *Arch Intern Med* 1940;**66**(5):1079–86.
38. Lonsdale D. A review of the biochemistry, metabolism and clinical benefits of thiamin(e) and its derivatives. *Evid based Complement Altern Med* 2006;**3**(1):49–59.
39. Casteels M, Sniekers M, Fraccascia P, Mannaerts GP, Van Veldhoven PP. The role of 2-hydroxyacyl-CoA lyase, a thiamin pyrophosphate-dependent enzyme, in the peroxisomal metabolism of 3-methyl-branched fatty acids and 2-hydroxy straight-chain fatty acids. *Biochem Soc Trans* 2007;**35**(5):876–80.
40. Shin BH, Choi SH, Cho EY, Shin MJ, Hwang KC, Cho HK, Chung JH, Jang Y. Thiamine attenuates hypoxia-induced cell death in cultured neonatal rat cardiomyocytes. *Mol Cells* 2004;**18**(2):133–40.
41. Banerjee PS, Ma J, Hart GW. Diabetes-associated dysregulation of O-GlcNAcylation in rat cardiac mitochondria. *Proc Natl Acad Sci USA* 2015;**112**(19):6050–5.
42. Giacco F, Brownlee M. Oxidative stress and diabetic complications. *Circ Res* 2010;**107**(9):1058–70.
43. Yu T, Robotham JL, Yoon Y. Increased production of reactive oxygen species in hyperglycemic conditions requires dynamic change of mitochondrial morphology. *Proc Natl Acad Sci USA* 2006;**103**(8):2653–8.
44. Lin Y, Berg AH, Iyengar P, Lam TK, Giacca A, Combs TP, Rajala MW, Du X, Rollman B, Li W, Hawkins M. The hyperglycemia-induced inflammatory response in adipocytes the role of reactive oxygen species. *J Biol Chem* 2005;**280**(6):4617–26.
45. Graves DT, Kayal RA. Diabetic complications and dysregulated innate immunity. *Front Biosci A J Virtual Libr* 2008;**13**:1227.
46. Xiu F, Stanojcic M, Diao L, Jeschke MG. Stress hyperglycemia, insulin treatment, and innate immune cells. *Int J Endocrinol* 2014;**2014**.
47. Manzanares W, Hardy G. Thiamine supplementation in the critically ill. *Curr Opin Clin Nutr Metab Care* 2011;**14**(6):610–7.
48. Crescenzo R, Bianco F, Mazzoli A, Giacco A, Liverini G, Iossa S. Mitochondrial efficiency and insulin resistance. *Front Physiol* 2015;**5**:512.

49. Hoehn KL, Salmon AB, Hohnen-Behrens C, Turner N, Hoy AJ, Maghzal GJ, Stocker R, Van Remmen H, Kraegen EW, Cooney GJ, Richardson AR. Insulin resistance is a cellular antioxidant defense mechanism. *Proc Natl Acad Sci USA* 2009;**106**(42): 17787–92.
50. Porta M, Toppila I, Sandholm N, Hosseini SM, Forsblom C, Hietala K, Borio L, Harjutsalo V, Klein BE, Klein R, Paterson AD. Variation in SLC19A3 and protection from microvascular damage in type 1 diabetes. *Diabetes* 2015:db151247.
51. Basciano H, Federico L, Adeli K. Fructose, insulin resistance, and metabolic dyslipidemia. *Nutr Metab* 2005;**2**(1):1.
52. Hirano T, Mamo JC, Furukawa S, Nagano S, Takahashi T. Effect of acute hyperglycemia on plasma triglyceride concentration and triglyceride secretion rate in non-fasted rats. *Diabetes Res Clin Pract* 1990;**9**(3):231–8.
53. Jung UJ, Choi MS. Obesity and its metabolic complications: the role of adipokines and the relationship between obesity, inflammation, insulin resistance, dyslipidemia and nonalcoholic fatty liver disease. *Int J Mol Sci* 2014;**15**(4):6184–223.
54. Birkenfeld AL, Shulman GI. Nonalcoholic fatty liver disease, hepatic insulin resistance, and type 2 diabetes. *Hepatology* 2014;**59**(2):713–23.
55. Pessayre D. Role of mitochondria in non-alcoholic fatty liver disease. *J Gastroenterol Hepatol* 2007;**22**(Suppl. 1):S20–7.
56. Carrodeguas L, Kaidar-Person O, Szomstein S, Antozzi P, Rosenthal R. Preoperative thiamine deficiency in obese population undergoing laparoscopic bariatric surgery. *Surg Obes Relat Dis* 2005;**1**(6):517–22.
57. Flancbaum L, Belsley S, Drake V, Colarusso T, Tayler E. Preoperative nutritional status of patients undergoing Roux-en-Y gastric bypass for morbid obesity. *J Gastrointest Surg* 2006;**10**(7):1033–7.
58. Liang X, Chien HC, Yee SW, Giacomini MM, Chen EC, Piao M, Hao J, Twelves J, Lepist EI, Ray AS, Giacomini KM. Metformin is a substrate and inhibitor of the human thiamine transporter, THTR-2 (SLC19A3). *Mol Pharm* 2015;**12**(12):4301–10.
59. Sharoff CG, Hagobian TA, Malin SK, Chipkin SR, Yu H, Hirshman MF, Goodyear LJ, Braun B. Combining short-term metformin treatment and one bout of exercise does not increase insulin action in insulin-resistant individuals. *Am J Physiol endocrinol Metab* 2010;**298**(4):E815–23.
60. Braun B, Eze P, Stephens BR, Hagobian TA, Sharoff CG, Chipkin SR, Goldstein B. Impact of metformin on peak aerobic capacity. *Appl Physiol Nutr Metab* 2008;**33**(1):61–7.
61. Wessels B, Ciapaite J, van den Broek NM, Nicolay K, Prompers JJ. Metformin impairs mitochondrial function in skeletal muscle of both lean and diabetic rats in a dose-dependent manner. *PLoS One* 2014;**9**(6):e100525.
62. De Jager J, Kooy A, Lehert P, Wulffelé MG, Van der Kolk J, Bets D, Verburg J, Donker AJ, Stehouwer CD. Long term treatment with metformin in patients with type 2 diabetes and risk of vitamin B-12 deficiency: randomised placebo controlled trial. *BmJ* 2010;**340**:c2181.
63. Chen L, Shu Y, Liang X, Chen EC, Yee SW, Zur AA, Li S, Xu L, Keshari KR, Lin MJ, Chien HC. OCT1 is a high-capacity thiamine transporter that regulates hepatic steatosis and is a target of metformin. *Proc Natl Acad Sci USA* 2014;**111**(27): 9983–8.
64. Gaggini M, Morelli M, Buzzigoli E, DeFronzo RA, Bugianesi E, Gastaldelli A. Non-alcoholic fatty liver disease (NAFLD) and its connection with insulin resistance, dyslipidemia, atherosclerosis and coronary heart disease. *Nutrients* 2013;**5**(5):1544–60.
65. Aasheim ET. Wernicke encephalopathy after bariatric surgery: a systematic review. *Ann Surg* 2008;**248**(5):714–20.
66. Gatenby RA, Gillies RJ. Why do cancers have high aerobic glycolysis? *Nat Rev Cancer* 2004;**4**(11):891–9.

67. Kim JW, Dang CV. Cancer's molecular sweet tooth and the Warburg effect. *Cancer Res* 2006;**66**(18):8927–30.
68. Senyilmaz D, Teleman AA. Chicken or the egg: Warburg effect and mitochondrial dysfunction. *F1000prime Rep* 2015;**7**.
69. Isenberg-Grzeda E, Shen MJ, Alici Y, Wills J, Nelson C, Breitbart W. High rate of thiamine deficiency among inpatients with cancer referred for psychiatric consultation: results of a single site prevalence study. *Psycho-oncology* 2016;**2**.
70. Duan W, Shen X, Lei J, Xu Q, Yu Y, Li R, Wu E, Ma Q. Hyperglycemia, a neglected factor during cancer progression. *BioMed Res Int* 2014;**2014**.
71. Picard M, Turnbull DM. Linking the metabolic state and mitochondrial DNA in chronic disease, health, and aging. *Diabetes* 2013;**62**(3):672–8.
72. Onodera Y, Nam JM, Bissell MJ. Increased sugar uptake promotes oncogenesis via EPAC/RAP1 and O-GlcNAc pathways. *J Clin Invest* 2014;**124**(1):367–84.
73. Lu'o'ng KVQ, Nguyễn LTH. The role of thiamine in cancer: possible genetic and cellular signaling mechanisms. *Cancer Genom Proteom* 2013;**10**(4):169–85.
74. Zastre JA, Sweet RL, Hanberry BS, Ye S. Linking vitamin B1 with cancer cell metabolism. *Cancer Metab* 2013;**1**(1):1.
75. Lonsdale D, Faulkner WR, Price JW, Smeby RR. Intermittent cerebellar ataxia associated with hyperpyruvic acidemia, hyperalaninemia, and hyperalaninuria. *Pediatrics* 1969;**43**(6):1025–34.
76. Massod MF, Mcguire SL, Werner KR. Analysis of blood transketolase activity. *Am J Clin Pathol* 1971;**55**(4):465–70.
77. Lonsdale D, Shamberger RJ, Audhya T. Treatment of autism spectrum children with thiamine tetrahydrofurfuryl disulfide: a pilot study. *Neuroendocrinol Lett* 2002;**23**(4):303–8.
78. Goldenthal MJ, Damle S, Sheth S, Shah N, Melvin J, Jethva R, Hardison H, Marks H, Legido A. Mitochondrial enzyme dysfunction in autism spectrum disorders; a novel biomarker revealed from buccal swab analysis. *Biomarkers* 2015;**9**(10):957–65.
79. Lonsdale D, Shamberger RJ, Obrenovich ME. Dysautonomia in autism spectrum disorder: case reports of a family with review of the literature. *Autism Res Treat* 2011;**2011**.
80. Shamberger RJ. Autism associated with B-Vitamin deficiency linked to sugar intake and alcohol consumption. *J Intellect Disabil Diagn Treat* 2015;**3**(1):7–12.
81. Blass JP, Gibson GE. Abnormality of a thiamine-requiring enzyme in patients with Wernicke-Korsakoff syndrome. *N Engl J Med* 1977;**297**(25):1367–70.
82. Rogers LE, Porter FS, Sidbury JB. Thiamine-responsive megaloblastic anemia. *J Pediatr* 1969;**74**(4):494–504.
83. Government Printing Office. *Sudden infant death syndrome: Selected Annotated Bibliography 1960-1971, us Dept of health, Education and Welfare publication No. (NIH) 73-237*. 1972.
84. Research planning workshop on the sudden infant death syndrome, US Dept of health, Education and Welfare publication nos (NIH) 74-582, 76–1014. Government Printing Office, Washington, DC, 20402.
85. Steinschneider A. Prolonged apnea and the sudden infant death syndrome: clinical and laboratory observations. *Pediatrics* 1972;**50**(4):646–54.
86. Salk L, Grellong BA, Dietrich J. Sudden infant death: normal cardiac habituation and poor autonomic control. *N Engl J Med* 1974;**291**(5):219–22.
87. Patural H, Goffaux P, Paricio C, Emeriaud G, Teyssier G, Barthelemy JC, Pichot V, Roche F. Infant botulism intoxication and autonomic nervous system dysfunction. *Anaerobe* 2009;**15**(5):197–200.
88. Berul CI. Neonatal long QT syndrome and sudden cardiac death. *Prog Pediatr Cardiol* 2000;**11**(1):47–54.
89. Lonsdale D. Sudden infant death syndrome and abnormal metabolism of thiamin. *Med Hypotheses* 2015;**85**(6):922–6.

90. Evans A, Bagnall RD, Duflou J, Semsarian C. Postmortem review and genetic analysis in sudden infant death syndrome: an 11-year review. *Hum Pathol* 2013;**44**(9):1730–6.
91. Hogan C. Socioeconomic factors affecting infant sleep-related deaths in St. Louis. *Public Health Nurs* 2014;**31**(1):10–8.
92. Li DK, Daling JR. Maternal smoking, low birth weight, and ethnicity in relation to sudden infant death syndrome. *Am J Epidemiol* 1991;**134**(9):958–64.
93. Douglas AS, Helms PJ, Jolliffe IT. Seasonality of sudden infant death syndrome (SIDS) by age at death. *Acta Paediatr* 1998;**87**(10):1033–8.
94. Goldstein RD, Trachtenberg FL, Sens MA, Harty BJ, Kinney HC. Overall postneonatal mortality and rates of SIDS. *Pediatrics* 2016;**137**(1):e20152298.
95. Naeye RL. Alveolar hypoventilation and cor pulmonale secondary to damage to the respiratory center. *Am J Cardiol* 1961;**8**(3):416–9.
96. Naeye RL. Pulmonary arterial abnormalities in the sudden-infant-death syndrome. *N Engl J Med* 1973;**289**(22):1167–70.
97. Naeye RL. Hypoxemia and the sudden infant death syndrome. *Science* 1974;**186**(4166):837–8.
98. Smeitink JAM, Fischer JC, Ruitenbeek W, Duran M, Hofkamp M, Bentlage HAJM, Poll-The BT. Sudden infant death associated with defective oxidative phosphorylation. *Lancet* 1993;**341**(8860):1601.
99. Davis RE, Icke GC, Hilton JM. High thiamine levels in sudden infant-death syndrome. *New Engl J Med* 1980;**303**(8):303–462.
100. Lonsdale D, Mercer RD. Primary hypoventilation syndrome. *Lancet* 1972;**300**(7775):487.
101. Lonsdale D, Nodar RH, Orlowski JP. The effects of thiamine on abnormal brainstem auditory evoked potentials. *Clevel Clin Q* 1978;**46**(3):83–8.
102. Read DJC. The aetiology of the sudden infant death syndrome: current ideas on breathing and sleep and possible links to deranged thiamine neurochemistry. *Aust N Z J Med* 1978;**8**(3):322–36.
103. Peterson DR, Labbe RF, van Belle G, Chinn NM. Erythrocyte transketolase activity and sudden infant death. *Am J Clin Nutr* 1981;**34**(1):65–7.
104. Barker JN, Jordan F, Hillman DE, Barlow O. Phrenic thiamin and neuropathy in sudden infant deaths. *Ann NY Acad Sci* 1982;**378**(1):449–52.
105. Gitlow SE, Bertani LM, Wilk E, Li BL, Dziedzic S. Excretion of catecholamine metabolites by children with familial dysautonomia. *Pediatrics* 1970;**46**(4):513–22.
106. Deleted in review.
107. Jeffrey HE, McCleary BV, Hensley WJ, Read DJC. Thiamine deficiency–a neglected problem of infants and mothers–possible relationships to sudden infant death syndrome. *Aust N Z J Obstet Gynaecol* 1985;**25**(3):198–202.
108. Pettigrew AG, Rahilly PM. Brainstem auditory evoked responses in infants at risk of sudden infant death. *Early Hum Dev* 1985;**11**(2):99–111.
109. Hunt NJ, Waters KA, Rodriguez ML, Machaalani R. Decreased orexin (hypocretin) immunoreactivity in the hypothalamus and pontine nuclei in sudden infant death syndrome. *Acta Neuropathol* 2015;**130**(2):185–98.
110. Liu ZW, Gan G, Suyama S, Gao XB. Intracellular energy status regulates activity in hypocretin/orexin neurones: a link between energy and behavioural states. *J Physiol* 2011;**589**(17):4157–66.
111. Date Y, Ueta Y, Yamashita H, Yamaguchi H, Matsukura S, Kangawa K, Sakurai T, Yanagisawa M, Nakazato M. Orexins, orexigenic hypothalamic peptides, interact with autonomic, neuroendocrine and neuroregulatory systems. *Proc Natl Acad Sci USA* 1999;**96**(2):748–53.
112. Dutschmann M, Dick TE. Pontine mechanisms of respiratory control. *Compr Physiol* 2012;**2**.
113. Girault EM, Yi CX, Fliers E, Kalsbeek A. Orexins, feeding, and energy balance. *Prog Brain Res* 2012;**198**:47–64.

114. Parsons MP, Belanger-Willoughby N, Linehan V, Hirasawa M. ATP-sensitive potassium channels mediate the thermosensory response of orexin neurons. *J Physiol* 2012;**590**(19):4707–15.
115. Aikawa H, Watanabe IS, Furuse T, Iwasaki Y, Satoyoshi E, Sumi T, Moroji T. Low energy levels in thiamine-deficient encephalopathy. *J Neuropathol Exp Neurol* 1984;**43**(3):276–87.
116. Riley CM, Moore RH. Familial dysautonomia differentiated from related disorders: case reports and discussions of current concepts. *Pediatrics* 1966;**37**(3):435–46.
117. Frank HJ, Frewin DB, Robinson SM, Wise PH. Cardiovascular responses in diabetic dysautonomia. *Aust N Z J Med* 1972;**2**(1):1–7.
118. Schiffman PL, Westlake RE, Santiago TV, Edelman NH. Ventilatory control in parents of victims of sudden-infant-death syndrome. *N Engl J Med* 1980;**302**(9):486–91.
119. Riley CM. Familial dysautonomia: clinical and pathophysiological aspects. *Ann N Y Acad Sci* 1974;**228**(1):283–7.
120. Okada F, Yamashita I, Suwa N. Two cases of acute pandysautonomia. *Arch Neurol* 1975;**32**(3):146–51.
121. Appenzeller O, Kornfeld M. Acute pandysautonomia: clinical and morphologic study. *Arch Neurol* 1973;**29**(5):334–9.
122. Kark RP, Brown WJ, Edgerton VR, Reynolds SF, Gibson G. Experimental thiamine deficiency: neuropathic and mitochondrial changes induced in rat muscle. *Arch Neurol* 1975;**32**(12):818–25.
123. Henriksson KG. Muscle pain in neuromuscular disorders and primary fibromyalgia. *Eur J Appl Physiol Occup Physiol* 1988;**57**(3):348–52.
124. Sato Y, Nakagawa M, Higuchi I, Osame M, Naito E, Oizumi K. Mitochondrial myopathy and familial thiamine deficiency. *Muscle Nerve* 2000;**23**(7):1069–75.
125. Čačić M, Wilichowski E, Mejaški-Bošnjak V, Fumić K, Lujić L, Marusić B, Marina D, Hanefeld F. Cytochrome c oxidase partial deficiency-associated Leigh disease presenting as an extrapyramidal syndrome. *J Child Neurol* 2001;**16**(8):616–9.
126. Marriage BJ, Clandinin MT, Macdonald IM, Glerum DM. Cofactor treatment improves ATP synthetic capacity in patients with oxidative phosphorylation disorders. *Mol Genet Metab* 2004;**81**(4):263–72.
127. Sumi K, Nagaura T, Itagaki Y, Inui K, Abe J. A case of MELAS (mitochondrial myopathy, encephalopathy, lactic acidosis and stroke-like episodes) with progressive cytochrome c oxidase deficiency. *Rinsho Shinkeigaku = Clin Neurol* 1989;**29**(7):901–8.
128. Chandra SR, Issac TG, Gayathri N, Gupta N, Abbas MM. A typical case of myoclonic epilepsy with ragged red fibers (MERRF) and the lessons learned. *J Postgraduate Med* 2015;**61**(3):200.
129. Li W, Zhang W, Li F, Wang C. Mitochondrial genetic analysis in a Chinese family suffering from both mitochondrial encephalomyopathy with lactic acidosis and stroke-like episodes and diabetes. *Int J Clin Exp Pathol* 2015;**8**(6):7022.
130. Wang YX, Le WD. Progress in diagnosing mitochondrial myopathy, encephalopathy, lactic acidosis, and stroke-like episodes. *Chin Med J* 2015;**128**(13):1820.
131. Kassem H, Wafaie A, Alsuhibani S, Farid T. Biotin-responsive basal ganglia disease: neuroimaging features before and after treatment. *Am J Neuroradiol* 2014;**35**(10):1990–5.
132. Coghlan HC, Phares P, Cowley M, Copley D, James TN. Dysautonomia in mitral valve prolapse. *Am J Med* 1979;**67**(2):236–44.
133. Mastrogiacomo F, Bettendorff L, Grisar T, Kish SJ. Brain thiamine, its phosphate esters, and its metabolizing enzymes in Alzheimer's disease. *Ann Neurol* 1996;**39**(5):585–91.
134. Gagnon JF, Postuma RB, Mazza S, Doyon J, Montplaisir J. Rapid-eye-movement sleep behaviour disorder and neurodegenerative diseases. *Lancet Neurol* 2006;**5**(5):424–32.
135. Costantini A, Pala MI, Grossi E, Mondonico S, Cardelli LE, Jenner C, Proietti S, Colangeli M, Fancellu R. Long-term treatment with high-dose thiamine in Parkinson disease: an open-label pilot study. *J Altern Comp Med* 2015;**21**(12):740–7.

136. Nguyễn LTH. Role of thiamine in Alzheimer's disease. *Am J Alzheimers Dis Other Demen* 2011;**26**(8):588–98.
137. Lonsdale D. Thiamine tetrahydrofurfuryl disulfide: a little known therapeutic agent. *Med Sci Monit* 2004;**10**(9):RA199–203.
138. Irwin JB. *The natural way to a trouble-free pregnancy: the toxemia/thiamine connection.* Fairfield, CT: Asian Publishing; 2008.
139. Dellon ES. Diagnosis and management of eosinophilic esophagitis. *Clin Gastroenterol Hepatol* 2012;**10**(10):1066–78.
140. Lonsdale D. Is eosinophilic esophagitis a sugar sensitive disease. *J Gastric Disord Ther* 2016;**2**(1).
141. Asher BF, Guilford FT. Oxidative stress and low glutathione in common ear, nose, and throat conditions: a systematic review. *Altern Ther Health Med* 2016;**22**(5):44.
142. Casciano J, Krishnan J, Dotiwala Z, Li C, Sun SX. Clinical and economic burden of elevated blood eosinophils in patients with and without uncontrolled asthma. *J Managed Care Spec Pharm* 2017;**23**(1):85–91.
143. Greer FR, Sicherer SH, Burks AW. Effects of early nutritional interventions on the development of atopic disease in infants and children: the role of maternal dietary restriction, breastfeeding, timing of introduction of complementary foods, and hydrolyzed formulas. *Pediatrics* 2008;**121**(1):183–91.
144. Cicek D, Kandi B, Berilgen MS, Bulut S, Tekatas A, Dertlioglu SB, Ozel S, Saral Y. Does autonomic dysfunction play a role in atopic dermatitis? *Br J Dermatol* 2008;**159**(4):834–8.
145. Zhang B, Alysandratos KD, Angelidou A, Asadi S, Sismanopoulos N, Delivanis DA, Weng Z, Miniati A, Vasiadi M, Katsarou-Katsari A, Miao B. Human mast cell degranulation and preformed TNF secretion require mitochondrial translocation to exocytosis sites: relevance to atopic dermatitis. *J Allergy Clin Immunol* 2011;**127**(6):1522–31.
146. Crook WG, Harrison WW, Crawford SE, Emerson BS. Systemic manifestation due to allergy, report of fifty patients and a review of the literature on the subject (sometimes referred to as allergic toxemia and the allergic tension-fatigue syndrome). *Pediatrics* 1961;**27**(5):790–9.
147. Huneycutt D, Folch E, Franco-Paredes C. Atypical manifestations of infections in patients with familial dysautonomia. *Am J Med* 2003;**115**(6):505–6.
148. Van den Bossche J, Baardman J, Otto NA, van der Velden S, Neele AE, van den Berg SM, Luque-Martin R, Chen HJ, Boshuizen MC, Ahmed M, Hoeksema MA. Mitochondrial dysfunction prevents repolarization of inflammatory macrophages. *Cell Rep* 2016;**17**(3):684–96.
149. Kominsky DJ, Campbell EL, Colgan SP. Metabolic shifts in immunity and inflammation. *J Immunol* 2010;**184**(8):4062–8.
150. Kawasaki T, Kosaki F, Okawa S, Shigematsu I, Yanagawa H. A new infantile acute febrile mucocutaneous lymph node syndrome (MLNS) prevailing in Japan. *Pediatrics* 1974;**54**(3):271–6.

# CHAPTER 7

# The Three Circles of Health

## Contents

| | |
|---|---|
| Of Stress and Stressors | 265 |
| Energy Metabolism Mediates the Stress Response | 268 |
|     The Hypoactive Stress Response | 269 |
|         *Genetic Variation in Stress Responsiveness* | *270* |
|     Hyperactive Stress Response | 270 |
|     Unbalanced or Oscillating Responses | 271 |
|     The Energy Equation | 272 |
| Reconsidering Stress and Stressors: Metabolic Mismatches and Autonomic Adaptations | 274 |
| Genetic Stressors | 276 |
|     Familial Genetic Liabilities and Thiamine With Alpha-1 Antitrypsin Deficiency | 277 |
|         *Points of Consideration* | *279* |
|         *Points of Consideration* | *282* |
|     Environmental Stressors | 282 |
|         *Points of Consideration* | *283* |
|         *Neurosis, Mitral Valve Prolapse, and Dysautonomia* | *284* |
|     Pharmaceutical Stressors | 285 |
|         *Points of Consideration* | *287* |
|     Disturbances of Energy Metabolism Cannot Be Diagnosed With Medical Hyperspecialization | 288 |
|         *Points of Consideration* | *294* |
| Conclusion | 297 |
| References | 299 |

The basic root of any disease could well be derived from three phenomena: genetic stressors, environmental stressors, and nutritional liabilities. To the extent those stressors can be effectively managed determines health. It is of course true that a genetic cause, the stress of an injury, or starvation may dominate, but the other two circles are always potentially present. The new science of epigenetics completely alters our previous concept that genes represent a fixed blueprint. We now know that they can be influenced by lifestyle and the quality of nutrition. Many common diseases can only be understood by considering all three components.

1. *Genetics*: This is viewed as inborn specifications derived from forebears and governed by an infinite number of permutations and combinations that create a unique individual. Certain design modalities emerge that may enable us to classify certain individuals within broad groups of similarity, now possible via DNA analysis. Such similarities may vary sufficiently within a family structure that a given member may respond to an inherent constitutional weakness differently from another family member. Thus it would become apparent that if one individual had psychosis and his brother had an organic disease, the two apparently clinically dissimilar conditions, their symptoms might be caused by the common characteristics of energy balance. The model allows for Mendelian inheritance as a direct cause of genetically determined disease but considers that genetic risk is but one determinant that may undergo clinical expression in relationship to the other two circles. In some instances the weakness within a given family may be a constitutional one brought about by a composite of gene action, rather than the sole influence of a single gene.
2. *Environment*: This is seen as the life journey and represents a potential for a lesser or greater degree of stress. Any one of the multiple environmental factors, whether it be infection, chemical, natural day-to-day weather conditions, or social circumstances, represents the forces that act upon, and are themselves independent of, the individual upon whom they act. Thus stress is considered to be a characteristic of the environment itself.
3. *Nutrition*: This is the fuel that provides the organized system with its raw materials. Very important questions have arisen as to whether the fuel can alter the functions of the machine and whether it truly differs from the effect of drugs, which are often considered to be highly specific. Recent work has shown that we are far from understanding the long-term implications of this, particularly with reference to our desire to maintain health rather than treat disease. For example, the work of Fernstrom and Wurtman showed that nutrition does indeed signal the brain[1] and the neurotransmission can be altered by nutrition.[2] The new science of epigenetics strongly supports this. Even the role of vitamin deficiency is clouded, since experimental work has shown the extraordinary diversity of response that can be seen, and we have not come to fully realize the implications of endogenous biochemical mechanisms in activating the ingested vitamins. Perhaps not surprisingly, there appears to be a fundamental relationship between the nature of the fuel and the capacity of the organism to oxidize it. But the results are not always predictable. For example, thiamine deficiency in rats may produce muricidal behavior[3] or may be associated with permanent penile erection,[4] not

usually considered to be classic symptoms of this deficiency. Iwata and associates reported results of animal experiments in relation to raised tissue catecholamine levels in thiamine-deficient rats.[5] It would certainly seem to be reasonably proven that an excess of simple carbohydrate can produce functional changes in the brain, but whether this applies to everyone is unknown, and it may well be shown that constitutional characteristics represent decisive factors in the nature of this response.

All three factors—genetics, environment, and diet—have to be considered at all times. Throughout the book we describe cases where one or other of the circles dominates the clinical picture, but the other two circles always appear to contribute. In fact, in some cases it was difficult to nominate the dominating circle. In the previous chapter, we demonstrated how high-calorie malnutrition can initiate new-onset disease processes or trigger latent disease of genetic origins. Similarly, we have demonstrated repeatedly how by correcting nutritional liabilities and supporting energy metabolism, disease processes, formerly thought intractable, become manageable and in some cases dissipate entirely. Here we will delve more deeply into the two remaining components of health, genetics, and environmental stressors, and show once again how nutritional capacity impacts stress response and adaptive ability.

## OF STRESS AND STRESSORS

The word "stress" is used today almost exclusively to indicate a mental response. Selye used it to indicate a physical force that requires a biological response of the organism. A successful response showed that the organism had adapted and its collapse indicated a failure of adaptation. One of Selye's students even published that the general adaptation syndrome could be induced by making animals thiamine deficient.[6] Our use of the word stress in humans is defining it as the physical (e.g., shoveling snow, virus infection) or mental (e.g., bad news, a divorce) force, initiating a message to the brain that demands an energy-consuming adaptive physical or mental reaction. A response to an acute stress input, organized and put into action by the lower, primitive brain, can be lifesaving with a genuinely critical danger.

If, on the other hand, the fight-or-flight reflex is initiated with only trivial reason because of brain pseudohypoxia and without the "advice and consent" of the higher brain, it can be bizarre. Since the reflex is below conscious level in its initiation and because sympathetic action is potentially linked to aggressiveness, a trivial grievance may perhaps explode in violence. The aggressive action may not even come to conscious notice and the affected person "sees red," a common word picture used to describe extreme anger. In Ohio a claim for temporary insanity can be used in court if the defense can provide proof that the criminal committed the crime because he or she could not help doing it. This became a law precedent in the so-called "Twinkie case" where the defense used the consumption of a sweet commercial "food" substance as the reason that murder had been committed.[7] Examples of such responses might explain some of the "inexplicable" recent events in our culture such as vandalism and even the school shootings. It is hypothesized that high-calorie malnutrition, such as alcohol, can cause a minor grievance to become inflated in an immature brain, inducing increased sympathetic brain balance. Selye throughout his writings emphasized energy as the decisive factor in the stress response. Perhaps that is the reason that British criminologists have classified current crime in the lower socioeconomic areas of Britain as a disease. It is also proposed in the action of a murderer in the famous novel by Dostoevsky, *Crime and Punishment*.

The history of early attempts to solve the problem of beriberi can tell us about the impact of stress upon a metabolic disease. As a reminder of this concept of stress, it is worth repeating the early history of the false solution to understanding the cause of beriberi. The workers in factories in Japan would take their lunch in the corridor between factory buildings in the summer months. Initially in the shade, the sun would shine into the corridor and several of the workers would get their first symptoms of the disease. Historical references also indicate that the first symptoms were often triggered by a simple infection such as a common cold. This was confusing to the investigators who naturally thought that the etiology was infectious. We now have to assume that the ultraviolet light or a virus infection acted as a "stress factor" that precipitated the first symptoms in individuals who either had minor symptoms or were asymptomatic prior to their exposure to sunlight or infection. The boy with beriberi-like disease discussed later in this chapter is an excellent example of sunlight stress induction into a situation that was inherently metabolic in character. A group of investigators in Japan have reported sympathetic nerve dysfunction in adolescent girls after immunization with human papillomavirus (HPV) vaccine.[8] There may be an indirect explanation for this. Perhaps the vaccine acted as a stress factor in a group of adolescents who either had mild nonspecific symptoms or were asymptomatic, but on the edge of a metabolic decline based on inadequate nutrition.

Table 7.1 Thiamine Deficiency and Solute Carrier (SLC) Mutations in Adolescents With Postural Orthostatic Tachycardia Syndrome (POTS)

| | Gardasil | POTS | TPPE | SLC19A2 | SLC19A3 | SLC25A19 |
|---|---|---|---|---|---|---|
| 1 | Yes | Yes | 49% | 5 | 14 | 1 |
| 2 | Yes | Yes | 48% | 9 | 16 | 6 |
| 3 | No | Yes | 25% | 9 | 16 | 6 |
| 4 | Yes | Yes | – | 5 | 17 | 0 |
| 5 | Yes | Yes | – | 5 | 8 | 0 |
| 6 | Yes | Yes | – | 9 | 15 | 6 |

Number of single-nucleotide polymorphisms recorded in the genomes of six adolescents, five of whom developed POTS immediately after receiving Gardasil vaccination and three of whom had proven thiamine deficiency. Subject #3 had POTS and proven thiamine deficiency but had not been vaccinated with Gardasil. The TPPE is acceptable between zero and 18%. *TPPE*, thiamine pyrophosphate effect.

We encountered a similar situation in a group of adolescents whose positive transketolase thiamine pyrophosphate effect (TPPE) indicated thiamine deficiency following their vaccination with HPV vaccine.[9] They were not patients, but had reached out via Internet resources. The mother of one of these young women reported that her daughter had developed postural orthostatic tachycardia syndrome (POTS) after receiving the HPV vaccine. POTS has since been recognized as a post-Gardasil reaction.[10,11] The mother had done her own research and had come to the conclusion that her daughter had beriberi. Although the daughter's transketolase activity (TKA) was in the normal range, the TPPE was strongly positive for thiamine deficiency. This mother knew of four other adolescents with POTS, three of whom had developed the condition after the HPV vaccine. Three of these adolescents had the erythrocyte transketolase test, all of which had a strongly positive TPPE. All had genetic testing and were found to have single-nucleotide polymorphisms (SNPs) in the solute carrier family of thiamine transporters (Table 7.1). From these data we hypothesized that the vaccination was a stress factor that initiated thiamine deficiency in the three individuals whose nutrition was marginally insufficient in thiamine, whereas the fourth had developed POTS from high-calorie malnutrition alone. The SNPs also indicated a genetically determined risk for thiamine. Two additional adolescents who had developed POTS after receiving the HPV vaccine subsequently reached out to us by email.

It may not be coincidental that all of these six young people were reported to Dr. Lonsdale as exceptional students and athletes before they developed POTS. We extended the hypothesis to suggest that a first-class brain requires first-class nutrition.[12] POTS has been reported following the

HPV vaccination.[13] Since POTS is one of the conditions grouped under dysautonomia, it is indistinguishable from early-stage beriberi and relies on finding evidence of thiamine deficiency for differential diagnosis.

This type of stress response is not uncommon. In type 1 diabetes, Huntington's chorea, and other diseases with well-documented genetically determined cause, the symptoms usually come on many years after birth. If the gene were the sole cause, one would expect the symptoms to show up at birth. This means that either slowing metabolism from age or some kind of unexpected stress factor contributes to onset of the disease. It is well known that diabetics often develop their first symptoms when the patient develops a virus infection such as a simple coryza acting as a stressor.[14] Now that thiamine deficiency has been documented in the course of diabetes[15] and a long list of other diseases,[16] nutrition emerges as a major contributing factor.

## ENERGY METABOLISM MEDIATES THE STRESS RESPONSE

Energy metabolism was seldom considered to be an important part of a disease process by the clinician until mitochondrial activity began to stimulate interest.[17–19] Nutritional disease other than starvation has not been prominent in the minds of clinicians, much less high-calorie malnutrition. In a highly developed society, it has been usually taken for granted that energy will always be available to an organ and almost no consideration has been given to the rate of utilization of high-energy phosphate bonds or how the stores are replaced. It is a simple fact that energy can only be created by using energy. Rolling a stone up a hill stores its potential energy, which is changed to kinetic energy as it rolls down. An archer will use the energy of his or her arm to pull back a bowstring. Energy expenditure takes place in cells to synthesize ATP. The process depends mostly upon the citric acid cycle, which provides the electron transfer chain with electrons. The coupling process that synthesizes ATP in the inner mitochondrial membrane depends upon the mechanical efficiency of the membrane itself. The storage of ATP in the form of creatine phosphate is its main source for muscle control. Thus an organ "called to action" through nervous impulses initiates ATP utilization.

It is hypothesized that the sensation of fatigue, whether it be localized to a single muscle, limb, or generalized, is through an input signal to the brain that indicates exhaustion of energy stores. Its survival value is that it warns the brain through a code that demands rest. It therefore subserves the whole organism, since the centrencephalic organization causes the system to rest either partially or totally. This is the proposal that was made by Selye, who suggested that disease was caused by a failure to adapt to a new situation brought about by stress. The advances in biochemistry made it possible to see how the energy of adaptation proposed by Selye is provided by the normal mechanism of oxidative phosphorylation, formation of ATP, and its expenditure in driving cellular mechanisms. From a clinical perspective we can consider three patterns of sympathetic function that might emerge from errant metabolism:

1. Hypoactive response with diminished sympathetic activation and/or increased parasympathetic responsiveness;
2. Hyperactive or excessive sympathetic response with diminished parasympathetic responsiveness;
3. Oscillating or unbalanced responses.

## The Hypoactive Stress Response

The following Case Example illustrates the failure of the brain to activate the vagus-mediated antiinflammatory reflex because of the patient's malnutrition and chronic long-term infection with tuberculosis.[20]

### Case Example 7.1 Sick Brain Syndrome

When I was a newly graduated resident in my teaching hospital in London in 1949, I had to admit a middle-aged man with pneumonia. He was also known to be a sufferer from chronic pulmonary tuberculosis. Patients were housed in multiple bed wards where every bed could be seen from the nurses' station at the entrance to the ward. In the morning I was waiting for my "chief," the physician with whom I was lucky enough to obtain employment. Unbeknown to me he was standing behind me and I heard him say, "Oh I see that you have a dying patient, Lonsdale." Of course, I turned around and asked him how he knew. He said, "See that patient over there who is picking at thin air with his fingers. That indicates a sick brain and he's going to die." He was pointing at my patient.

Well, of course, he died and at the autopsy not only did he have pulmonary tuberculosis but every tissue in the body and brain was filled with microabscesses caused by staphylococcal infection. The astute clinical observation made by my chief provided me with the first indication of how the brain commands the defense mechanisms of the body. From malnutrition and poverty, so common in the East End of London at that time, the capacity of his brain to dictate the necessary bodily functions was so undermined, infection was overwhelming. He never showed a rise in body temperature and his white cell count was in the normal range. In fact, there was no indication whatsoever from the laboratory of the serious nature of the disease.

*Continued*

**Case Example 7.1 Sick Brain Syndrome—Cont'd**
A few years later I was in practice in a Midlands city and was called to see a middle-aged man by two of his daughters. When I asked them what the problem was they said that he had had a cough for about 10 days and they desired a house call. When I entered the house I was confronted by the sight of this man, kneeling on all fours and extending one of his hands, picking at thin air with his fingers. He died in hospital from meningitis caused by a pneumococcus, an unusual organism for that disease. I concluded that the 10-day cough had represented an unrecognized case of pneumococcal pneumonia. The bodily defenses, undermined by lack of command from a "sick brain," had allowed the organism to spread to the meninges. Similar to the patient described earlier, he died from overwhelming infection.

*Genetic Variation in Stress Responsiveness*

An individual whose oxidative process is slow for any of multiple reasons is a hypometabolic subject, as Lejeune[21] proposed for Down's syndrome. Lejeune pointed out that patients with Down's syndrome had normal adrenergic but weak cholinergic responses, and compared the syndrome with homocystinuria—which he suggested was a hypermetabolic state. It is not illogical to consider that homocystinuria occurs when the transmethylation or transulfuration mechanisms are overwhelmed, perhaps by a fast oxidative drive. Such a condition is considered only in relationship to a specific enzyme defect on pure Mendelian lines, and perhaps this is indeed the only way that homocysteine may actually appear as an abnormal product of metabolism, and therefore perhaps an oxidative overflow marker. The important aspect may well be how fast and overactive overall sulfur metabolism is in such an individual. Folate-responsive schizophrenia has been reported[22] and this is consistent with the hypothesis that the devious behavior in such an individual might be derived from an overwhelmed transmethylation mechanism, resulting in abnormal neurotransmitter metabolism.

## Hyperactive Stress Response

If fever is a normal response to infection, what is fever in the absence of infection? In an earlier chapter we saw that fever without infection was directly related to insufficient energy metabolism, linked to nutrient deficiency. If we map that response through the autonomic system we see that the fever is centrencephalically controlled.[23] Perhaps it is the result of a false signal to the brain (metabolically influenced pseudohypoxia). It has been suggested that an infection is merely a form of stress, indicating that any other form of attack might generate the same response if the brain-controlling mechanism is hypersensitive to an endogenous signal. The possibility of psychosomatic fever would then have to be considered as a distorted and abnormal response in a patient with a continuously stressful life situation. It would be difficult to accept this with present concepts of psychogenic versus organic disease, but if it were true it could be extended to consider that leukocytosis might be possible under similar circumstances. Such a phenomenon represents a hyperactive stage in hypothalamic control. Selye's experiments certainly showed that leukocytosis was a familiar stress response in his experimental animals.[24]

## Unbalanced or Oscillating Responses

Normal defense is considered to be mediated through a reflex combination of sympathetic and parasympathetic balance with the required system dominating according to necessity. It is possible to consider that such a system might be warped either temporarily or permanently so that there might exist a state of parasympathetic or sympathetic dominance activated under stress conditions or that these two states might oscillate. In Case Example 7.2 we see how two, seemingly unrelated, disease processes, psychosis and Crohn's disease, oscillate in the same patient, suggesting insufficient energy metabolism to maintain remission in both processes simultaneously.

> **Case Example 7.2 Alternating Psychosis and Crohn's Disease**
> A young man was incarcerated in a psychiatric locked ward. He had Crohn's disease and psychosis, although the two conditions alternated. When the mental component was successfully treated, the bowel symptoms increased. When the physical aspect of his condition was treated and improved, psychotic symptoms returned. Surely, both conditions were merely complementary to each other, since they may well have been produced by the same basic cause affecting different aspects of the complete physiologic system.

POTS, mentioned earlier, is a common manifestation of dysautonomic function and we believe that we have shown that it can be initiated by a stress factor. Since it occurs as an early manifestation of thiamine deficiency, it could be cautiously assumed that energy metabolism is marginal and overwhelmed when an adaptive response is required as a result of the stress.

## The Energy Equation

Overall, physical and mental well-being represents an equation between the rate at which energy can be produced and the rate at which it is expended. Energy production depends on a number of consecutive biochemical links, each one of which would have the same net effect if it broke down. If oxidative metabolism were slow, there would be slow production of high-energy phosphate bonds, but also a fast rate of metabolism would depend upon a proper alignment of the coupling mechanisms to produce ATP. If uncoupling took place from damage to the inner mitochondrial membrane, for example, there would be rapid conversion of oxygen to water and increased heat production. Such a physiologic situation is seen in the thermogenic effect of uncoupled metabolism in brown fat,[25] which is known to be responsive to sympathetic stimulation. One can easily perceive the value of such a mechanism in maintaining normal body habitus. Excess calories can be burned off simply by applying a sympathetic signal to brown fat. Evidence has suggested that obese subjects fail to engender this normal response when injected intravenously with norepinephrine and thus they lose a significant mechanism for balancing their energy equation.[26] Since depression might be considered to be a failure of normal neurotransmission, it would provide a theoretical link between obesity and the well-known personality changes usually associated with it. It would even provide a theoretical basis for explaining the close association between obesity, diabetes, and hypertension. We have already pointed out that there is autonomic neuropathy in diabetes, and that insulinopenia is seen in familial dysautonomia.[27]

If this concept is true, it demands considerable practical knowledge of the biochemical relationships for a physician to interpret pathophysiologic mechanisms. It no longer becomes necessary to remember that a given symptom might occur in a given disease, but only how the symptom arises. For example, it would not be necessary to remember that gastroesophageal reflux is associated with the syndrome of sudden infant death—among other conditions. One could reason that the association in a particular case depended upon failure of parasympathetic action on the esophageal peristalsis, since the esophagus has no sympathetic innervation. Similarly, the erythematous rash seen on the neck and chest in nervous people can be visualized as the same rash that occurs in familial dysautonomia. It was pointed out that this rash occurred in familial dysautonomia after eating and when the patient is emotionally excited. Eating requires integrated autonomic reflex action and emotional stimulus results in reflex neurotransmission. It is deductive reasoning that suggests that the rash represents a spotty vascular response involving dilatation of some skin vessels and failure to dilate in others. It is much harder to project organ disease as a long-term result of functional dysautonomic neurotransmission but an example of this might be given from our own experience.

### Case Example 7.3 Vomiting, Psychiatric Symptoms, Atonic Bowel, and Fatty Liver

A 40-year-old woman was in hospital under the care of other physicians with a combination of vomiting and psychiatric symptoms. Studies carried out extensively and repeatedly showed that her entire bowel was atonic but that each sphincter that was visualized was in spasm. Her liver biopsy revealed extensive fatty infiltration.

The kind of fatty infiltration of liver observed in Case Example 7.3 is regarded as nonspecific but it is also seen in experimental choline deficiency.[28] Since choline is derived from the diet she could have been nutritionally deprived. If other nutritional elements were missing, for example, folate, she would be unable to transmethylate endogenous ethanolamine to form choline. She would then be unable to synthesize acetylcholine and her bowel would be under unilateral sympathetic action. Physiologically, we know that adrenergic neurotransmission will cause decreased peristaltic action and closure of sphincters, which was the chronic state of her bowel. Unfortunately, her gastroenterologist was unable to perceive the possibility of a nutritional link between "mental" and "physical" so the total medical condition was beyond interpretation by using our present orthodox medical thinking. We would suggest that this patient's erratic and hostile personality, identifying her as a "psychiatric" case by the conventional model, was caused by acetylcholine deficiency. It is obvious that her "mental" state could not be dissociated from her "physical" state, and that each was a part of a disease that was biologic in nature.

We have already discussed the emerging role of nutrition in neurotransmission[29] and it would seem that greater consideration must be given to all its aspects in both the prevention and treatment of disease in humans. If we are able to accelerate or decelerate metabolic function by appropriate mixing of caloric and noncaloric nutrients, and if the recipe produces valid

effects on the "balance" of neurotransmission, then we must concentrate on a number of related factors:
1. The physiologic balance of neurotransmission within a genetically determined individual;
2. Further information on how diet has its effect on that balance;
3. The application of broad nutritional principles to suit the genetically determined characteristics of either sympathetic or parasympathetic dominance on a "preventive" basis;
4. The application of highly specific principles of vitamins, minerals, and caloric intake to apply correction when a long-term chronic state of abnormal neurotransmission has been in effect for some time.

This overall concept suggests that appropriate nutrition is the only means we have to attempt to prevent disease. It is understood that avoidance of toxic chemicals is the other preventive that we can use, but in a world that depends so much upon industry, that is virtually impossible. It also seems that the weakness of humans lies in their voracious appetite for addictive substance over which they apparently lose control, and these are apparently harmful in much the same way. It suggests also that all is not lost if the disease process is under way, and that healing regeneration can occur if the pathophysiology can be "coerced" back into a state of normal balance. Using vitamins or other nutrients in larger than physiologic dose converts them from being purely nutrients to becoming drugs, since they are then being used to change the "balance" of neurotransmission.

On the other hand, it is also important to consider that such nutrients might be used at an excessive rate, as has been suggested in the case of vitamin C deficiency in Australian aboriginal children,[30] or that biochemical deactivation might occur, as has been suggested for thiamine in some victims of sudden infant death.[31] Indeed, there are many different ways in which effective deficiency may occur. It would seem that any disease process could be considered only in the light of genetics, environment, and nutrition, as we have tried to demonstrate.

## RECONSIDERING STRESS AND STRESSORS: METABOLIC MISMATCHES AND AUTONOMIC ADAPTATIONS

All things, both animate and inanimate, are stressed by simply being. All animals, including humans, survive by adapting to environmental changes. These are manifested by sensory information that must be analyzed and interpreted for meaning by the brain. The result, whether it be a thought process involving a decision or physical action, requires the expenditure of energy. This might explain why a complicated divorce or a failed business transaction results in some form of mental/physical illness in people that are unable to muster the necessary energy, while another person finds it merely challenging. From a metabolic perspective, a stressor exerted on the organism requires energy to withstand or reconcile. There is no distinction between a psychological stressor and a physical one. Each requires some units of metabolic energy to power a coordinated autonomic response. Absent the appropriate energy, dysautonomic responses emerge.

Although a complete collapse of energy metabolism is lethal, it is the more subtle aberrations in energetics with which we concern ourselves. A loss of efficiency in mitochondrial function that results from mild hypoxia or pseudohypoxia impacts the brain and everyday health. The automatic reaction is sympathetic dominance by the autonomic nervous system; a reaction designed to initiate activity in the face of threat. The commonest manifestations might be anxiety, accompanied by physical symptoms such as cardiac palpitations or unusual sweating. These are the normal physical reactions of the fight-or-flight reflex. The point at issue is that the reflex is initiated by mild hypoxia or pseudohypoxia[32] simply because the brain is issuing a warning of danger to its owner. In the short term, this state is beneficial, serves a purpose, and can be managed, provided the stressor does not overwhelm the organism's ability to respond and the requisite fuel stores are available. In the long term, however, and in the case where deficiencies or other stressors are present, what is originally adaptive becomes deleterious to health and survival. It is at this point we get disease.

From Selye's perspective,[33] latent disease is triggered and new-onset disease processes induced when metabolic stores are depleted in the face of ongoing or severe stressors. Whether the stressor is genetic, psychosocial, as in a stressful circumstance, or physical, as in the case of an infection, is unimportant. All stress responses demand energy.[34] Energy metabolism thus becomes the most fundamental of survival mechanisms, guided first by mitochondrial adaptations[35] and then by the higher-order adaptations in the brain and other systems. An organism's response to stress, or more specifically stressors, in many ways suggests overall health. With insufficient or inflexible metabolic capacity, the organism's response to stressors becomes disjointed and mismatched to the situation at hand. The mismatch manifests in dysautonomic symptoms, e.g., a disintegrated stress response. Autonomic perturbations thus are among the clearest representations of metabolic distress. Moreover, no matter the origins of the metabolic distress, energy metabolism can be supported and improved by modifying what is modifiable in the environment.

## GENETIC STRESSORS

Genetic risk accounts for a very small percentage of the total risk for disease onset.[36] Far from being hardwired predictors of ultimate health or disease, we find that genes, in general, are not predictive of disease and may be more appropriately considered stressors. The potential for epigenetic variation within an individual or family is such that disease expression is highly varied.[37] The discordance between genotype and phenotype is particularly broad with mitochondrial diseases[38] and when we add the possibility of *de novo mutations*,[39] the schism grows immensely. If we consider genetic health a stressor, instead of a hardwired predictor of disease, it opens the possibility that health and disease are malleable, that weaknesses can be supported or compensated. From this perspective, genetics offers clues regarding possible disease expression, but only when considered among a totality of risks that include environmental stressors and nutritional liabilities and only when considered with regard to how a particular mutation or set of mutations alters the functional capacity of the organism. Ultimately, we would argue, how the organism responds to stressors tells the tale of their health, not necessarily the particular diagnostic category within which their disease falls.

Consider the case histories that follow. The father of the first series was homozygous for alpha-1 antitrypsin (AAT) deficiency, an uncommon heritable disorder occurring in 1 in 1500 to 1 in 3500 in populations of European descent, which causes lung and/or liver disease.[40] The children were heterozygous. They all exhibited an array of autonomic disturbances, not consistent with AAT phenotype per se, but indicative of adaptive and maladaptive processes to a genetic stressor, with environmental and nutrition stressors superimposed. Each, it could be argued, exhibited a reduced capacity to meet the energetic demands of their environment. When the energetic deficiencies were remediated, that is, when the environmental stressors were reduced and nutritional support offered, symptoms improved. We see a similarly anomalous family history replete with unexplained illnesses associated with Case Example 7.4, a child with evidence of AAT deficiency. In each of these cases, symptom reduction was achieved by simple dietary remediation suggesting, even with diseases of genetic origins, energy metabolism matters. To the extent energy metabolism is supported, health improves.

## Familial Genetic Liabilities and Thiamine With Alpha-1 Antitrypsin Deficiency

### Case Example 7.4 Thirty-Eight-Year-Old Male Homozygous for Alpha-1 Antitrypsin Deficiency

A.F.R. was first examined at the age of 38 years because of extreme dyspnea and inability to function. Symptoms had been increasingly severe for 11 years and were exacerbated by air pollution. He had smoked cigarettes for 14 years but had given this up for 1 year. Pulmonary function studies showed evidence of chronic obstructive emphysema. The serum trypsin inhibitory capacity (STIC) and protease inhibitor (Pi) phenotype were characteristic of the homozygous state of AAT deficiency. He was the father of four children, Case Examples 7.5 through 7.8.

### Case Example 7.5 AAT Carrier With Fatigue, Recurrent Abdominal Pain, Dermographia

M.T.R. was the oldest of four siblings and was brought for STIC and Pi phenotyping at the age of 17½ years because of the father's condition. Both were typical for the carrier state for AAT deficiency. She complained of excessive fatigue and an increased sleep requirement. Past history revealed that she had been born prematurely with a birth weight of 2.1 kg. General health had been good until the age of 16 when there was marked increase in her sleep requirement from an average of 7– 8 h a night to 10–12 h, and she usually awakened with a sense of fatigue. The mother noted that she would return from school looking extremely tired and she would retire to bed. She had recurrent abdominal pain above the right iliac crest. Menses were irregular and associated with cramps. She experienced unusual intolerance to cold.

On examination she was pale. There was widespread hypertrichosis and the left breast was visibly smaller than the right. The pulse was regular at 52 bpm. Deep tendon patellar reflexes were unobtainable without reinforcement and there was moderate dermographia on light stroking of the skin of the legs. Red cell TKA was low and TPPE increased. Because of this she received a supplement of thiamine, although she ingested it irregularly. Three months later, TKA had increased and TPPE was in the normal range. She noticed less fatigue and felt better. She volunteered the fact that she appeared to have more energy and less fatigue when she was taking the supplement regularly.

### Case Example 7.6 Fifteen-Year-Old Girl With a History of Syncope, Headaches, Dizziness, Heterozygous AAT Deficiency

R.A.R. was first examined at the age of 15 years and 10 months. She was brought also for STIC and Pi phenotyping, which were characteristic of the heterozygous state for AAT deficiency. Past history revealed that at the age of 3 years she had had several episodes of syncope, each associated with a slight injury, a hot environment, or inoculation. At the age of 14 years she began to have recurrent headaches and spells of dizziness when she described herself as "nearly blacking out." Apart from the irregular menses, there were no other symptoms. Red cell TKA was normal. At the age of 16 years she consulted again because of near-fainting episodes, insomnia, tachycardia, and intermittently swollen right ankle. Physical examination was normal. She exhibited profound dermographia on light stroking of the legs.

### Case Example 7.7 Dramatic Personality Change, Nocturnal Sweating, Anorexia in 9-Year-Old Boy, Heterozygous AAT Deficiency

J.M.R. was 9 years of age when first examined because of a rather dramatic change in personality. Past history revealed that both early development and school performance had been normal. On a visit to a dentist he complained of abdominal pain and extreme fear. The dental examination had to be cut short because of his total lack of cooperation, which his parents felt was quite out of character. After this incident he became increasingly worried by trivialities. Two months later he had an illness involving vomiting and diarrhea for 3 days, followed by rather abrupt change in personality. His parents felt that before this incident he had been more self-assured and confident but he became hesitant and cried easily. There were repeated episodes of periumbilical pain and he became persistently anorexic in contrast to his former appetite, which had been excellent. After relatively mild exercise he was heard to gasp for air, and this also occurred during sleep. During sleep he also sweated profusely and exhibited extreme restlessness, occasionally awakening and entering his parents' room. He was reported to consume a considerable amount of candy and sweet beverages. Because of abnormal TKA he received a clinical trial using a supplement of thiamine hydrochloride in a dose of 150 mg per day. Two months later he was greatly improved, regaining his former personality traits. Craving for sweets had diminished and his normal appetite had returned. Unpleasant dreams and occasional night terrors still occurred. Profuse nocturnal sweating had decreased. After an initial weight loss of 0.3 kg he gained 2.5 kg in the next 2 months and appeared to be in good health. The red cell TKA was normal.

## Case Example 7.7 Dramatic Personality Change, Nocturnal Sweating, Anorexia in 9-Year-Old Boy, Heterozygous AAT Deficiency—Cont'd

Three years after this he witnessed a serious accident to a friend and a similar change in personality occurred. Although there was some increase in TPPE, it was still in the normal range. Physical examination was normal, although he was considered to be immature for his age. His mother reported that he was always better in his general health and behavior when he was receiving a regular supplement of the vitamin.

## Case Example 7.8 Recurrent Febrile Asthma, Dermatitis, Fatigue, Heterozygous AAT Deficiency

J.A.R. was first examined by an allergist at the age of 2 years because of atopic dermatitis, which was particularly sensitive to peanuts, chocolate, and eggs. He had recurrent episodes of febrile asthmatic bronchitis, which was responsive to epinephrine.

At the age of 10 years and 7 months he complained of extreme fatigue, sleeping as long as 12 h. He complained of irritation of the eyes, nasal congestion, intermittent cough, and nocturnal wheezing. He had demonstrated a recent tendency to crave chocolate and iced tea. Although red cell TKA was normal, it was still considered to be worth providing him with a thiamine supplement because of the improvement that occurred in his brother. When seen again 4 months later his general health was excellent. Fatigue had disappeared and he had not experienced any more asthmatic wheezing.

### *Points of Consideration*

The father in this family was homozygously affected for the ZZ phenotype, AAT deficiency, which was presumably related to his severe pulmonary disease, although smoking likely contributed. His four children were heterozygously affected since their Pi and STIC test results were compatible with the MZ phenotype (Table 7.2).

By the use of red cell transketolase studies, two of the four children were shown to be deficient in thiamine pyrophosphate (TPP) and responded symptomatically to supplementation with thiamine hydrochloride. This abnormality apparently could not be linked directly with the genetic trait since the father (A.F.R.) had the clinical manifestations of the ZZ phenotype, but whose TKA was normal. Two of the siblings with abnormal TKA

**Table 7.2** Pedigree of Alpha-1 Antitrypsin (AAT) Family

| Family Member | STIC | Pi Phenotype | Date | TKA | TPPE |
|---|---|---|---|---|---|
| A.F.R. | 0.2 | ZZ | | 70.3 | 0% |
| M.T.R. | 0.99 | MZ | July 1980 | 48.8 | 30.70% |
| | | | October 1980 | 70.3 | 0% |
| | | | January 1981 | 85.9 | 7.50% |
| R.A.R. | 0.89 | MZ | | 65.3 | 3.00% |
| J.M.R. | 0.98 | MZ | July 1976 | 64.4 | 23.70% |
| | | | November 1976 | 72.2 | 0.50% |
| | | | September 1979 | 76.1 | 11.90% |
| J.A.R. | 0.95 | MZ | | 57.1 | 11.20% |

Results of STIC, Pi phenotyping, red cell transketolase activity (TKA), and thiamine pyrophosphate percentage effect (TPPE) on Case Examples 7.8–7.12. *STIC*, serum trypsin inhibitory capacity ($N = 1.2$–$5.0$ mg/mL); *Pi phenotype*, serum-crossed immunoelectrophoretic pattern for AAT phenotype. Normal = MM heterozygous = MZ homozygous = ZZ normal TKA = 42.1–86.1 mU/L/min. Normal TPPE = 0–17.4%. Determination of STIC and Pi phenotype performed by Dr. Rynbrandt at St. Luke's Hospital, Cleveland, Ohio.

were shown to have normal TPPE and increased TKA after thiamine supplementation and their symptoms coincidentally improved. One of the siblings (J.A.R.) had symptoms that were generally similar to those of M.T.R. and J.M.R., but TKA and TPPE were in the normal range.

The important question, which cannot be answered, is whether the transketolase observations were merely coincidental or whether it indicated a biochemical relationship with the primary genetic disease. Perhaps the genetic abnormality that was so clearly expressed in this family placed a physiological burden that made them more susceptible to normal environmental stressors and/or nutrient deficiency. If this concept is extended, the logical interpretation would state that the only defense against this would be in recognition of a unique nutritional need and that this need would be more valuable when any such stress was applied. If so, then functional changes in personality might be seen only under certain circumstances and not during others, depending upon (1) individual variation within family members, (2) degree of stress imposed, and (3) quality of nutrition.

Persons heterozygous for Z, S, and rare AAT polymorphisms are often considered to be "silent" carriers with increased vulnerability to environmentally modulated liver and lung disease. They may have significantly more anxiety and bipolar spectrum disorders, nutritional compromise, and white matter disease. One thousand, five hundred and thirty-seven consecutive persons aged 16–90 years received comprehensive evaluation including testing for AAT phenotype and nutritional factors. Persons with non-MM genotype had a significantly higher proportion of thiamine deficiency.[41] White matter diseases include the Zellweger spectrum disorders, a group of diseases caused by genetic disorders in the peroxisome. Common polymorphisms that affect cell injury and inflammation include AAT. In consideration of these disorders, attention needs to be given to comorbid illnesses such as alcohol use, nutritional deficiencies, and sleep disorders.[42] TPP has been found to be the cofactor for 2-hydroxyacyl-CoA lyase, a peroxisomal enzyme involved in alpha-oxidation of phytanic acid and 2-hydroxy straight-chain fatty acids.[43] The downstream effects of a mutation in this enzyme, not yet reported, would have a devastating effect on brain metabolism. On the other hand, cofactor deficiency might be expected to produce similar effects, perhaps in lesser degree, depending on the severity of the deficiency. For example, our clinical and laboratory experience with erythrocyte transketolase has suggested that the TPPE on enzyme activity (TKA) recognizes increasingly severe thiamine deficiency in proportion to the percentage increase in its activity over baseline. It represents a shift from thiamine adequacy to deficiency. After therapeutic doses of thiamine, the TKA increases and the TPPE decreases, often to zero, indicating cofactor saturation of the enzyme. This may alter our perspective toward the effect of thiamine deficiency and may explain why all the heterozygotes in the R family had normal TKA and variable TPPE, in spite of their obvious clinical response.

### Case Example 7.9 Severe Asthma, Allergies, and Alpha-1 Antitrypsin in an 8¼-Year-Old Girl

An African American girl aged 8¼ years had a 4-year history of increasingly severe asthma and many episodes of bronchitis. Skin testing revealed multiple sensitivities. The episodes of asthma increased in severity and began to occur nightly. An attack would begin in the late evening, become worse during the night, and gradually subside throughout the following day. Occasionally, there was associated fever and at least one of these had been accompanied by a headache, intractable vomiting, and sweating. Family history revealed that the maternal grandmother had chronic asthma and liver disease of unknown cause. Examination of lungs revealed audible high-pitched expiratory wheezing, evanescent scattered expiratory sybilant rhonchi, and crepitant rales by auscultation. There was widespread piloerection on the trunk. Chest roentgenogram showed no organic changes and immunoglobulins were in the normal range. Serum AAT assay revealed a concentration of 394 mEq/mL (0–400 mcg/mL=homozygous range of deficiency). Symptomatic therapy was continued as required and a clinical trial with 150 mg of thiamine hydrochloride begun. During the next 5 months she experienced only two mild attacks of asthma and her weight had increased by 6.4 kg. The lungs were clear by auscultation and serum AAT assay revealed a concentration of 1786 mcg/mL, an increase of more than four times the former concentration.

## Points of Consideration

It is difficult to prove a cause-and-effect relationship here, but the symptomatic improvement was obvious and physical examination normal after thiamine supplementation. The change in serum antitryptic activity, performed in the same laboratory, was striking although no suggestion is made for the mechanism by which this test gave such radically different results. It is possible that the clinical improvement was brought about by modification of overly sensitive autonomic reflex pathways, improved oxidative metabolism, or membrane function (Fig. 7.1).

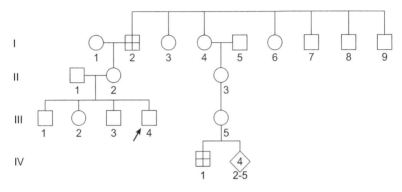

Figure 7.1 Family pedigree of Case Example 7.10 with dysautonomic trends: I—2 died: amyotrophic lateral sclerosis; I—4 diabetes; I—5 diabetes; II—3 breast cancer; IV—1 died: crib death; III—1,2,3,4 recurrent croup.

The cases represented here do not conform to our present ideas about genetic disease entities. The physical complaints are inextricably related to a loss of energy metabolism and reflect its effects on the brain, particularly limbic system and brain stem. The clinical response to vitamin therapy in most of these patients appears to indicate that defective energy metabolism, with its related inability to meet the stresses of daily living, is a common cause of disease. Genetic risk appears to be more important than a pure genetic determination. Epigenetics is seen to be increasingly vital to a better understanding of the relationship between genetics, nutrition, and lifestyle.

## Environmental Stressors

Conceptually, any force that exerts stress on an organism requiring a response should be considered an environmental stressor. This includes environmental[44] and pharmaceutical chemicals,[45,46] lifestyle variables,[47,48] and psychosocial stressors.[49] From a metabolic standpoint, each requires energy to adapt and manage. Deficient oxidative metabolism reduces adaptive capacity resulting ultimately in autonomic lability. Autonomic disturbances affect whole body physiology and thus manifest broadly. Absent an understanding of oxidative metabolism and the sequelae chemistry, too many patients are ascribed the depreciative and ill-considered psychosomatic or neurotic diagnoses. Case Example 7.10 demonstrates how a stressor, in this case an injury, sets off a cascade of seemingly unrelated symptoms that can be traced back to deficient oxidative metabolism. The autonomic response was ill adapted and in this case represented a hypometabolic response. An important point to consider is that absent an understanding of oxidative metabolism, nutrition, and the autonomic stress response, each of the symptoms would be considered as discrete disease processes if they were considered seriously at all and not designated as psychosomatic.

### Case Example 7.10 Anorexia, Crohn's Disease, Reynaud's, and Arthritis in a Teenage Girl

An adolescent girl gave a history of being well until 3 years before she presented with typical anorexia nervosa. Her symptoms began after an abdominal injury when she developed vascular changes in the legs and arthritis in several joints. Later she developed Crohn's disease, Reynaud's disease, and then the personality change and loss of weight of anorexia nervosa. Her heart rate was 48 per min and her skin was dry and cold. Capillary skin circulation in the legs was poor and she complained of feeling cold all the time.

### *Points of Consideration*

There is no medical model for connecting Case Example 7.10's inflammatory joint disease with her bowel disease, except that we know that this relationship is common in Crohn's disease. It is not possible to connect this aspect of her condition with anorexia nervosa, and so she appears to have two diseases. Using the proposed model it is possible to put it together to make one disease process. We know that reflex sympathetic dystrophy[50] (now known as complex regional pain syndrome) occurs after injury and that this condition starts with sympathetically dominant activity, which may be followed by painful swelling of joints and even lead to bone changes, including Sudeck's atrophy.[51] The reflex mechanisms then begin to affect the bowel vasculature and the patient develops Crohn's disease. The complex associations of neurotransmission led to chronic loss of appetite, characteristic personality changes, and profound weight loss as the patient becomes progressively more hypometabolic.

This patient makes an excellent example for the interpretation of the proposed hypothesis. It is true that she was under family stress of a psychologic nature and she was subjected to unforeseen physical stress, which may have created an overload in her response mechanisms, so we certainly can perceive the stress element. Her constitution, genetically determined, provided her with certain energy limitations that have to be protected by appropriate nutrition. The vicious cycle is completed by the advent of anorexia, considered to be part of the sympathetic mechanism. This, in turn, leads to nausea at the sight of food and she will get most of her survival calories from liquids, which, because of their carbohydrate nature, cause more sympathetic activity; a compensatory response to the high-calorie nutrient deficiency imperiling mitochondrial metabolism. It is of considerable importance that the only controllable condition is nutrition. Her disease, starting as an autonomic response to stress, had gradually led her to a condition that endangered her life and that had all the elements of "organic" as well as "psychiatric" effect.

From a molecular standpoint, the illness cascades are clear. Hypometabolism can be considered both a cause and consequence of the anorexia and the other symptoms. Recall that the will to eat is modified by the orexin system,[52] which is acutely sensitive to diminishing ATP concentrations.[53] When ATP stores decline, orexin neurons cease firing, inducing sleep and anorexia.[54] Receptors for the neuropeptide dynorphin, which is responsible for pain and analgesia, are colocated on orexin neurons.[55] Stress activates dynorphin[56] and dynorphin reduces orexin firing by as much as 50%.[57] Finally, orexin firing is further diminished with hyperglycemia.[58] The net result is increased pain,[59] reduced appetite, and increased need for sleep. Any suggestion that this girl's symptoms were simply psychosomatic fails to recognize the chemistry involved in human health and behavior.

### *Neurosis, Mitral Valve Prolapse, and Dysautonomia*

The diagnosis of psychosomatic disease is an all-too-common occurrence with dysautonomic and mitochondrial diseases. Dating back decades, complicated diseases, even those with clear physical measures, have been relegated to annals of neurotic conditions. In 1979, for example, Coghlan recognized the association of mitral valve prolapse with dysautonomia,[60] and this condition was designated "the cardiac disease of the decade." It has since been reported that it occurs in about 10% of the US population.[61] It is fascinating to read the important information that is to be found in these two papers, one delivered in the austere tones of the medical scientist writing for his medical colleagues, the other one more freely presented for nonmedical readers. In the second paper, the author noted that the condition had often been endured by patients after a diagnosis of neurosis had been made, in spite of the fact that some of them died suddenly, suffered documented heart attacks, or were admitted to coronary care units with severe chest pain "almost indistinguishable from the pain of severe coronary artery disease."

Coghlan noted that his own research suggested very strongly that there was failure of the "central computer" located in the midbrain, which acts as if it is unable to interpret the incoming messages accurately or unable to modulate or control the activity of the sympathetic and parasympathetic systems within an appropriate balance. He and his associates described the technicalities of their research,[60] and several interesting comments were made that are compellingly supportive of some of the ideas in this book. They listed a number of clinical abnormalities in these patients that included easy fatigability, asthenia, reduced effort tolerance, vasomotor instability, inappropriate heart response during general anesthesia, and excessive bradycardia.

Changes in the electrocardiogram included ST segment depression during submaximal treadmill testing, despite demonstrated normal coronary arteriograms and normal thallium 201 uptake by the myocardium. The defects in autonomic reflexes reported are similar to those discussed in Chapter 2 and emphasize again the widespread association of autonomic dysfunction with human disease. The symptoms are also those described in the various forms of beriberi, the prototype for autonomic dysfunction. These phenomena were discussed in Chapter 3 when beriberi was compared and contrasted with manifestations of the general adaptation syndrome resulting in animals from experimental stress. The association of mitral valve prolapse with dysautonomia has been recognized recently,[62] but we suspect has yet to be fully appreciated in clinical care.

## Pharmaceutical Stressors

Pharmaceuticals represent one of the largest categories of mitochondrial stressors in modern medicine. Most, if not all, medications and vaccines damage the mitochondria and reduce oxidative metabolism.[63–65] Some of the most commonly prescribed medications including psychotropics,[66,67] antibiotics,[68,69] statins,[70–72] and diabetic medications,[73,74] and vaccines, because of their adjuvants,[75–78] are among the worst offenders. The collateral damage to mitochondria has only recently begun to be appreciated in research circles. In clinical care, however, medication induced-mitochondrial damage remains largely unrecognized. It is quite possible that a large number of medication and vaccine adverse reactions are attributable to mitochondrial distress, particularly those reactions that appear unrelated to the drug's expected pharmacodynamic influence.

## Case Example 7.11 Vaccine-Induced Hypersomnia, Hashimoto's, POTS, and Cerebral Salt Wasting

In 2008, 26-year-old G.C.,[79] a previously healthy, athletic young woman, finishing a Master's program in finance, received the three injections of the Gardasil vaccine. It bears mentioning that 2 years prior she received several travel-related vaccines including diphtheria, typhoid, yellow fever, hepatitis A and B, the flu vaccine, and a tetanus boost and suffered no apparent ill effects.

After the second injection of Gardasil she experienced a flu-like episode with high fever lasting over a week. Full-blown hypersomnia manifested shortly thereafter and worsened to the point where she was able to sustain wakefulness for only 45 min to a maximum of 3 h per day. She experienced fatigue, muscle weakness, and dizziness. Over the next several months she developed tachycardia, intense salt cravings, with concurrent dizziness and thirst. The salt cravings led to blackouts and as she described "waves of extreme somnolence" that included slurred speech, lack of coordination, and imbalance. She learned to keep salt with her at all times. Both physical (e.g., walking, standing up, cooking) and mental exertion were profoundly draining. She reported that if she became angry or experienced any emotional event, she would immediately fall asleep. Multiple doctors had been seen and tests completed. By 2010, only low levels of vitamin D had been recognized.

In late 2010, the fifth physician seen, it was diagnosed as narcolepsy without cataplexy–hypersomnia. She was prescribed 300 mg per day of Modiodal (Modafinil, Australia; Provigil, United States). Wakefulness increased, but she was still dizzy and required multiple hour naps after any exertion. She returned to working out. By the end of 2010 she began a PhD program and was determined to "power through." She found that exercise, though difficult, allowed her to avoid blackouts. Of note, cardio-type workouts provided respite from the dizziness for 4–6 h, whereas weight-lifting netted 24 h without dizziness. Similarly, she observed that if she ate simple sugars or carbohydrates the dizziness and blackouts would return.

Six months after beginning Modiodal her health continued to decline despite experiencing greater wakefulness. She developed severe noise and light sensitivity, continued to experience dizziness, and required excessive amounts of sleep, sea salt, and water. She developed a thick, dry, painful scale on her scalp. Another series of doctors could offer nothing and suggested the illness was in her head, inferring that she "needed to pull herself together." Despite her health issues she defended her PhD in July 2013.

By October 2013 she had seen 10 physicians as her health continued to decline. She read our work on post-Gardasil thyroid dysfunction[80–82] and other adverse reactions and requested additional testing. Hashimoto's, hypogammaglobulinemia, vitamin B deficiencies, and low potassium levels were identified. On several occasions she attempted to get transketolase testing but was unsuccessful. In Nov. 2013 she decided to treat empirically beginning with 100 mg thiamine tetrahydrofurfuryl disulfide (TTFD). She subsequently developed the paradoxical reactions discussed in Chapter 4, with her symptoms worsening.

### Case Example 7.11 Vaccine-Induced Hypersomnia, Hashimoto's, POTS, and Cerebral Salt Wasting—Cont'd

With the dizziness and increased heart rate she reduced her dose to 50 mg of TTFD. Over the course of the next 5 weeks, the tachycardia landed her in hospital on four occasions. By December 2013 her body adjusted to the dosage of TTFD and the tachycardia and dizziness subsided. This is important to note. Long-term dysfunction of this nature requires new knowledge from the physician. Though not damaging to the patient it is regarded as "side effects" and either the patient or the physician stops the treatment. This effect was known to the ancient Chinese and regarded as examples of yin and yang by acupuncturists.

Over the course of the 5 years of progressively declining health she saw a total of 24 doctors. None of whom was able to identify or treat what was ultimately a metabolic disturbance brought on by thiamine deficiency that was likely triggered by the vaccine. Her final diagnoses included cerebral salt wasting, POTS, beriberi, hypersomnia, and Hashimoto's. Arguably, the thiamine deficiency and the mitochondrial damage that ensued were at the root of each of these diagnoses.

Since 2013 she has continued to maintain her health with thiamine, magnesium, and a cocktail of other mitochondrial supplements (which included very high doses of coenzyme Q10), along with thyroxine for Hashimoto's and Modiodal to treat the somnolence. As of this writing she is doing well, training in various Asian forms of kickboxing daily and working full time. Without the balance of heavy training, the cocktail of supplements, the Modiodal, and thyroxine, her symptoms reappear. It is a brilliant management system of the underlying condition that she was able to develop overtime. She indicates that she is unable to carry a pregnancy through because of the difficulty in energy management and the potential toxicity to a fetus of the Modiodal, without which she cannot function.

### *Points of Consideration*

This is an example of cerebral salt-wasting disease, one of the rare manifestations of dysautonomia. After the second injection of the vaccine she developed fever that lasted for a week and this is not an uncommon association with this vaccine, suggesting the first stress impact on the brain. This was soon followed by extreme hypersomnia, indicating failure of the hypocretin/orexin system. What followed was years of polysymptomatic disease and it is not surprising that the various doctors had repeatedly told her that it was "all in her head," because they had a complete lack of understanding concerning the reality of the pathophysiological situation. Because hypersomnia was initiated by some emotional event and blackouts could occur if she was unable to satisfy her salt craving, medical ignorance tended to confirm in their minds that this was psychosomatic. Notice that the dizziness and blackouts would return if she consumed sugar, strongly suggesting the catatorulin effect described by Peters.[83] Although she was never able to prove thiamine deficiency or lack of homeostasis, her response to TTFD suggested its implication and its potential benefit in what surely amounts to an exhibition of a stress insult causing mitochondrial dysfunction. We have mentioned previously that a high rate of intelligence, because of the energy requirement of the brain, is an additional risk factor. This woman is known to be a world traveler in the field of finance and economics.

## Disturbances of Energy Metabolism Cannot Be Diagnosed With Medical Hyperspecialization

Part of the difficulty in recognizing metabolic disorders is the current overspecialization of medical practice that forces us to compartmentalize disease to the affected tissues. When a patient visits his or her physician because of periodic heart palpitations, the physician's emphasis is placed on the heart as the seat of the problem, often without considering that the heart is innervated by the autonomic nervous system that could be the underlying cause. It is treated as a symptom and a medication is offered. Even if a diet history is taken by the physician, including alcohol consumption, the patient is seldom asked specifically about his or her ingestion of sugar, carbonated beverages, candy, or doughnuts. These are often consumed as an accompaniment to social activities and may in some cases be the source of high-calorie malnutrition.

Physical examination includes blood pressure, almost invariably taken on one arm only. Dysautonomic function, caused by inefficient oxidative metabolism, can produce widely different brachial blood pressures in the two arms when measured simultaneously by two operators. In fact, it would suggest that if the blood pressure were measured on one arm, the patient would leave the office with antihypertensive medication, whereas if it were measured on the other arm, no such medication would be prescribed.

Hyperexcitable deep tendon reflexes or their absence, being common findings in dysautonomia, might well lead to extensive neurological testing. A simple test is by eliciting an axon reflex. In many cases of dysautonomia seen by Dr. Lonsdale, a stroke of the inner side of the thigh and lower leg with the tip of a finger would cause blanching in the track of the finger that could be easily seen as white dermographia. It would last for a few minutes and gradually fade. In many cases the femoral artery could be heard by auscultation over the inguinal ligament.

Supposing the primary doctor finds evidence of neurological disease, the patient is referred to a neurologist. The patient volunteers the information that he also has diarrhea. The neurologist will say that this is out of his expertise and the patient is referred to a gastroenterologist. This shifting of medical responsibility often confuses the issue and adds to the mounting expense of practice. Importantly, it enforces an artificial compartmentalization of disease that is fundamentally incapable of recognizing causative factors spanning multiple organ systems; factors like a deficient oxidative metabolism that present as dysautonomic chaos. Consider the preceding case, perhaps one of the most troubling cases of Dr. Lonsdale's career.

### Case Example 7.12 Shoshin Beriberi and Cardiac Collapse in a Teenage Boy

The following case needs an introduction. The child was a puzzle from birth. It was only later in retrospect that Dr. Lonsdale was able to perceive the polysymptomatic nature of thiamine deficiency or abnormal homeostasis. The repeated episodes of gastroenteritis throughout childhood were metabolic in nature and if they had been treated with thiamine at that stage the later symptomatic disasters could have been avoided. It must be emphasized that after one of these episodes at the age of 16 years, now adolescent, his parents took him on a picnic in mountainous terrain where there would be a depreciation in oxygen concentration. It was the combination of this and his exposure to sunshine (ultraviolet stress) that caused the onset of hemiplegia, marking the first evidence of energy deficiency in the brain.

Notice that in our description of beriberi symptoms in a previous chapter, groups of workers developed their first symptoms of beriberi when suddenly exposed to sunlight. Also notice that he recovered the hemiplegia on his way to the hospital when he was exposed to the comfort of an air-conditioned car. On his arrival at the hospital they were surprised to find a grossly enlarged heart, obviously a cause of confusion in view of the history of a sudden self-resolving hemiplegia. He was transferred to Cleveland Clinic where the cardiologists refused to consider Dr. Lonsdale's startling diagnosis of beriberi. His initial response to an injection of thiamine hydrochloride was ignored by the cardiologists who were treating him with standard care drugs, to which they owed his improvement next day. Even when his response to TTFD later showed normalization of the heart shadow, there was still no interest by them. Yes, his final cardiac relapse from what appeared to be TTFD resistance remained a mystery, but in retrospect it may well have been that magnesium was required to complete the cofactorship. This child died because of collective ignorance. However, his death was not in vain because of the knowledge gained from the course of his disease. Here is the case report.

A 6-year-old white male was examined because of poor motor coordination. At birth the maternal liquor had been meconium stained (evidence of hypoxia). His birth weight was 2.5 kg. Spontaneous respirations were delayed and cyanosis was noted initially. Throughout the neonatal period he was irritable; he sat up at

*Continued*

### Case Example 7.12 Shoshin Beriberi and Cardiac Collapse in a Teenage Boy—Cont'd

10 months, walked at 22 months, and talked indistinctly at 2 years. Hyperactivity, short attention span, sound sensitivity, and periodic asthmatic wheezing became apparent in early childhood (all evidence of lower brain dysfunction). Family history revealed that the paternal grandmother was diabetic (?genetic effect). On examination the child overreacted to all stimuli. Echolalia and hyperactive deep tendon reflexes were observed, and psychological examination revealed an IQ of 73 on the Stanford–Binet Form L-M.

At the age of 12 years he was examined again because of coughing and coffee-ground vomiting (evidence of beriberi). Previous history disclosed similar episodes for the previous 2 years and for which no cause had been determined. Malena and hematemesis were reported in one of these. On examination the pulse was 100 and blood pressure 140/90. There was a grade II systolic murmur at the pulmonic base. There was a striking lack of body hair, a morbilliform rash (dysautonomia) on the anterior chest, and some well-marked dermographia. No ulceration of the bowel could be detected by roentgenography. Some increase in ground-glass clotting time was revealed, but it was not studied further, and glucose tolerance showed a fasting concentration of 114 mg/100 mL, 170 at 1 h and 150 mg/100 at 2 h (hyperglycemia). There was no glycosuria. The electroencephalogram was nonspecifically abnormal. Chest roentgenogram revealed a normal heart shadow.

At 16 years of age he was admitted to a hospital with a transient right hemiplegia. Two weeks previously he had had a severe episode of anorexia, lethargy, diarrhea, vomiting, abdominal pain, and cardiac palpitations. Ten days later, recovery seemed complete and a family picnic took him into mountainous terrain. He complained of malaise, and while sitting at a table in hot sunshine he suddenly complained of feeling dizzy and tried to stand up. Slurred speech, oculogyria, and ataxia (beriberi) were described. Weakness in the right arm and leg were accompanied by left facial weakness and drooling. During transmission to hospital in an air-conditioned car the hemiplegia disappeared within 20 min. While in hospital he was febrile and developed generalized giant urticaria. An enlarged heart was revealed by roentgenography. He was discharged home after 3 days but complained of a severe "pinching" in the chest, and so the parents brought him to Cleveland Clinic for further examination. On examination he was acutely ill and orthopneic. There was intermittent dilatation of alae nasi and a repetitive dry cough (hypoxic accentuated reflex). Respirations were 40 and pulse 140 per min with many dropped beats. Auscultation of the heart revealed muffled heart sounds and gallop rhythm. Roentgenography revealed cardiomegaly (Fig. 7.2A).

Thiamine-deficient beriberi should be considered a "great imitator" of diseases because it results in energy deficit and dysautonomia in its early stages. Thiamine enters into the pathology of many neurodegenerative diseases. It may represent the underlying cause of permanent damage when the early manifestations are treated symptomatically without recognizing their basic etiology.

## Case Example 7.12 Shoshin Beriberi and Cardiac Collapse in a Teenage Boy—Cont'd

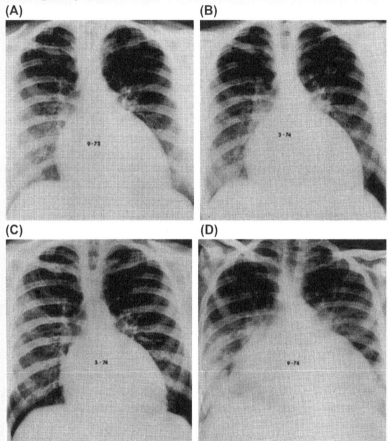

**Figure 7.2** (A) September 1973, PA chest demonstrating generalized cardiomegaly (Case Example 7.12). (B) March 1974, PA chest demonstrating further cardiac enlargement, small right-sided pleural effusion and prominence of pulmonary vasculature. (C) May 1974, PA chest demonstrating decrease in cardiac size and less vascular engorgement 2 months after commencing thiamine tetrahydrofurfuryl disulfide (TTFD). (D) September 1974, portable AP supine chest demonstrating massive cardiomegaly and pulmonary edema. *AP*, anterior-posterior; *PA*, posterior-anterior (Case Example 7.12).

There is little doubt that this boy represented an unknown disease, possibly inherited or acquired and severely affecting energy metabolism. Because the cardiac condition was mindful of beriberi, 100 mg of thiamine hydrochloride was given by intramuscular injection as well as the usual treatment from a

*Continued*

## Case Example 7.12 Shoshin Beriberi and Cardiac Collapse in a Teenage Boy—Cont'd

cardiologist with digitalis and diuretic. On the following day, respirations were 36 per min and the pulse 100 to 130 per min and regular. He was less distressed. Improvement was accompanied by diuresis. During the next few days he improved steadily and he was discharged from hospital without further study.

He returned 2 weeks later with the main complaint of recurrent acute "pinching" chest pain. He had experienced increased sweating and orthopnea. He was apprehensive, wheezing, and pitting edema was observed over the sacrum and ankles. The fingernail beds were cyanotic. Electrocardiography revealed myocardial changes (Fig. 7.2B). During the next few months there were repeated admissions to hospital. He complained increasingly of a "thumping" epigastric pain, nausea, vomiting, intermittent diarrhea, and sweating, and it was apparent that his cardiac condition was slowly progressive. Hypokalemia was frequent and potassium supplements were given (hypokalemia occurs in thiamine deficiency). In spite of an improved appetite he lost 7 kg in weight (loss of edema). He continued to experience premature auricular contractions and the pulse was bigeminal. After 6 months there was rapid clinical deterioration. Recurrent episodes of chest and epigastric pain, vomiting, diarrhea, constant sweating, and irritating cough were accompanied by increasing heart size (Fig. 7.3A). Gallop rhythm, hepatomegaly, peripheral cyanosis, and edema testified to the cardiac status. The constant state of anxiety and sensitivity to sound prevailed. Hemoglobin concentration was 17.2 gm/100 mL and hypokalemia was persistent. All relevant laboratory studies are shown in Tables 7.2 and 7.3. Viral studies were negative.

Within a month the patient's condition was critical again. He had massive carotid pulsation in the neck, audible sounds by auscultation of the femoral artery in the inguinal region, and pounding of the chest wall. Dyspnea and extreme restlessness of the patient were typical of the Shoshin form of beriberi. The parents gave informed consent for the use of TTFD and the drug was started in a dose of 150 mg a day. His general condition rapidly improved. Carotid pulsations ceased and there was no dyspnea or restlessness within several days. Diuresis occurred and there was a striking loss of weight. This therapeutic response suggested that the disease had a metabolic etiology related to thiamine metabolism. Electromyography showed diffuse muscle irritability or active denervation in almost every muscle in the lower extremity, much more abundant in the vastus lateralis and in two proximal upper extremity muscles. The changes suggested a combination of chronic neurogenic and upper motor neuron abnormality, although there were spotty changes in a few lower extremity muscles, which appeared to be those of myopathy. A muscle biopsy from the right biceps showed a group (denervation) atrophy. There was some decrease in the number of fibers in the intramuscular nerves and increased connective

## Case Example 7.12 Shoshin Beriberi and Cardiac Collapse in a Teenage Boy—Cont'd

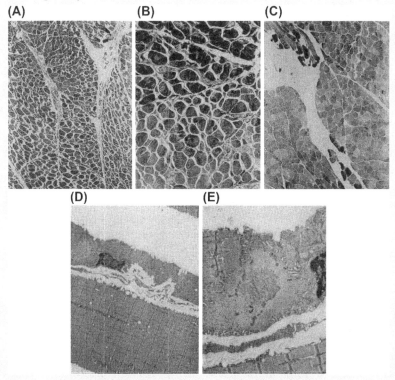

**Figure 7.3** (A) Right biceps muscle biopsy: small group and perifascicular muscle fiber atrophy (paraffin, H&E, original magnification ×64). (B) Right biceps muscle biopsy: small group and single muscle fiber atrophy. Intramuscular nerve twigs show increased endoneurial connective tissue (paraffin, H&E, original magnification ×160). (C) Right biceps muscle biopsy: glycolytic enzyme histochemistry. Note that the small angular fibers are both Type I and Type II (frozen section, phosphorylase.). (D) Right biceps muscle biopsy: longitudinal section of two myofibers. The atrophic fiber above shows mild dilatation of the SR-T system and a cytoplasmic body (left upper margin). The fiber below is small and relatively normal (original magnification ×7, 850). (E) Right biceps muscle biopsy: high magnification of cytoplasmic body showing its apparent origin from Z-band streaming and disorganized myofilaments (original magnification ×20, 200).

tissue, indicating a neuromyopathic cause (Fig. 7.3A–E). There were no pathologic changes in the retina.

One week later he had another episode of abdominal pain and nausea, accompanied by intense anxiety, and TTFD was increased to 450 mg per day. All

*Continued*

## Case Example 7.12 Shoshin Beriberi and Cardiac Collapse in a Teenage Boy—Cont'd

symptoms disappeared and after 3 more weeks he claimed that he felt better than he had for several years.

Fig. 7.2 shows the appearance of the heart by roentgenogram, which revealed some reduction in overall size. The laboratory studies shown in Table 7.3 were much improved. In the next 2 months his weight increased by 2.7 kg and there was some visible increase in muscle tissue, but blood pressure remained labile. Pulsus alternans and cardiac gallop rhythm reappeared intermittently. He began to have renewed episodes of "thumping" epigastric pain associated with a sense of nervousness (typical beriberi). Respiratory and cardiac rate steadily increased and he was readmitted to hospital 6 months after beginning TTFD. Examination revealed acute distress, cyanotic lips, hyperdynamic precordium, carotid pulsation, sweating, dyspnea, hepatomegaly, and edema resistant to all therapeutic measures. Cardiac size by roentgenography had increased (Fig. 7.2). A 24-h urine revealed 900 mg of creatine per 24 h and 700 mg of creatinine per 24 h—a ratio of 1.3. He expired 2 weeks after readmission to hospital. Autopsy was refused.

## *Points of Consideration*

There was a history of probable hypoxic birth. The infant was irritable, cried endlessly, and was unusually sensitive to sound (mild hypoxia or pseudohypoxia). Neurologic, psychologic, and cardiac disease were associated with episodes of vomiting, diarrhea, acute abdominal pain, and bowel hemorrhage of unknown cause (but typical of beriberi). Autopsy may have ultimately shed further light on the mechanism. Throughout life he had never been normal. His sensitivity to sound was remarkable, particularly in the final stages of his disease, when the exploding of a firecracker caused extreme palpitations, sweating, and unusual fear (typical fight-or-flight). Hemoglobin concentration and physical signs of hypoxia suggested that there were endogenous attempts unsuccessfully to adapt to the physical environment that would be encountered on a high mountain, the equivalent of high-altitude sickness. This may have been important in reference to the seizure-like episode that occurred in mountainous terrain on a hot day, the ultraviolet light exposure being an additional stress factor. Repeated episodes of vomiting, diarrhea, and abdominal pain indicated abnormal brain stem hypoxic or pseudohypoxic reactions. This is similar to the clinical course of Leigh's disease, already discussed in detail, in which the histopathology is similar to Wernicke's disease. His clinical and laboratory imitation of beriberi was

**Table 7.3** Laboratory Results for Case Example 7.12

| Age/Date | Test | Result | Normal Range |
|---|---|---|---|
| Age 12 years | | | |
| 2/11/1969 | Ground-glass clot time | 145, 145, 150 s | 90–130 s |
| 2/12/1969 | Glucose tolerance | | 60–105 mg/100 mL |
| | Fasting blood sugar | 114 mg/100 mL | |
| | 1 h blood sugar | 170 mg/100 mL | |
| | 2 h blood sugar | 154 mg/100 mL | |
| 9/8/1973 | SGOT | 64 U | <40 U |
| | SGPT | 80 U | 0–40 U Karmen units |
| | LDH | 150 U | 30–120 U |
| Age 16 years | | | |
| 11/8/1973 | Serum potassium | 3.8 mEq/L | 4–5.6 mEq/L |
| 12/8/1973 | Serum uric acid | 10 mg/100 mL | 2.5–8 mg/100 mL |
| 12/4/1973 | Serum potassium | 2.9 mEq/L | 4–5.6 mEq/L |
| 3/11/1974 | CPK | 1090 mU/mL | 28–145 mU/mL |
| | LDH | 370 mU/mL | 100–225 mU/mL |
| | SGOT | 106 mU/mL | 7–40 mU/mL |
| 3/11/1974 | Arterial $O_2$ tension | 64 mm Hg | 90 mm Hg |
| | Arterial $O_2$ saturation | 96% | >95% |
| | Serum lactate | 84 mg/100 mL | 3–12 mg/100 mL |
| | Serum pyruvate | 0.4 mg/100 mL | 0.3–0.7 mg/100 mL |
| 3/21/1974 | Urine pyruvate | Night 7.6 mg/12 h<br>Day 8.6 mg/12 h | <5 mg/12 h |
| | Urine alpha keto glutarate | 1.6 mg/100 mL | <2.5 mg/100 mL |
| 3/24/1974 | Serum $CO_2$ | 28.5 mEq/L | 22/27 mEq/L |
| | Serum chloride | <90 mEq/L | 95–195 mEq/L |

*Continued*

**Table 7.3** Laboratory Results for Case Example 7.12—cont'd

| Age/Date | Test | Result | Normal Range |
|---|---|---|---|
| 3/25/1974 | Serum sodium | 125 mEq/L | 130–150 mEq/L |
|  | Serum potassium | 4.3 mEq/L | 4–5.6 mEq/L |
|  | Serum BUN | 30 mg/100 mL | 10–20 mg/100 mL |
| 3/28/1974 | Serum carotene | 25 µg/100 mL | 50/250 µg/100 mL |
|  |  | TTFD started |  |
| 4/5/1974 | CPK | 80 mU/mL | 28–145 mU/mL |
| 7/10/1974 | SGOT | 15 mU/mL | <40 mU/mL |
|  | LDH | 215 mU/mL | 100–225 mU/mL |
|  | CPK | 150 mU/mL | 28–145 mU/mL |
| 9/12/1974 | Urine pyruvate | Night 9.0 mg/12 h | <5 mg/12 h |
|  |  | Day 9.2 mg/12 h |  |
|  | Urine alpha keto glutarate | 0.7 mg/100 mL | <2.5 mg/100 mL |
| 9/13/1974 | RBC transketolase | 71 mU/L/min | 42.1–86.1 mU/L/min |
|  | TPP uptake (in vitro) | 10.80% | 0%–17.4% |
|  | SGOT | 70 mU/mL | 7–40 mU/mL |
|  | CPK | 390 mU/mL | 23–145 mU/mL |
|  | LDH | 380 mU/mL | 100–225 mU/mL |
| 9/18/1974 | A.m. plasma cortisol 407.7 µg/100 mL | 6–26 µg/100 mL |  |
|  | Urine creatine | 900 mg/24 h | 0–50 mg/24 h |
|  | Urine creatinine | 700 mg/24 h | 1060–1590 mg/24 h |
| 9/18/1974 | Capillary blood gases |  |  |
|  | pH | 7.5 | 7.35–7.45 |
|  | $CO_2$ content | 35 mEq/L | 23–27 mEq/L |
|  | $CO_2$ tension | 36.2 mm Hg | 34–46 mm Hg |
|  | $O_2$ tension | 46 mm Hg | 85–95 mm Hg |
|  | $O_2$ saturation | 90% | 90%–98% |

*CPK*, creatine phosphokinase; *LDH*, lactate dehydrogenase; *RBC*, red blood cell; *SGOT*, serum glutamic oxaloacetic transaminase; *SPGT*, serum glutamic pyruvic transaminase; *TTP*, thiamine triphosphate.

exact and possibly indicated a genetically determined abnormality in thiamine metabolism. His temporary response to TTFD is also similar to that seen in Leigh's disease in which "resistance" develops and symptoms and signs of the disease reappear.[21] In the preterminal stage there was marked creatinuria, also suggestive of beriberi. Urinary creatinine concentration was 200 mg less than that of creatine, resulting in a high ratio of creatine to creatinine. If pseudohypoxic metabolic function of brain could have been proved it might have provided an adequate etiology. No thiamine triphosphate inhibitory substance was found in the urine. In retrospect there was a possibility that the large dose of TTFD created an imbalance between thiamine and magnesium, both of which are essential to entry of glucose into the citric acid cycle.

## CONCLUSION

Just as in any artificial machine, there must be energy supply and its consumption for function. Oxidative metabolism depends upon the citric acid cycle and the electron transport chain for energy synthesis. All other metabolic pathways are energy dependent. Health is maintained by a lock-step equation between supply and demand. Hence all disease is related to a loss of balance between energy synthesis and functional demand. Any form of genetic or environmental stress, mental or physical, automatically increases demand and energy synthesis must accelerate to compensate. It is only recently that therapeutic doses of cofactor have been found to stimulate their respective enzymes and the new science of epigenetics has shown that in many cases genetic abnormality can be corrected. The ultimate diagnosis of ongoing chronic disease must be made by defining the biochemical lesion. It is no longer sufficient to make a diagnosis in descriptive terms since recent research has shown that there is an overlap of symptomology and physical findings between various conditions long thought to be distinctive diseases. It would explain why a metabolic abnormality might be sufficient to maintain a degree of health, but be inadequate to meet the stress response of a relatively mild insult such as an infection, mild trauma, or even an inoculation.

Throughout this book, thiamine and its therapeutic derivatives have been on center stage. It is not intended to imply that thiamine is the only nutrient that has been used therapeutically by the authors or by preventive physicians. On the other hand, the experience of the authors has slowly accumulated an absolute conviction that many of the common diseases in advanced society are caused by energy-related failures of adaptation, exactly as was proclaimed by Selye. In the last analysis we are getting to grips with the complicated mechanisms of redox, the ability to convert fuel to energy. In other words, the optimum efficiency of utilization of oxygen must be the one factor that would enable us to judge whether a human body is working up to top capacity if there is no genetic influence.

Since thiamine is a catalyst that is linked to citric acid cycle function as well as its possible role in cell membranes—and hence its potential regulation of electron transfer in producing ATP—it certainly stands astride the fundamental mechanisms of energy metabolism. However, a number of examples have been provided in attempting to show that this vitamin is closely related to all other vitamin and mineral functions in their catalytic role.

It is suggested that traditionally diagnosed "functional" or "neurotic" manifestations are merely the reactions of a brain that is chronically starved of oxidative metabolism. In a sense, it can be viewed as a biochemical distortion that is epitomized by the early behavioral changes in both beriberi and experimental thiamine deficiency, even though there are definite differences between the two conditions as epitomized by Williams et al. in 1943.[84] It must alter medical perspective toward psychosomatic disease. We must begin to realize that our traditional approaches may be catastrophically wrong and that there is no artificial separation of mental from physical. The psychiatrist, like the internist, may have to stop being concerned about the descriptive diagnosis and begin to probe the total individual for determining the biochemical lesion.

The very interesting observation that a given nutrient (thiamine) can be used in the treatment of 250 different conditions does not imply that the symptomatic representation is always caused by the same biochemical lesion.[85] For example, a patient with rheumatoid arthritis may have the same biochemical cause, which in another individual results in depression. Therefore both would be treated in the same way in that instance. By the same token, three patients with the same disease, diagnosed in descriptive terms, may have three different biochemical causes. Hence each may have to be treated by applying differently selected nutritional therapy. Even cancer has moved into scientific thought as a possibly nutritionally related disease, and there seems to be little doubt that the science of nutrition is on the eve of a massive renaissance.

To come even close to understanding the basic nature of the disease process, a physician requires a very broad base of knowledge of the mechanics of the "machine" that he is servicing. His or her handmaiden must therefore be biochemistry, and how it relates to the synthesis of neurotransmitters. For example, the esophagus has only a parasympathetic supply and we can assume that the autonomic neurotransmitter to that organ is unequivocally cholinergic. Knowing that sympathetic action in the heart is different, according to which sympathetic chain delivers the signal, helps us to understand the peculiarities that are represented in the prolonged Q-T syndrome.[86] Most of all it provides a basic view of the relationship between mental and physical, since all controls are central and the body is merely the target. However, the brain is also part of that total body and is activated by the same neurotransmitters. Hence behavior is a composite of brain/body interplay.

## REFERENCES

1. Fernstrom MH, Kety DS. *Nutrition and the brain*. Nestlé Nutrition Services: Nestec; 1977.
2. Kolata GB. Brain biochemistry: effects of diet. *Science* 1976;**192**(4234):41–2.
3. Onodera K, Tadano T, Sakai K, Kisara K, Ogura Y. Muricide induced by thiamine deficiency in the rats (author's transl). *Nihon yakurigaku zasshi. Folia Pharmacol Jap* 1978;**74**(5):641–8.
4. Onodera K, Tadano T, Kisara K, Kimura Y, Ogura Y. Persistent erection in thiamine-deficient rats. *Andrologia* 1978;**10**(6):467–72.
5. Iwata H, Watanabe K, Nishikawa T, Ohashi M. Effects of drugs on behavior, heart rate and catecholamine levels in thiamine-deficient rats. *Eur J Pharmacol* 1969;**6**(2):83–9.
6. Skelton FR. Some specific and non-specific effects of thiamine deficiency in the rat. *Exp Biol Med* 1950;**73**(3):516–9.
7. Pogash C. *Myth of the 'Twinkie defense': the verdict in the Dan White case wasn't based on his ingestion of junk food*. San Francisco Chronicle, 23. 2003.
8. Kinoshita T, Abe RT, Hineno A, Tsunekawa K, Nakane S, Ikeda SI. Peripheral sympathetic nerve dysfunction in adolescent Japanese girls following immunization with the human papillomavirus vaccine. *Intern Med* 2014;**53**(19):2185–200.
9. Lonsdale D. Thiamine and magnesium deficiencies: keys to disease. *Med Hypotheses* 2015;**84**(2):129–34.
10. Tomljenovic L, Colafrancesco S, Perricone C, Shoenfeld Y. Postural orthostatic tachycardia with chronic fatigue after HPV vaccination as part of the "Autoimmune/Autoinflammatory Syndrome Induced by Adjuvants" case report and literature review. *J Invest Med High Impact Case Rep* 2014;**2**(1). 2324709614527812.
11. Brinth LS, Pors K, Theibel AC, Mehlsen J. Orthostatic intolerance and postural tachycardia syndrome as suspected adverse effects of vaccination against human papilloma virus. *Vaccine* 2015;**33**(22):2602–5.
12. Lonsdale D. Thiamine and magnesium deficiencies: keys to disease. *Med Hypotheses* 2015;**84**(2):129–34.
13. Blitshteyn S. Postural tachycardia syndrome following human papillomavirus vaccination. *Eur J Neurol* 2014;**21**(1):135–9.
14. Puig-Perez S, Hackett RA, Salvador A, Steptoe A. Optimism moderates psychophysiological responses to stress in older people with Type 2 diabetes. *Psychophysiology* 2016. http://dx.doi.org/10.1111/psyp.12806.

15. Pácal L, Kuricová K, Kaňková K. Evidence for altered thiamine metabolism in diabetes: is there a potential to oppose gluco-and lipotoxicity by rational supplementation. *World J Diabetes* 2014;**5**(3):288–95.
16. Frank LL. Thiamin in clinical practice. *J Parenter Enteral Nutr* 2015;**39**(5):503–20.
17. Auger C, Alhasawi A, Contavadoo M, Appanna VD. Dysfunctional mitochondrial bioenergetics and the pathogenesis of hepatic disorders. *Front Cell Dev Biol* 2015;**3**.
18. Appanna VD, Auger C, Lemire J. Energy, the driving force behind good and ill health. *Front Cell Dev Biol* 2014;**2**.
19. Ren J, Pulakat L, Whaley-Connell A, Sowers JR. Mitochondrial biogenesis in the metabolic syndrome and cardiovascular disease. *J Mol Med* 2010;**88**(10):993–1001.
20. Reardon C. Neuro-immune interactions in the cholinergic anti-inflammatory reflex. *Immunol Lett* 2016;**178**:92–6.
21. Lejeune J. On the mechanism of mental deficiency in chromosomal diseases. *Hereditas* 1977;**86**(1):9–14.
22. Freeman JM, Finkelstein JD, Mudd SH. Folate-responsive homocystinuria and schizophrenia: a defect in methylation due to deficient 5, 10–methylenetetrahydrofolate reductase activity. *N Engl J Med* 1975;**292**(10):491–6.
23. Zhao ZD, Yang WZ, Gao C, Fu X, Zhang W, Zhou Q, Chen W, Ni X, Lin JK, Yang J, Xu XH. A hypothalamic circuit that controls body temperature. *Proc Natl Acad Sci USA* 2017:201616255.
24. Selye H. The general adaptation syndrome and the diseases of adaptation 1. *J Clin Endocrinol Metab* 1946;**6**(2):117–230.
25. Nicholls DG. The bioenergetics of brown adipose tissue mitochondria. *FEBS lett* 1976;**61**(2):103–10.
26. James WPT, Sahakian BJ. Overgrowth: energetic significance in relation to obesity. *Nutr Child Health* 1981.
27. Cole HS. The demonstration of insulinopenia in familial dysautonomia. *Pediatrics* 1973;**52**(1):137–9.
28. Wilgram GF, Holoway CF, Kennedy EP. The content of cytidine diphosphate choline in the livers of normal and cholinedeficient rats. *J Biol Chem* 1960;**235**:37–9.
29. Bizon-Zygmańska D, Jankowska-Kulawy A, Bielarczyk H, Pawełczyk T, Ronowska A, Marszałł M, Szutowicz A. Acetyl-CoA metabolism in amprolium-evoked thiamine pyrophosphate deficits in cholinergic SN56 neuroblastoma cells. *Neurochem Int* 2011;**59**(2):208–16.
30. Kalokerinos A. *Every second child*. Melbourne: Nelson; 1974.
31. Davis RE, Icke GC, Hilton JM. High thiamine levels in sudden infant-death syndrome. *New Engl J Med* 1980;**303**(8):462.
32. Struzik L, Katzman M, Vijay N, Coonerty-Femiano A, Mahamed S, Duffin J. Central and peripheral chemoreflex characteristics: panic disorder patients vs. healthy volunteers. In: *Frontiers in modeling and control of breathing*. 2001. p. 435–7. [Springer US].
33. Selye H. Stress and the general adaptation syndrome. *Br Med J* 1950;**1**(4667):1383.
34. Yalamanchili N, Kriete A, Alfego D, Danowski KM, Kari C, Rodeck U. Distinct cell stress responses induced by ATP restriction in quiescent human fibroblasts. *Front Genet* 2016;**7**.
35. Barbour JA, Turner N. Mitochondrial stress signaling promotes cellular adaptations. *Int J Cell Biol* 2014;**2014**.
36. Rappaport SM. Genetic factors are not the major causes of chronic diseases. *PLoS One* 2016;**11**(4):e0154387.
37. Wong AH, Gottesman II, Petronis A. Phenotypic differences in genetically identical organisms: the epigenetic perspective. *Hum Mol Genet* 2005;**14**(Suppl. 1):R11–8.
38. Wallace DC, Chalkia D. Mitochondrial DNA genetics and the heteroplasmy conundrum in evolution and disease. *Cold Spring Harbor Perspect Biol* 2013;**5**(11):a021220.

39. Iossifov I, O'Roak BJ, Sanders SJ, Ronemus M, Krumm N, Levy D, Stessman HA, Witherspoon KT, Vives L, Patterson KE, Smith JD. The contribution of de novo coding mutations to autism spectrum disorder. *Nature* 2014;**515**(7526):216–21.
40. https://ghr.nlm.nih.gov/condition/alpha-1-antitrypsin-deficiency.
41. Schmechel DE. Art, alpha-1-antitrypsin polymorphisms and intense creative energy: blessing or curse? *Neurotoxicology* 2007;**28**(5):899–914.
42. Schmechel DE, Browndyke J, Ghio A. Strategies for dissecting genetic-environmental interactions in neurodegenerative disorders. *Neurotoxicology* 2006;**27**(5):637–57.
43. Casteels M, Sniekers M, Fraccascia P, Mannaerts GP, Van Veldhoven PP. The role of 2-hydroxyacyl-CoA lyase, a thiamin pyrophosphate-dependent enzyme, in the peroxisomal metabolism of 3-methyl-branched fatty acids and 2-hydroxy straight-chain fatty acids. *Biochem Soc Trans* 2007;**35**(5):876–80.
44. Meyer JN, Leung MC, Rooney JP, Sendoel A, Hengartner MO, Kisby GE, Bess AS. Mitochondria as a target of environmental toxicants. *Toxic Sci* 2013;**134**(1):1–17.
45. Neustadt J, Pieczenik SR. Medication-induced mitochondrial damage and disease. *Mol Nutr Food Res* 2008;**52**(7):780–8.
46. Wallace KB. Drug-induced mitochondrial neuropathy in children: a conceptual framework for critical windows of development. *J Child Neurol* 2014. 0883073814538510.
47. Apabhai S, Gorman GS, Sutton L, Elson JL, Plötz T, Turnbull DM, Trenell MI. Habitual physical activity in mitochondrial disease. *PLoS One* 2011;**6**(7):e22294.
48. Safdar A, Bourgeois JM, Ogborn DI, Little JP, Hettinga BP, Akhtar M, Thompson JE, Melov S, Mocellin NJ, Kujoth GC, Prolla TA. Endurance exercise rescues progeroid aging and induces systemic mitochondrial rejuvenation in mtDNA mutator mice. *Proc Natl Acad Sci USA* 2011;**108**(10):4135–40.
49. Picard M, McManus MJ, Gray JD, Nasca C, Moffat C, Kopinski PK, Seifert EL, McEwen BS, Wallace DC. Mitochondrial functions modulate neuroendocrine, metabolic, inflammatory, and transcriptional responses to acute psychological stress. *Proc Natl Acad Sci USA* 2015;**112**(48):E6614–23.
50. Fermaglich DR. Reflex syrnpathetic dystrophy in children. *Pediatrics* 1977;**60**(6):881.
51. Kozin F, Haughton V, Ryan L. The reflex sympathetic dystrophy syndrome in a child. *J Pediatr* 1977;**90**(3):417–9.
52. Rodgers RJ, Ishii Y, Halford JCG, Blundell JE. Orexins and appetite regulation. *Neuropeptides* 2002;**36**(5):303–25.
53. Liu ZW, Gan G, Suyama S, Gao XB. Intracellular energy status regulates activity in hypocretin/orexin neurones: a link between energy and behavioural states. *J Physiol* 2011;**589**(17):4157–66.
54. Tsujino N, Sakurai T. Orexin/hypocretin: a neuropeptide at the interface of sleep, energy homeostasis, and reward system. *Pharmacol Rev* 2009;**61**(2):162–76.
55. Chou TC, Lee CE, Lu J, Elmquist JK, Hara J, Willie JT, Beuckmann CT, Chemelli RM, Sakurai T, Yanagisawa M, Saper CB. Orexin (hypocretin) neurons contain dynorphin. *J Neurosci* 2001;**21**(19):1–6.
56. Land BB, Bruchas MR, Lemos JC, Xu M, Melief EJ, Chavkin C. The dysphoric component of stress is encoded by activation of the dynorphin κ-opioid system. *J Neurosci* 2008;**28**(2):407–14.
57. Pasternak GW, editor. *The opiate receptors*. Springer Science + Business Media, LLC; 2011.
58. Yamanaka A, Beuckmann CT, Willie JT, Hara J, Tsujino N, Mieda M, Tominaga M, Yagami KI, Sugiyama F, Goto K, Yanagisawa M. Hypothalamic orexin neurons regulate arousal according to energy balance in mice. *Neuron* 2003;**38**(5):701–13.
59. Inutsuka A, Yamashita A, Chowdhury S, Nakai J, Ohkura M, Taguchi T, Yamanaka A. The integrative role of orexin/hypocretin neurons in nociceptive perception and analgesic regulation. *Sci Rep* 2016;**6**.

60. Coghlan HC, Phares P, Cowley M, Copley D, James TN. Dysautonomia in mitral valve prolapse. *Am J Med* 1979;**67**(2):236–44.
61. Coghlan HC. Mitral valve prolapse: is it a problem with the patient's computer?. In: *Presented at the American Heart Association's Eighth Science Writer's Forum, Tucson, Az*. 1981.
62. Orhan AL, Sayar N, Nurkalem Z, Uslu N, Erdem I, Erdem EC, Erer HB, Soylu Ö, Emre A, Sayar K, Eren M. Assessment of autonomic dysfunction and anxiety levels in patients with mitral valve prolapse. *Turk Kardiyol Dern Ars* 2009;**37**(4):226–33.
63. Will Y, Dykens J. Mitochondrial toxicity assessment in industry–a decade of technology development and insight. *Expert Opin Drug Metab Toxicol* 2014;**10**(8):1061–7.
64. Scatena R, Bottoni P, Botta G, Martorana GE, Giardina B. The role of mitochondria in pharmacotoxicology: a reevaluation of an old, newly emerging topic. *Am J Physiol Cell Physiol* 2007;**293**(1):C12–21.
65. Varga ZV, Ferdinandy P, Liaudet L, Pacher P. Drug-induced mitochondrial dysfunction and cardiotoxicity. *Am J Physiol Heart Circ Physiol* 2015;**309**(9):H1453–67.
66. Neustadt J, Pieczenik SR. Medication-induced mitochondrial damage and disease. *Mol Nutr Food Res* 2008;**52**(7):780–8.
67. Finsterer J. Mitochondrion-toxic drugs given to patients with mitochondrial psychoses. *Behav Brain Func* 2012;**8**(1):1.
68. Kalghatgi S, Spina CS, Costello JC, Liesa M, Morones-Ramirez JR, Slomovic S, Molina A, Shirihai OS, Collins JJ. Bactericidal antibiotics induce mitochondrial dysfunction and oxidative damage in mammalian cells. *Sci Transl Med* 2013;**5**(192):192ra85.
69. Barnhill AE, Brewer MT, Carlson SA. Adverse effects of antimicrobials via predictable or idiosyncratic inhibition of host mitochondrial components. *Antimicrob Agents Chemother* 2012;**56**(8):4046–51.
70. Neale R, Reynolds TM, Saweirs W. Statin precipitated lactic acidosis? *J Clin Pathol* 2004;**57**(9):989–90.
71. Okuyama H, Langsjoen PH, Hamazaki T, Ogushi Y, Hama R, Kobayashi T, Uchino H. Statins stimulate atherosclerosis and heart failure: pharmacological mechanisms. *Expert Rev Clin Pharmacol* 2015;**8**(2):189–99.
72. Golomb BA, Evans MA. Statin adverse effects. *Am J Cardiovasc Drugs* 2008;**8**(6):373–418.
73. Wessels B, Ciapaite J, van den Broek NM, Nicolay K, Prompers JJ. Metformin impairs mitochondrial function in skeletal muscle of both lean and diabetic rats in a dose-dependent manner. *PLoS One* 2014;**9**(6):e100525.
74. Liang X, Chien HC, Yee SW, Giacomini MM, Chen EC, Piao M, Hao J, Twelves J, Lepist EI, Ray AS, Giacomini KM. Metformin is a substrate and inhibitor of the human thiamine transporter, THTR-2 (SLC19A3). *Mol Pharm* 2015;**12**(12):4301–10.
75. Niu PY, Niu Q, Zhang QL, Wang LP, He SC, Wu TC, Conti P, Di Gioacchino M, Boscolo P. Aluminum impairs rat neural cell mitochondria in vitro. *Int J Immunopathol Pharmacol* 2005;**18**(4):683–9.
76. Niu PY, Niu Q, Zhang QL, Wang LP, He SC, Wu TC, Conti P, Di Gioacchino M, Boscolo P. Aluminum impairs rat neural cell mitochondria in vitro. *Int J Immunopathol Pharmacol* 2005;**18**(4):683–9.
77. Murakami K, Yoshino M. Aluminum decreases the glutathione regeneration by the inhibition of NADP-isocitrate dehydrogenase in mitochondria. *J Cell Biochem* 2004;**93**(6):1267–71.
78. Sharpe MA, Livingston AD, Baskin DS. Thimerosal-derived ethylmercury is a mitochondrial toxin in human astrocytes: possible role of fenton chemistry in the oxidation and breakage of mtDNA. *J Toxicol* 2012;**2012**.
79. Chow G. *Five years after Gardasil: nursing my mitochondria*. 2014. Hormones Matter. https://www.hormonesmatter.com/five-years-gardasil-nursing-mitochondria/.

80. Marrs C. *Thyroid dysfunction with medication or vaccine induced demyelinating diseases.* 2013. Hormones Matter. https://www.hormonesmatter.com/thyroid-medication-vaccine-induced-demyelination/.
81. Marrs C. *Cerebellar ataxia and the HPV vaccine – connection and treatment.* 2013. Hormones Matter. https://www.hormonesmatter.com/cerebellar-ataxia-hpv-vaccine-connection-treatment/.
82. Marrs C. *Adverse reactions, Hashimoto's thyroiditis, gait, balance and tremors.* 2013. Hormones Matter. https://www.hormonesmatter.com/adverse-reactions-hashimotos-thyroiditis-gait-balance-tremors/.
83. Peters RA. The catatorulin test for vitamin B1. *Biochem J* 1938;**32**(11):2031.
84. Williams RD, Mason HL, Power MH, Wilder RM. Induced thiamine (vitamin B1) deficiency in man: relation of depletion of thiamine to development of biochemical defect and of polyneuropathy. *Arch Intern Med* 1943;**71**(1):38–53.
85. Zbinden G. Therapeutic use of vitamin B1 in diseases other than beriberi. *Ann NY Acad Sci* 1962;**98**(2):550–61.
86. Wilde AA, Moss AJ, Kaufman ES, Shimizu W, Peterson DR, Benhorin J, Lopes C, Towbin JA, Spazzolini C, Crotti L, Zareba W. Clinical aspects of type 3 long QT syndrome: an international multicenter study. *Circulation* 2016. CIRCULATIONAHA-116.

CHAPTER 8

# Energy Metabolism in a Revised Medical Model

## Contents

| | |
|---|---|
| Malnutrition in the Face of Obesity: Economics Versus Chemistry | 307 |
| Medically Unexplained Symptoms | 309 |
| Chemistry, Energy, and Metabolism | 311 |
| Beyond Cartesian Dualism | 313 |
| Iatrogenesis and Medically Unexplained Symptoms: Two Sides of the Same Question? | 314 |
| Return of the Case Study and N-of-1 in Clinical Care and Research | 316 |
| Next Time the Labs are Negative | 317 |
| Why Thiamine? Why Now? | 318 |
| Those Who Have the Privilege to Know Have the Duty to Act | 320 |
| References | 321 |

Throughout this book we have challenged the predominant notion that nutrition has little bearing on, or role in, modern medicine. We provided epidemiological, clinical, and biochemical evidence connecting nutrient status to health and disease. This evidence is not new. Physicians and researchers have been presenting these data for generations, and for generations commercial interests that no doubt align squarely with our innate human desires to have everything but risk nothing, have belied these data. What is new, however, is the recognition that high-calorie malnutrition, just as clearly as genetic predispositions, can induce functional dysautonomias that emanate from thiamine-deficient and distressed mitochondria. A review of mitochondrial chemistry shows us that micronutrients are critical components of energy metabolism,[1,2] while the review of dietary data shows that those micronutrients are often missing from the modern diet, with large swathes of the population deficient in one or more micronutrients.[3,4] Finally, the clinical research and case studies presented herein demonstrate that thiamine can be used pharmacologically to treat dysautonomic symptoms safely and effectively, often where other treatments had failed.

Although the seeds for these connections were planted decades ago, they have been mostly dismissed or forgotten altogether. The idea that nutrient deficiencies could develop where food was abundantly available was considered ludicrous; even more so was the idea that a mere vitamin could reset metabolism and become a curative agent. It remains so today. Over the years the notion that we can eat anything, that the type of calories do not matter, only that there are calories has become so deeply ingrained that when faced with evidence to the contrary it is viewed suspiciously. "Nutrition is something only those alternative medicine folks consider. It is not real medicine," we think to ourselves. It is a convenient dissonance that energy metabolism will continue unaltered absent critical substrates and in the face of significant stressors. We tell ourselves that the food we eat, the drugs we consume, the environmental toxicants we are exposed to, and the lifestyles we engage in somehow magically dissipate once absorbed by human physiology. When diseases of metabolic origin predominate the landscape of modern medicine[5,6] diseases that modern medical treatments are incapable of treating except by an ever-increasing reliance on polypharmacy that renders the patient sicker, it should not be unreasonable to consider other options, and yet, by far and away, it is.

To consider nutrition as medicine is to commit professional suicide. It should not be, but it is. We all know physicians who have used vitamins and minerals preferentially to medication. We have all read articles about conventional physicians who move over to what is derisively called "alternative" medicine. Many had to leave their practices, their hospital, or university appointments to practice this type of medicine and conduct this type of research. Dr. Lonsdale was one of those doctors. Many of the successful treatments reported in this book were achieved at Cleveland Clinic. What surprised him was that each case was viewed by his colleagues as spontaneous remission with no consideration given at all to the possibility that vitamins used under these circumstances had any valid effect. There was only one possibility for him, to join a like-minded physician who had already begun a private practice specializing in nutrient therapy. Dr. Marrs, too, made a conscious decision to follow a different path and to pursue a more thorough understanding of health and disease. Although this choice was far from easy for either of us, resulting in loss of colleague respect and friendships, we both have witnessed such remarkable benefits in the treatment of patients; we have no regrets.

To admit that nutrients matter, to point out the supporting biochemistry, and to demonstrate clinical effectiveness goes against decades of medical dogma that has convinced itself of the primacy of pharmaceutical and surgical interventions. This in part is because of a tacit assumption in modern medicine that food availability equates with nutritional competence and in part because the economics of health care coincide with the current disease model of medicine;

neither will be disentangled from the other easily, but if we are to help patients live healthier lives, we must. This means that we must begin to respect the role of nutrition in prevention and the therapeutic properties of nutrients. By all accounts the current medical model, despite all of its technological brilliance, is producing a population that is living sicker and dying younger.[7]

## MALNUTRITION IN THE FACE OF OBESITY: ECONOMICS VERSUS CHEMISTRY

On the surface, and to the extent Western societies are plagued with epidemics of obesity and overconsumption, the idea that malnutrition is possible seems laughable. Indeed, the scientific literature is rife with terms such as overnutrition,[8,9] suggesting that not only are we getting sufficient nutrients, but in fact modern illness emanates from an overabundance of nutrients. Some of the most advanced mitochondrial research links overnutrition with myriad degenerative disorders.[10,11] The absolute absurdity of the notion of population-wide overnutrition implies an excess of both macro- and micronutrients. The epidemiological evidence indicates, however, that a good percentage of the population, especially those with weight problems, is deficient in many critical vitamins and minerals.[12,13] The acceptable notion of overnutrition rests entirely on an overly simplistic black-box model of mitochondrial metabolism; one where no matter what goes in, ATP comes out. As we illustrated in Chapter 3, macronutrients are not the same as micronutrients. Respiration requires molecular oxygen, which requires micronutrients[14–16] as do each of the enzymatic reactions that convert macronutrients into ATP[17] and the redox cycles responsible for clearing and recycling byproducts and toxicants.[18–20] An overabundance of macronutrients paired with low micronutrients or high-calorie malnutrition overloads mitochondrial capacity, setting off the cascades linked to illness.[21] Indeed, metabolic flexibility is conferred by micronutrient status, even in the face of excess macronutrients, explaining to a large degree why the diseases of obesity are not necessarily linear.[22] Recognizing these fallacies, however, requires equal parts chemistry and courage and no small amount of time and energy for very little of this information is taught in medical school. It must be learned independently.

In today's hurried medical practice, it is so much easier to reach for the prescription pad than address root causes. The textbooks support this approach. Medical economics support this approach, and corporate interests, whether hospital, pharmaceutical, or insurer, support this approach.

Diagnostic and billing codes are based upon identifying a discrete diagnosis or multiple overlapping diagnoses and applying the appropriate billable intervention(s). They are procedural in nature, meant to streamline processes and maximize efficiencies. For the conscientious physician this becomes an increasingly difficult model to uphold, particularly in the face of chronic suffering. For the patient plagued with complex multisystem disease processes, the current model is untenable. Chronic suffering that falls beyond the current diagnostic modalities and is completely intractable to modern therapeutics force many to look beyond conventional approaches and return to the basics of chemistry. Therein lie the professional difficulties. To approach basic biochemistry as something that should be supported works against the current medical model for the practitioner.

Human illness, however, does not emanate from a shortage of pharmaceuticals. It begins and ends with oxidative capacity. How well mitochondria process energy and how effectively they sense and signal danger,[23–25] clear toxicants,[26] manage steroidogenesis,[27] sequester $Ca^{2+}$,[28,29] and how flexibly they adapt to stressors[30] determine health or disease. Recognizing that each of these functions is intensely energy dependent, to the extent any one of these processes is deranged, we must address disturbed energetic capacity first and foremost. This leads us to two questions: (1) what does the body require for efficient oxidative metabolism and (2) is the patient meeting those requirements? Chances are the answer to question number two is no, otherwise he or she would not be seeking treatment. If we ignore these questions, no matter how many medical or surgical interventions are applied, health will not be achieved and we risk the very real possibility of death.

Whether cause or consequence, pathogenic or simply pathological, mitochondria sit at the nexus of disease. Oxidative metabolism, the most basic unit of health, can be either supported or diminished depending upon the treatments offered. All pharmaceuticals damage mitochondria by one mechanism or another[31–35] as do all industrial[36,37] and environmental chemicals[36,37] including agricultural chemicals[38–40] and the bevy of chemicals used in processing, preserving,[41,42] and packaging foodstuffs.[43–45] The degree to which an individual can eliminate or manage these exposures metabolically determines his or her capacity to maintain health and survive the stress of illness. Recognizing that medications are often necessary and worth the risk of damage to the mitochondria, it is important to consider how to offset this damage by offering mitochondrial support.[46] Failing to support mitochondrial health in the face of critical or even chronic illness risks severe injury and death. This has been evidenced repeatedly in critical care patients where life or death was predicated on nutrient status in general[47] and thiamine status in particular.[48–50]

In primary care, where chronic illness predominates, the use of medications for what are essentially the manifestations of nutrient deficiencies is foolhardy, bordering on negligent. Cardiovascular disease comes to mind. Fully 80% of cardiovascular disease is attributable to lifestyle variables,[51] of which nutrition, or lack thereof, plays an enormous role.[52] As one cardiologist suggested:

> I believe the collective denial of lifestyle disease is the reason cardiology is in an innovation rut. This denial is not active or overt. It is indolent and apathetic… This is how I see modern cardiology. Our tricks can no longer overcome eating too much and moving too little. We approach health but never get there. If you waddle, snore at night, and cannot see your toes while standing, how much will a statin or ACE inhibitor or even LCZ696 help?[53]

No medication can correct high-calorie malnutrition and unless and until those dietary toxicants and deficiencies are dealt with, the condition for which the patient is seeking treatment will continue to worsen. From an economic standpoint, as crass as it seems, continued care is beneficial, but is that really what medicine is about? Isn't our job as physicians and researchers to help people feel better, to live better? Shouldn't our goal be to reduce the burden of suffering, even if doing so requires speaking hard truths, e.g., that diet matters? Reconsider the case studies presented throughout this text. Each patient saw many physicians, was given multiple discrete and sometimes contradictory diagnoses, and offered many medications but became progressively worse, until dietary changes were made and thiamine and other nutrient deficiencies were recognized. How can we tell ourselves that we are providing good medical care if we dismiss the core constituents of organismal health?

## MEDICALLY UNEXPLAINED SYMPTOMS

Perhaps a more prescient indication of the inherent limitations in the current medical model are the data on medically unexplained symptoms, defined as symptoms having no organic origin or falling beyond the boundaries of an organic disease process. They constitute 25%–75% of the symptoms reported in outpatient settings, often involving pain and inevitably designated as somatic or psychiatric.[54] These are disturbing numbers. Even at the lower end of this range they speak directly to the need for a new model. How is it that a field that prides itself on its technological and diagnostic modernity ascribes 25%–75% of the symptoms presented by patients to the categorical equivalent of hysterical? Does this statistic not suggest that the current understanding of disease is flawed and that the diagnostics upon which we rely so heavily might be incomplete or incorrect?

Let us reconsider a few of the cases of thiamine-deficient dysautonomic function presented throughout this text. Perhaps the one that comes to mind and is worth repeating is the case of an 18-month-old girl who was admitted to hospital in a coma and diagnosed as Reye's syndrome. She never responded to the conventional treatment used at that time and with fixed and dilated pupils and decerebrate posture she was judged to be in a terminal state. One week after admission there was no change and all treatment other than normal life support was withdrawn. Intravenous and oral thiamine tetrahydrofurfuryl disulfide (TTFD) in a total dose of 750 mg per 24 h was administered and after passing through a state of coma vigilum, consciousness returned and she eventually walked out of the hospital. Although this is an isolated case described much more fully in a previous chapter, it demonstrates the lack of toxicity of TTFD and its potential for revival of oxidative metabolism.

In yet another less serious case, Dr. Lonsdale was confronted with a middle-aged woman who had been crying constantly day and night for 3 weeks without any observable cause. A series of intravenous water-soluble vitamins was given to her with complete recovery from what appeared to be an emotional storm. This was contingent on the knowledge that emotions are initiated in the lower brain that is extremely susceptible to thiamine deficiency. Thiamine does not function on its own. It is a member of a complex team, but its position in so many aspects of energy metabolism makes it vitally important. Dr. Lonsdale also successfully treated several patients with sleep apnea, using 150 mg per day of TTFD, on the basis that automatic breathing is controlled in the brain stem where function is so easily damaged by thiamine deficiency. We have no doubt that an explanation offered by others for the repeated clinical benefits we have shown in these pages would be based on the placebo effect and Dr. Lonsdale remained conscious of this throughout his career. Since the placebo effect must somehow be initiated by the brain, it is entirely possible that some of the beneficial effect of nutrients is because they initiate this unknown mechanism. However, there is little doubt that identifying the biochemical lesion as a nutrient deficiency gives direct information on the underlying cause of symptoms. There is also no doubt that further research is necessary but this can only happen when the principle of defective oxidative metabolism as the underlying etiology of many, if not all, diseases is accepted.

## CHEMISTRY, ENERGY, AND METABOLISM

It seems so obvious that we should consider mitochondrial functioning as the foundation of human health and by association medical treatments should be sought that restore and/or support mitochondrial energetics. Energy, after all, is the basis for survival. Among the difficulties in accepting mitochondrial health as requisite for human health, however, resides in the nature of mitochondrial distress itself. Mitochondrial illness shatters the very constructs we hold dear in modern medicine–that of discrete disease processes with clearly compartmentalized symptom expression and easy, one-to-one correlations with available diagnostic tests.

If mitochondrial dysfunction and the subsequent disorder in stress responsiveness teach us anything, it is that this is no longer a valid approach to medicine, if it ever was. Throughout the book we have illustrated the diversity of symptoms indicative of disturbed oxidative metabolism. One patient might present with photophobia, fatigue, gastroparesis, postural orthostatic tachycardia syndrome, and ataxia, while another will present with hypersomnia, salt cravings, blepharospasm, and muscle weakness, and yet another with migraines, diabetes, anxiety, and insomnia. Children may present with any combination of symptoms, including esophagitis, hyperactivity, night terrors, unexplained fevers, or cyclic vomiting. Even cancer, dogmatically attributed to genetic origins, appears to emanate not from mutated oncogenes and tumor suppressor genes, but from disturbed oxidative metabolism. That is, mitochondrial metabolism determines whether oncogenes and failure of tumor suppressor genes induce cancer. Cancer cells transplanted to media with healthy mitochondria suppress tumorogenesis while healthy cells with unhealthy mitochondria induce cancer.[55] Perhaps Warburg was correct[56] and cancer[57] and indeed, all illness begins and ends with respiratory insufficiency and disturbed oxidative metabolism. What disturbs oxidative metabolism? High-calorie malnutrition, genetic risk, chronic stress (including microorganisms), and toxicant exposures.

Using the current medical model, metabolic insufficiency can neither be comprehended nor treated because each set of symptoms necessitates its own diagnosis and specialist, and presumably, separate, medications. If we step back, however, and recognize the fundamental requirement of energy to fuel adaptive autonomic responses, disordered responses, no matter what organ or tissue they emanate from or in what form they present, are easily identified and sometimes easily remedied. The specialization required? Chemistry, with an eye toward nutrition.

Addressing the chemistry and working our way up through the systems likely to be disturbed by deficient oxidative metabolism provides an effective lens through which to view health and disease, particularly with complex cases. It is a framework that relies less on the rote memorization of discrete symptoms and more on understanding human health. Central to this framework is the recognition that organismal survival is a lifelong battle between the environment and the constitutional design of the organism. The environment is entirely modifiable and, as the field of epigenetics is showing us, so too is constitutional design.[58]

How we modify those variables, however, demands reconsideration. The current model that seeks only to "kill the enemy" and suppress or otherwise alter a particular signal transduction pathway without recognition that we are simply overriding innate survival processes adds undue stress to an already stressed system. The limitations of our current approach become manifest in the ever-increasing problem of antibiotic resistance[59,60] and the simultaneous increase in chronic treatment of refractory illnesses.[61] We have spent decades killing the enemy with very little attention to supporting host defenses. While killing the enemy is necessary in many contexts, to do so without offering proper support for host defenses is shortsighted.

Louis Pasteur discovered that organisms, only visible with a microscope, caused disease. It became the first paradigm in medicine, accepted by all eventually. Pasteur spent 80% of his professional life trying to persuade the medical establishment of this finding. What would he have accomplished in addition to these discoveries if they had been more readily accepted? It is interesting to note, however, that on his deathbed he reportedly said "I was wrong: it is the defenses of the body that really matter." Pasteur's contemporary and friend, the physiologist Claude Bernard (1813–78), argued instead for the importance of balance in the body's internal environment—what he called *le milieu interior.* "The constancy of the interior environment is the condition for a free and independent life." Bernard saw that the body became susceptible to infectious agents only if the internal balance—or homeostasis as we now call it—is disturbed.[62] Did Pasteur and Bernard, in fact, provide us with a concept leading to a second paradigm in medicine, one that we have yet to accept after almost 200 years, that maintaining host defenses and homeostatic balance matters as much as killing the pathogenic invaders?

Using the war analogy, one can only push troops so far without the food or armament required to defend against encroaching invaders. Any general knows that to send a starving and ill-equipped army into battle is suicide. Yet, that is exactly the current approach to medicine. Battles are fought without the necessary resources, and the expectation is that somehow the individual will not only survive but also thrive as long as the enemy is kept at bay. The survival instinct is strong, but not that strong. Survival requires energy. Energy requires micronutrients.

Extending the analogy a little further: an army that goes into battle without a functional command structure is also doomed to fail. The hypothalamic–endocrine–autonomic axis is that command structure. When the energy wanes and hypoxic manifestations begin, the command structure falters. Processes that were previously automatic, organized, and structured become disturbed, disjointed, and chaotic. Neurological integrity requires oxidative sufficiency.[63] Oxidative sufficiency requires efficient mitochondrial metabolism.[64] Efficient mitochondrial metabolism requires thiamine and other nutrients.[65] Killing the enemy without regard to supporting host defenses is misguided and illogical.

## BEYOND CARTESIAN DUALISM

If autonomic dysfunction is the cardinal expression of oxidative insufficiency, and we believe it is, then the long-held dichotomies between the brain and body and the body and environment dissolve. The human organism is no more separate from itself than are its interactions distinct from the environment within which it resides. It is one organism among many. Like the quorum-sensing bacterial biofilms that have come to the forefront of medical research,[66] the human organism is a multilayered ecosystem of bidirectional communication signals and adaptive mechanisms dedicated entirely to survival. The reductionist approach to study or treat an inherently complex and dynamic system, while necessary when medicine began to understand the intricacies of anatomy and physiology, is no longer valid. The mind/body dualism, the compartmentalization of body parts, and subsequent hyperspecialization of physicians and researchers are insufficient to recognize disease processes that span the entire organism, those that reflect insufficient mitochondrial capacity. With metabolic diseases, no compartment is privileged, especially the brain.[67]

No matter from whence a stressor originates, internally or externally or what form it takes, psychological, viral, dietary, or other, an autonomic response is necessitated. The organization of that response, though guided by genetics, is predicated ultimately on oxidative capacity. In that regard, psychosocial stressors[68] influence physiological functioning just as surely as viral stressors. Each requires energy to respond. Absent the available resources, the response will be ineffective or aberrant. Inasmuch as the brain represents only 2% of the total body weight but consumes about 20% of the metabolic energy produced,[69] it is not difficult to suggest that neuropsychiatric symptoms can be a consequence of disturbed oxidative metabolism. Without the arbitrary divisions that segregate the brain from body, what we currently label as comorbid, the separate but cooccurring disease processes that arise with complex illness can be unified. When metabolism is destabilized, so too is autonomic integrity. Neuropsychiatric symptoms should be expected along with the array of body-wide symptoms such as gastrointestinal dysmotility,[70] neuropathic[71] or neuromuscular pain,[72] and diabetes,[72] to name but a few. These are not necessarily discrete pathologies and perhaps should not be treated as such.

A growing body of evidence links mitochondrial mechanisms to psychiatric illness.[73–79] The current standard of care recommends psychotropic medications for psychiatric illness. All psychotropic medications damage mitochondria.[31,80] If psychiatric illness represents one of the many manifestations of insufficient oxidative metabolism, it would seem reasonable to consider supporting mitochondrial insufficiencies in psychiatric care, particularly when comorbid disorders are present and dietary issues are evident. By considering mitochondrial functioning first, the therapeutic goal becomes minimizing the mitochondrial damage,[81] restoring and supporting mitochondrial function. Central to this approach is nutrition. Returning to the two questions asked at the beginning of the chapter—what is required for efficient oxidative metabolism and is the patient meeting those requirements?—we have even suggested that marginal malnutrition can create criminal behavior like in the novel *Crime and Punishment* by Dostoyevsky. Perhaps a nursed grievance can explode into violence when brain metabolism is marginally inefficient.

## IATROGENESIS AND MEDICALLY UNEXPLAINED SYMPTOMS: TWO SIDES OF THE SAME QUESTION?

According to some statistics, iatrogenic death represents the third leading cause of death in the United States.[82,83] Although the data are widely disputed and reflect mostly medical error, the estimated death rate from iatrogenic means ranges from 200,000 to 400,000 annually. Some suggest the numbers significantly underrepresent the true incidence because of the methods used to tabulate these deaths.[84] While others argue that the numbers are overrepresented by a particular class of medications and/or interventions and thus appear much higher than they are.[85] The high rate of medically unexplained symptoms, the data suggesting that we are living sicker, dying younger,[7] and the increased reliance on medications (70% of adults take one medication chronically, 50% take two, and 20% take five or more medications[86]), together suggest iatrogenesis is real and perhaps underestimated. Just how many medically unexplained illnesses are potentially iatrogenic no one knows, but if we look at the rate of adverse drug events (ADRs) for drugs that were prescribed appropriately, we find that an exceptionally high rate of illnesses are potentially caused by common medical treatments.

A systematic review of patient hospitalizations in the United States from 1964 to 1995 found that 6.8% of cases were attributable to an ADR. This included reactions that precipitated the hospital admission (4.7%) and those that occurred during hospitalizations (2.1%). A 1-year analysis conducted in 2011 of ADR data reported to the Food and Drug Administration (FDA) corroborated the early findings suggesting that annually from 2.1 to 2.7 million Americans experience a serious, drug-related adverse reaction with 128,000 resulting in death.[87] Clinical Evidence, a project of the *British Medical Journal*, reports that of the 3000 common therapeutic interventions evaluated to date, only 11% had evidence of efficacy, another 35% were likely to be beneficial but not proven, and a whopping 50% of treatments currently used by practitioners are completely unproven.[88] Considering that pharmaceuticals damage the mitochondria, and thus are major contributing factors in defective oxidative metabolism, leading to both morbidity and mortality, as damning as these numbers are, it is very likely that they represent only a fraction of the illnesses evoked.

Mitochondrial damage is not on the FDA's radar. Assessment is not a preapproval requirement or even a consideration in postmarket safety studies[32] and so the rate of iatrogenic illness induced by mitochondrial damage is truly unknown. Even if mitochondrial damage were on the FDA's radar, the very nature of mitochondrial illness makes it difficult to calculate incidence. The expression of mitochondrial illness does not comport with the linear dose–response models of modern toxicology.[89] The symptoms are diverse and thus fall outside our current disease classification system. Though temporally related to the medication or vaccine, the symptom onset time varies because of the individual's metabolic flexibility at the time of administration and other cooccurring stressors. The dosages that evoke the reactions also vary, with some patients able to withstand multiple rounds of a particular medication while others develop symptoms immediately, after only a few pills. Finally, pharmacologically distinct entities seem to evoke similar patterns of symptoms, at least to the extent that mitochondrial symptoms can be considered similar. Although the evidence that pharmaceuticals damage mitochondria is clear, whether, when, and in what conformation an individual develops symptoms attributable to that damage is difficult to delineate using the currently favored research design methods. Population studies, case control, and the favorite among biomedical researchers, the double-blind randomized clinical trial, obfuscate what are essentially individual responses embedded within a highly complex and dynamic system of adaptations; adaptations that vary depending upon both intrinsic and extrinsic factors.[90] A more appropriate approach, at least until the math and modeling catch up, would be to return to the classical case studies, the N-of-1. It is here where the physician can truly determine whether and how a treatment works in his/her patients.

## RETURN OF THE CASE STUDY AND N-OF-1 IN CLINICAL CARE AND RESEARCH

As a physician, Dr. Lonsdale is perfectly aware that case reports are generally considered to be of little or no value. He and Dr. Marrs vehemently disagree. With mitochondrial illness, the symptomology is so diverse that it is the constellation of symptoms that gives pointers to the underlying biochemical lesion. Turning once again to the patient with eosinophilic esophagitis, presented in an earlier chapter, the esophagitis had been seen for many years as a diseased organ and hence considered to be the seat of the disease. The so-called psychosomatic issues that preceded the discovery of esophagitis were regarded as a separate issue. The case report makes it clear that the mental (psychosomatic) symptoms were caused by adverse biochemistry in the brain. The erythrocyte transketolase proved a defect in thiamine homeostasis, leading to solving the biochemical lesion. Knowing that the hindbrain is highly sensitive to thiamine deficiency, that thiamine is central to the production of acetylcholine, and that the vagus nerve suppresses the inflammatory response,[91] it is possible to unite the mental with the physical and explain how the brain plays its part in causing the pathology. Since physicians are trying to repair an electrochemical machine, it would seem necessary that the biochemistry learned in medical school should be retained, built upon, and used by the practicing physician. In this context, we believe that case reports are valuable in showing the complexity of brain–body interrelationships. Unfortunately, the practicing physician has been relegated to becoming a pen-pushing technician. Case reports encourage documentation of simple clinical observations that should be the province of a lifetime spent in clinical medicine. We would like to see physicians returning to the use of their training. It cuts both ways since reports of observations help the patient and increase the interest and excitement of being a physician.

## NEXT TIME THE LABS ARE NEGATIVE

If standard laboratory assessments are negative, too often a "real" disease is considered to be nonexistent. This is a remnant from the Flexner report of 1910 that adopted the laboratory as the definitive proof of disease. It was a laudable goal as medicine moved toward standardization in the early part of the 20th century, but one with significant limitations nevertheless. For there to be laboratory confirmation we have to presume that we know all there is to know about human health and illness, that the current body of diagnostic tests can accurately identify those disease processes, and that the practitioner will order those tests and interpret them correctly. Given the embarrassingly high rate of medically unexplained symptoms and the high rate of ADRs, which go largely unrecognized by most practitioners, this is clearly not the case.

If we assume the patient's suffering is real, that his symptoms represent some form of illness, and likewise that our understanding of illness is incomplete, negative labs suggest only that the more common culprits might be ruled out; no more, no less. Negative labs in the face of obvious illness suggest that either disease classifications or associated laboratory tests are incomplete or incorrect and that we have to look elsewhere for the answers. This may mean expanding the scope of analytes measured or measuring the analytes differently. Recall the discussion in Chapter 4 about how to assess thiamine. The most commonly used laboratory tests, free thiamine in blood or plasma are incapable of identifying deficiency in all but the most severe deficiencies.[92] Similarly, insufficient laboratory methodologies are common across clinical chemistry,[93] a fact that must be recognized before ruling out organic disease. Of course, one has to test for these micronutrient deficiencies first before one can rule out organic disease. For all intents and purposes, testing for micronutrient deficiencies does not occur with any regularity in primary or critical care, even when there are clear indications of deficiency. Wernicke's encephalopathy in alcoholics, the symptoms of which are taught from undergrad through medical school, is missed 80% of the time.[94] If the most obvious and well-articulated syndrome related to thiamine deficiency goes unrecognized 80% of the time, how can we so cavalierly dismiss a patient's suffering as "psychosomatic"?

## WHY THIAMINE? WHY NOW?

We began the book with these questions. Why thiamine? Why now? To reiterate our answer, thiamine plays a fundamental role in energy metabolism, one that has been ignored. As a rate-limiting cofactor in oxidative metabolism, it is easy to see how even slight deficiencies can evoke illness and we have provided ample evidence that those deficiencies exist. There is an obvious disconnect, however, between what the data demonstrate and what reaches clinical care. Organized medicine firmly believes that vitamin deficiency disease has been conquered. As a result, the symptoms that would have been readily recognized 70 or 80 years ago are attributed to other causes. Vitamin deficiency never enters the differential diagnosis. Research in genetics has dominated the overall picture without sufficiently considering the role of epigenetics. Because nutrition has long been considered to play a minor role in disease, we have not paid attention to the overwhelming malnutrition produced by the widespread consumption of empty carbohydrate and fat calories. We have shown throughout the book that thiamine is vital to the processing of glucose and that recent research has revealed its importance in the oxidation of fats. Because the hindbrain is particularly sensitive to thiamine deficiency we have shown that the principles of adaptation to environmental stressors through the hypothalamic–autonomic–endocrine axis easily become distorted. We have tried to show that this has behavioral consequences as well as producing traditional psychosomatic symptoms. Emphasis has been placed on the relationship between genetics, environmental stress, and nutrition in that they each contribute to the etiology of most diseases. Nutrition as the source of energy emerges with vital importance as a major factor. We ignore this to our own and our patient's peril.

With thiamine and other nutrient deficiencies, laboratory confirmation is not always available, in large part because of weaknesses in laboratory methodologies. Sometimes the determination of thiamine deficiency must be made empirically or clinically. Methods for doing so were provided in Chapter 4. Many of the assessments can be performed in the office quickly, sometimes requiring no more than observation and inquiry, but only if the clinician considers the possibility of nutrient deficiency. Nutrient deficiency is rarely considered in either routine or acute care. It should be. Indeed, we believe it should be among the first and most routinely assessed markers of health.

One of the more peculiar aspects of thiamine deficiency is that it can result in minor symptoms, none of which is pathognomonic. It can affect the patient for years, producing what is perceived by many physicians as the classic "problem patient." Problem patients, those with an inordinately large number of unrelated and treatment refractory symptoms, have become increasingly common in primary care. We would argue that perhaps the problem resides not with the patient but with us and our failure to recognize the obvious. Our concept of disease under the present medical model has become extremely familiar to all of us and thus we do not see its limitations. As Devisch and Murray wrote:

> *There is something sinister about familiar concepts ... The more familiar or "natural" they appear, the less we wonder what they mean; but because they are widespread and well-known, we tend to act as if we know what we mean when we use them.*[95]

To make a diagnosis is in the forefront of trying to solve the problem, regarding each disease entity as having a roughly similar course and for which there must be a specific treatment for that disease. In light of everything that was presented in this text, can we honestly say that current disease classifications, diagnostics, and treatment modalities fully capture the totality of human illness? If this is the case then we are justified in willfully dismissing the conditions not identified by our labs or resistant to our treatments as medically unexplained symptoms, unimportant or psychosomatic. If we trust in the infallibility of medical science as it currently stands, what we do not know can be attributed to the idiopathy of random chance, as these and so many other researchers and physicians have.

> *These results suggest that only a third of the variation in cancer risk among tissues is attributable to environmental factors or inherited predispositions. The majority is due to "bad luck," that is, random mutations arising during DNA replication in normal, noncancerous stem cells.*[96]

If what we do not understand is random chance, there is no need to question the model or methods from which such high rates of unexplained or random chance events occur. It is simply fate, something more akin to religion than science. For some of us, however, it is difficult to reconcile medicine as a *fete accompli*. It is difficult not to ask whether those are really the only choices available: that the patient standing before us, suffering immensely, is either imagining or fabricating his/her ill health or simply unlucky. Do we believe so strongly in the infallibility of the current medical model and our own diagnostic acumen that when a treatment fails it is the patient's fault and not ours? We should not, but if we are honest with ourselves that is exactly what we do when we dismiss the patient's suffering and when we dismiss nutrition, lifestyle, and other environmental factors in the onset and maintenance of disease. That is exactly what we do when we repeat the same familiar labs with the expectation that we are correctly measuring all there is to measure of a given disease process. That is exactly what we are doing when we offer the same familiar treatment approaches to a suffering patient for whom all other drugs in that class, or even in other classes, have not worked. What is it about familiarity with a given protocol that breeds a willful ignorance about the limits of our own understanding?

There is another option, however, but it requires going against convention into what are essentially uncharted and unsupported territories. It requires accepting that the patient's suffering is real and perhaps falls outside current diagnostic classification systems. Indeed, recognizing diseases of mitochondrial metabolism will shatter the current differentials. Most importantly, however, it requires admitting that for all of our technological sophistication and medical brilliance, we still have much to learn about health and disease.

## THOSE WHO HAVE THE PRIVILEGE TO KNOW HAVE THE DUTY TO ACT

The idea of nutrient deficiency as a cause of disease is hardly new. Hippocrates wrote "let food be your medicine and let medicine be your food" in 400 BCE. Medical science has all but ignored that admonition and now we find ourselves in a near-perfect storm of environmental factors that preferentially damage mitochondria coalescing simultaneously with widespread nutrient deficiency. The result is a dizzying array of complex and seemingly unrelated but comorbid diseases in Westernized cultures. For clinical medicine to evolve we must recognize basic deficiencies in our collective understanding. The belief that nutrients are sufficiently available in a diet consisting of highly processed foodstuffs is ludicrous. The assumption that everyday exposures to both environmental and pharmaceutical chemicals have no bearing on human health requires a degree of cognitive dissonance unbefitting the practitioner of medical science. While the notion that the patient standing before us, suffering, is fabricating or exaggerating denigrates our very humanity. Einstein said "those who have the privilege to know have the duty to act." The symptoms caused by aberrant metabolism are fully correctable once recognized. It is time we start recognizing.

## REFERENCES

1. Ames BN. Low micronutrient intake may accelerate the degenerative diseases of aging through allocation of scarce micronutrients by triage. *Proc Natl Acad Sci USA* 2006;**103**(47):17589–94.
2. Gomes A, Sengupta J, Datta P, Ghosh S, Gomes A. Physiological interactions of nanoparticles in energy metabolism, immune function and their biosafety: a review. *J Nanosci Nanotechnol* 2016;**16**(1):92–116.
3. Ames BN. DNA damage from micronutrient deficiencies is likely to be a major cause of cancer. *Mutat Res* 2001;**475**(1):7–20.
4. Allen LH. Current information gaps in micronutrient research, programs and policy: how can we fill them?. In: *Hidden Hunger*, ;**115**. Karger Publishers; 2016. p. 109–17.
5. Aguilar M, Bhuket T, Torres S, Liu B, Wong RJ. Prevalence of the metabolic syndrome in the United States, 2003–2012. *Jama* 2015;**313**(19):1973–4.
6. Karolina P, Agnieszka P, Barbara SA, Jerzy C, Alicja KR, Aleksandra S, Jean-Pierre M, Tomasz G. Clustering of geriatric deficits emerges to be an essential feature of ageing-results of a cross-sectional study in Poland. *Aging (Albany NY)* 2016;**8**(10):2437.
7. National Research Council, Committee on Population. *US health in international perspective: shorter lives, poorer health*. National Academies Press; 2013.
8. Chopra M, Galbraith S, Darnton-Hill I. A global response to a global problem: the epidemic of overnutrition. *Bull World Health Organ* 2002;**80**(12):952–8.
9. Scholz GH, Hanefeld M. Metabolic vascular syndrome: new insights into a multidimensional network of risk factors and diseases. *Visceral Medicine* 2016;**35**.
10. Picard M, Turnbull DM. Linking the metabolic state and mitochondrial DNA in chronic disease, health, and aging. *Diabetes* 2013;**62**(3):672–8.
11. Varlamov O. Western-style diet, sex steroids and metabolism. *Biochim Biophys Acta (BBA)-Molecular Basis of Disease* 2016. http://dx.doi.org/10.1016/j.bbadis.2016.05.025.
12. Via M. The malnutrition of obesity: micronutrient deficiencies that promote diabetes. *ISRN Endocrinol* 2012;**2012**.
13. Shah A, Shah FU, Khan SUD, Rana UA, Khan MS, Ahmad Z. Impact of micronutrient malnutrition on the health of preschool children: a cross-sectional Study. International journal for vitamin and nutrition research. Internationale Zeitschrift fü̈r Vitamin-und Erna''hrungsforschung. *J Int Vitam Nutr* 2015;**85**(1–2):31.
14. Sweet RL, Zastre JA. HIF1-α-Mediated gene expression induced by vitamin B. *Int J Vitam Nutr Res* 2013;**83**(3):188–97.
15. Ishimaru T, Yata T, Hatanaka-Ikeno S. Hemodynamic response of the frontal cortex elicited by intravenous thiamine propyldisulphide administration. *Chem Senses* 2004;**29**(3):247–51.
16. Lindenbaum GA, Larrieu AJ, Carroll SF, Kapusnick RA. Effect of cocarboxylase in dogs subjected to experimental septic shock. *Crit Care Med* 1989;**17**(10):1036–40.
17. Ma Y, Ordovas JM. The integration of epigenetics and genetics in nutrition research for CVD risk factors. *Proc Nutr Soc* 2016:1–14.

18. Lobo V, Patil A, Phatak A, Chandra N. Free radicals, antioxidants and functional foods: impact on human health. *Pharmacogn Rev* 2010;**4**(8):118.
19. Datta S, Sahdeo S, Gray JA, Morriseau C, Hammock BD, Cortopassi G. A high-throughput screen for mitochondrial function reveals known and novel mitochondrial toxicants in a library of environmental agents. *Mitochondrion* 2016;**31**:79–83.
20. Kasahara T, Kato T. Nutritional biochemistry: a new redox-cofactor vitamin for mammals. *Nature* 2003;**422**(6934):832.
21. Troesch B, Biesalski HK, Bos R, Buskens E, Calder PC, Saris WH, Spieldenner J, Verkade HJ, Weber P, Eggersdorfer M. Increased intake of foods with high nutrient density can help to break the intergenerational cycle of malnutrition and obesity. *Nutrients* 2015;**7**(7):6016–37.
22. Hainer V, Aldhoon-Hainerová I. Obesity paradox does exist. *Diabetes Care* 2013;**36**(Suppl. 2):S276–81.
23. Maeda A, Fadeel B. Mitochondria released by cells undergoing TNF-α-induced necroptosis act as danger signals. *Cell Death Dis* 2014;**5**(7):e1312.
24. Galluzzi L, Kepp O, Kroemer G. Mitochondria: master regulators of danger signalling. *Nat Rev Mol Cell Biol* 2012;**13**(12):780–8.
25. Naviaux RK. Metabolic features of the cell danger response. *Mitochondrion* 2014;**16**:7–17.
26. Caito SW, Aschner M. Mitochondrial redox dysfunction and environmental exposures. *Antioxid Redox Signal* 2015;**23**(6):578–95.
27. Chien Y, Rosal K, Chung BC. Function of CYP11A1 in the mitochondria. *Mol Cell Endocrinol* 2017;**441**:55–61.
28. Rizzuto R, De Stefani D, Raffaello A, Mammucari C. Mitochondria as sensors and regulators of calcium signalling. *Nat Rev Mol Cell Biol* 2012;**13**(9):566–78.
29. Kohlhaas M, Nickel AG, Maack C. Mitochondrial energetics and calcium coupling in the heart. *J Physiol* 2017. http://dx.doi.org/10.1113/JP273609c.
30. Xiao A, Gan X, Chen R, Ren Y, Yu H, You C. The cyclophilin D/Drp1 axis regulates mitochondrial fission contributing to oxidative stress-induced mitochondrial dysfunctions in SH-SY5Y cells. *Biochem Biophys Res Commun* 2016;**483**.
31. Neustadt J, Pieczenik SR. Medication-induced mitochondrial damage and disease. *Mol Nutr Food Res* 2008;**52**(7):780–8.
32. Will Y, Dykens J. Mitochondrial toxicity assessment in industry–a decade of technology development and insight. *Expert Opin Drug Metab Toxicol* 2014;**10**.
33. Wallace KB. Drug-induced mitochondrial neuropathy in children: a conceptual framework for critical windows of development. *J Child Neurol* 2014. 0883073814538510.
34. Kang SWS, Haydar G, Taniane C, Farrell G, Arias IM, Lippincott-Schwartz J, Fu D. AMPK activation prevents and reverses drug-induced mitochondrial and hepatocyte injury by promoting mitochondrial fusion and function. *PLoS One* 2016;**11**(10):e0165638.
35. Oliveira MA, Machado N, Bernardo T, Sardao V. *Mitochondria as a biosensor for drug-induced toxicity-is it really relevant?*. INTECH Open Access Publisher; 2011.
36. Potera C. Potential mitochondrial toxicants: Tox21 screen identifies structures of interest. *Environ Health Perspect* 2015;**123**(1):A23.
37. Attene-Ramos MS, Huang R, Sakamuru S, Witt KL, Beeson GC, Shou L, Schnellmann RG, Beeson CC, Tice RR, Austin CP, Xia M. Systematic study of mitochondrial toxicity of environmental chemicals using quantitative high throughput screening. *Chem Res Toxicol* 2013;**26**(9):1323–32.
38. Møller P, Jacobsen NR, Folkmann JK, Danielsen PH, Mikkelsen L, Hemmingsen JG, Vesterdal LK, Forchhammer L, Wallin H, Loft S. Role of oxidative damage in toxicity of particulates. *Free Rad Res* 2010;**44**(1):1–46.
39. Peixoto F. Comparative effects of the Roundup and glyphosate on mitochondrial oxidative phosphorylation. *Chemosphere* 2005;**61**(8):1115–22.

40. Lim S, Ahn SY, Song IC, Chung MH, Jang HC, Park KS, Lee KU, Pak YK, Lee HK. Chronic exposure to the herbicide, atrazine, causes mitochondrial dysfunction and insulin resistance. *PLoS One* 2009;**4**(4):e5186.
41. Park HW, Park EH, YUN HM, Rhim H. Sodium bezoate-mediated cytotoxicity in mammalian cells. *J Food Biochem* 2011;**35**(4):1034–46.
42. MacFabe DF. Enteric short-chain fatty acids: microbial messengers of metabolism, mitochondria, and mind: implications in autism spectrum disorders. *Microb Ecol Health Dis* 2015;**26**.
43. Pierzchalska M, Grabacka M. The potential role of some phytochemicals in recognition of mitochondrial damage-associated molecular patterns. *Mitochondrion* 2016;**30**:24–34.
44. Jiang Y, Liu J, Li Y, Chang H, Li G, Xu B, Chen X, Li W, Xia W, Xu S. Prenatal exposure to bisphenol A at the reference dose impairs mitochondria in the heart of neonatal rats. *J Appl Toxicol* 2014;**34**(9):1012–22.
45. Moon MK, Kim MJ, Jung IK, Koo YD, Ann HY, Lee KJ, Kim SH, Yoon YC, Cho BJ, Park KS, Jang HC. Bisphenol A impairs mitochondrial function in the liver at doses below the no observed adverse effect level. *J Korean Med Sci* 2012;**27**(6):644–52.
46. Parikh S, Saneto R, Falk MJ, Anselm I, Cohen BH, Haas R. A modern approach to the treatment of mitochondrial disease. *Curr Treatment Options Neurol* 2009;**11**(6):414.
47. Fernández-Ortega JF, Meseguer JH, García PM. Guidelines for specialized nutritional and metabolic support in the critically-ill patient. Update. Consensus SEMICYUC-SENPE: indications, timing and routes of nutrient delivery. *Nutr Hosp* 2011;**26**(Suppl. 2):7–11.
48. Mallat J, Lemyze M, Thevenin D. Do not forget to give thiamine to your septic shock patient!. *J Thorac Dis* 2016;**8**(6):1062.
49. Manzanares W, Hardy G. Thiamine supplementation in the critically ill. *Curr Opin Clin Nutr Metab Care* 2011;**14**(6):610–7.
50. Donnino MW, Carney E, Cocchi MN, Barbash I, Chase M, Joyce N, Chou PP, Ngo L. Thiamine deficiency in critically ill patients with sepsis. *J Crit Care* 2010;**25**(4):576–81.
51. Åkesson A, Larsson SC, Discacciati A, Wolk A. Low-risk diet and lifestyle habits in the primary prevention of myocardial infarction in men: a population-based prospective cohort study. *J Am Coll Cardiol* 2014;**64**(13):1299–306.
52. Teigen LM, Twernbold DD, Miller WL. Prevalence of thiamine deficiency in a stable heart failure outpatient cohort on standard loop diuretic therapy. *Clin Nutr* 2016;**35**(6):1323–7.
53. Mandrola J. Heart disease and lifestyle: why are doctors in denial? *Medscape* 2015. http://www.medscape.com/viewarticle/837945.
54. Smith RC, Dwamena FC. Classification and diagnosis of patients with medically unexplained symptoms. *J Gen Intern Med* 2007;**22**(5):685–91.
55. Kaipparettu BA, Ma Y, Park JH, Lee TL, Zhang Y, Yotnda P, Creighton CJ, Chan WY, Wong LJC. Crosstalk from non-cancerous mitochondria can inhibit tumor properties of metastatic cells by suppressing oncogenic pathways. *PLoS One* 2013;**8**(5):e61747.
56. Warburg O. On the origin of cancer cells. *Science* 1956;**123**(3191):309–14.
57. Seyfried TN. Cancer as a mitochondrial metabolic disease. *Front Cell Dev Biol* 2015;**3**:43.
58. Marsit CJ. Influence of environmental exposure on human epigenetic regulation. *J Exp Biol* 2015;**218**(1):71–9.
59. Ventola CL. The antibiotic resistance crisis: part 1: causes and threats. *Pharm Ther* 2015;**40**(4):277.
60. Schroeder M, Brooks BD, Brooks AE. The complex relationship between virulence and antibiotic resistance. *Genes* 2017;**8**(1):39.
61. Center for Disease Control and Prevention. 2015. Chronic disease overview. Elsea, S.H., McGUIRK, P.R., Gootz, T.D., Moynihan, M. and Osheroff, N., 1993. Drug features that contribute to the activity of quinolones against mammalian topoisomerase II and cultured cells: correlation between enhancement of enzyme-mediated DNA cleavage in vitro and cytotoxic potential. Antimicrob Agents Chemother 37(10), 2179–2186. http://www.cdc.gov/chronicdisease/overview/.

62. ralphmetznerblog.com.
63. Magistretti PJ, Allaman I. A cellular perspective on brain energy metabolism and functional imaging. *Neuron* 2015;**86**(4):883–901.
64. Solaini G, Baracca A, Lenaz G, Sgarbi G. Hypoxia and mitochondrial oxidative metabolism. *Biochim Biophys Acta (BBA)-Bioenergetics* 2010;**1797**(6):1171–7.
65. Subramanian VS, Nabokina SM, Lin-Moshier Y, Marchant JS, Said HM. Mitochondrial uptake of thiamin pyrophosphate: physiological and cell biological aspects. *PLoS One* 2013;**8**(8):e73503.
66. Prindle A, Liu J, Asally M, Ly S, Garcia-Ojalvo J, Süel GM. Ion channels enable electrical communication in bacterial communities. *Nature* 2015;**527**(7576):59–63.
67. Louveau A, Smirnov I, Keyes TJ, Eccles JD, Rouhani SJ, Peske JD, Derecki NC, Castle D, Mandell JW, Lee KS, Harris TH. Structural and functional features of central nervous system lymphatic vessels. *Nature* 2015;**523**(7560):337–41.
68. Picard M, McManus MJ, Gray JD, Nasca C, Moffat C, Kopinski PK, Seifert EL, McEwen BS, Wallace DC. Mitochondrial functions modulate neuroendocrine, metabolic, inflammatory, and transcriptional responses to acute psychological stress. *Proc Natl Acad Sci USA* 2015;**112**(48):E6614–23.
69. Raichle ME, Gusnard DA. Appraising the brain's energy budget. *Proc Natl Acad Sci USA* 2002;**99**(16):10237–9.
70. Shah E, Rezaie A, Riddle M, Pimentel M. Psychological disorders in gastrointestinal disease: epiphenomenon, cause or consequence? *Annals Gastroenterol* 2014;**27**(3):224.
71. Argoff CE. The coexistence of neuropathic pain, sleep, and psychiatric disorders: a novel treatment approach. *Clin J Pain* 2007;**23**(1):15–22.
72. Meltzer HY. Neuromuscular abnormalities in the major mental illnesses. I. Serum enzyme studies. *Res Publ Assoc Res Nerv Mental Dis* 1974;**54**:165–88.
73. Marrs C. Micronutrient deficiencies and mitochondrial dysfunction. In: *Integrative therapies for depression: redefining models for assessment, Treatment Prev*. CRC Press; 2015. p. 73–95.
74. Fattal O, Link J, Quinn K, Cohen BH, Franco K. Psychiatric comorbidity in 36 adults with mitochondrial cytopathies. *CNS Spectr* 2007;**12**(6):429–38.
75. Lakhan SE, Vieira KF. Nutritional therapies for mental disorders. *Nutr J* 2008;**7**(1):2.
76. Anglin RE, Tarnopolsky MA, Mazurek MF, Rosebush PI. The psychiatric presentation of mitochondrial disorders in adults. *J Neuropsychiatry Clin Neurosci* 2012;**24**(4):394–409.
77. Clay HB, Sillivan S, Konradi C. Mitochondrial dysfunction and pathology in bipolar disorder and schizophrenia. *Int J Dev Neurosci* 2011;**29**(3):311–24.
78. Shao L, Martin MV, Watson SJ, Schatzberg A, Akil H, Myers RM, Jones EG, Bunney WE, Vawter MP. Mitochondrial involvement in psychiatric disorders. *Ann Med* 2008;**40**(4):281–95.
79. Burnett BB, Gardner A, Boles RG. Mitochondrial inheritance in depression, dysmotility and migraine? *J Affect Disord* 2005;**88**(1):109–16.
80. Finsterer J. Mitochondrion-toxic drugs given to patients with mitochondrial psychoses. *Behav Brain Func* 2012;**8**(1):45.
81. Cornish S, Mehl-Madrona L. The role of vitamins and minerals in psychiatry. *Integr Med Insights* 2008;**3**:33.
82. James JT. A new, evidence-based estimate of patient harms associated with hospital care. *J Patient Safety* 2013;**9**(3):122–8.
83. Null G, Dean C, Feldman M, Rasio D. Death by medicine. *J Orthomol Med* 2005;**20**(1):21–34.
84. Makary MA, Daniel M. Medical error—the third leading cause of death in the US. *Bmj* 2016;**353**:i2139.

85. Stokowski LA. Who believes that medical error is the third leading cause of hospital deaths. *Medscape* May 26, 2016.
86. Clinic M. Nearly 7 in 10 Americans are on prescription drugs. *ScienceDaily* 2013. www.sciencedaily.com/releases/2013/06/130619132352.htm.
87. Light DW, Lexchin J, Darrow JJ. Institutional corruption of pharmaceuticals and the myth of safe and effective drugs. *J Law Med Ethics* 2013;**41**.
88. British Medical Journal. What conclusions has Clinical Evidence drawn about what works, what doesn't based on randomised controlled trial evidence? http://clinicalevidence.bmj.com/x/set/static/cms/efficacy-categorisations.html.
89. Lagarde F, Beausoleil C, Belcher SM, Belzunces LP, Emond C, Guerbet M, Rousselle C. Non-monotonic dose-response relationships and endocrine disruptors: a qualitative method of assessment. *Environ Health* 2015;**14**(1):13.
90. Monteiro JP, Kussmann M, Kaput J. The genomics of micronutrient requirements. *Genes Nutr* 2015;**10**(4):1–10.
91. Rosas-Ballina M, Tracey KJ. The neurology of the immune system: neural reflexes regulate immunity. *Neuron* 2009;**64**(1):28–32.
92. Prinzo ZW. Thiamine deficiency and its prevention and control in major emergencies. In: *Micronutrient series. World health organization (WHO)*. Department of Nutrition for Health and Development; Office of the United Nations High Commissioner for Refugees (UNHCR); 1999.
93. Wayne P. *Defining, establishing, and verifying reference intervals in the clinical laboratory: approved guideline third edition*. CLSI documalet C28-A3c. 3rd ed. Wayne, PA: Clinical and Laboratory Standards Institute; 2008.
94. Harper CG, Giles M, Finlay-Jones R. Clinical signs in the Wernicke-Korsakoff complex: a retrospective analysis of 131 cases diagnosed at necropsy. *J Neurol Neurosurg Psychiatry* 1986;**49**(4):341–5.
95. Devisch I, Murray SJ. 'We hold these truths to be self-evident': deconstructing 'evidence-based'medical practice. *J Eval Clin Pract* 2009;**15**(6):950–4.
96. Tomasetti C, Vogelstein B. Variation in cancer risk among tissues can be explained by the number of stem cell divisions. *Science* 2015;**347**(6217):78–81.

# INDEX

'*Note*: Page numbers followed by "f" indicate figures, "t" indicate tables, and "b" indicate boxes.'

## A

AAT. *See* Alpha-1 antitrypsin (AAT)
Acetylcholine (ACh), 36–37, 41
Acetyl-CoA synthesis, 68
ACTH. *See* Adrenocorticotropin releasing hormone (ACTH)
Acute blepharospasm, 44–46
Adrenaline, 41–42
Adrenergic receptors, 37–38
Adrenocortical tract, of autonomic response
    brainstem, 33–34
    hypothalamus, 32–33
    prefrontal cortex (PFC), 34
Adrenocorticotropin releasing hormone (ACTH), 32
Adrenomedullary tract, 31–32
A3243G mutation, 237
Allergies, 281b
Allicin, 132
Alpha-1 antitrypsin (AAT), 276–282, 277b–279b, 281b
Altered respiratory function, 5
Alternating psychosis, 271b
"Alternative" medicine, 306
Alzheimer's disease, 239–240
Aminoaciduria, 122–123
Angioedema, 243–245
Anorexia, 81, 129–130, 175–177, 176b–177b, 278b–279b, 283b
Anorexia nervosa, 175b
ANS. *See* Autonomic nervous system (ANS)
Antiberiberi factor, 3
Apnea, 173b–174b
Arthritis, 283b
ASD. *See* Autism spectrum disorder (ASD)
Aspartic acid, 121
Asthma, 281b
Atonic bowel, 273b

Attentional deficits, 181–183
Autism spectrum disorder (ASD), 220–222
Autonomic adaptations, 274–276
Autonomic balance, 17–23
    energy production and consumption, 20–21
    nutritional *vs.* pharmaceutical therapies, 22–23
    oxidative metabolism, 21–22
    stress and nutrient demands, 19–20
Autonomic chemistry, 35–41
Autonomic dysfunction, 15–17, 44–52
    acute blepharospasm, 44–46
    bladder and bowel dysfunction, 49–50
    cognitive and mental health symptoms, 50–52
    gastrointestinal dysmotility syndromes, 49
    heart rate and rhythm, 46–48
    muscle weakness, 48–49
    neuropathy, 48–49
    pressure dysregulation, 46–48
    sexual and reproductive abnormalities, 50
    skin disorders and balance, 48–49
    sweating, 44–46
Autonomic function, 126–130
Autonomic imbalance, 52–53
Autonomic nervous system (ANS), 5, 11–12
    autonomic chemistry/neurotransmission, 35–41
        acetylcholine and receptors, 36–37
        adrenergic receptors and response, 37–38
        ANS modulators, 40–41
        hormones and receptors, stress response of, 38–40
    autonomic dysfunction. *See* Autonomic dysfunction
    autonomic imbalance, 52–53

Autonomic nervous system (*Continued*)
  autonomic signaling, 29–35
    adrenocortical tract, 32–35
    adrenomedullary tract, 31–32
    general arrangement and function, 28–29
      enteric nervous system, 29
      sympathetic and parasympathetic divisions, 29, 30f
    linearity and symmetry, 43–44
      asymmetrical autonomic innervation patterns, 42–44, 42t
      nonlinear dose-response actions, 41–42
Autonomic reflex, 31–32
Autonomic signaling, 29–35
  adrenocortical tract, 32–35
  adrenomedullary tract, 31–32

# B

*Bacillus thiaminolyticus*, 84
Bender-Gestalt test, 144f
Beriberi, 6b, 44, 163–165
  autonomic chaos, 9–12
  in children
    infantile beriberi, 6–7
    juvenile beriberi, 7
  clinical features, 3–4
  dysautonomia, 13–15
  Kakke, 1–6
  with methylation issues, 147–148
  and naked calories, 82b
  newer classifications, 8, 9t
  stress and autonomic regulation, 12–13
  symptoms
    appearance, 4
    cardiovascular/respiratory disturbances, 4–5
    gastrointestinal dysmotility, 5
    nervous system disruption, 5–6
  thiamine deficiency, 9–12
  wet and dry beriberi, 7–8
Beta oxidation, 68
Bilateral cortical necrosis, 84–85
Bladder, 49–50
Blepharospasm, 46b
Blood oxygenation, 10b
Blood pressure, 5

Bowel dysfunction, 49–50
Brainstem, 33–34
Bruising, 244b–245b

# C

Cancer, 218–220
Cardiac collapse, 289b–294b, 291f, 293f
Cardiomyopathy, 4
Cardiovascular disease, 216–218
Catatorulin effect, 3
Cellular respiration, 65–67, 187
Cerebellar dysfunction, 129
Cerebellar functioning, 127–129
Cerebral lactate doublets, 115–116
Cerebral salt wasting, 286b–287b
Cervical lymphadenopathy, 184b–185b
Childhood hyperactivity, 182b
Cholinesterase, 41
Chromosomal abnormality, 173b
*Clostridium sporogenes*, 84
*Clostridium thiaminolyticum*, 84
Cocarboxylase, 65–66
Coenzyme Q (CoQ), 69
Cognitive disturbances, 50–51
Coma, 187b–189b
Complex regional pain syndrome, 170–172, 177b–178b
Corticotropin releasing hormone (CRH), 32
Creatine/creatinine metabolism, 117, 117f
Creatinuria
  in adults, 118–119
  in children, 119
CRH. *See* Corticotropin releasing hormone (CRH)
Crohn's disease, 271b, 283b
Cuban molasses disease, 83
CVS. *See* Cyclic vomiting syndrome (CVS)
Cyanosis, 191b–192b, 231b
Cyclic vomiting syndrome (CVS), 177–181, 179b–180b, 181f
  with complex regional pain and sleep irregularities, 177b–178b

# D

Dermatitis, 243–245, 279b
Dermographia, 277b
Developmental delay, 175b

Diaphoresis, 191b–192b
Diarrhea, 193b
Diet-driven thiamine deficiency, 17b–18b
Diet-induced thiamine deficiency, 168–170
Dihydroxyphenylalanine (DOPA), 225
Dizziness, 244b–245b, 278b
Down's syndrome, 270
Dramatic personality change, 278b–279b
Dry beriberi, 7–8
Dysautonomia, 13–15, 14b, 163–165, 175b, 202b–203b
  environmental stressors, 284–285
  familial dysautonomia
    molecular components, 206–207
    symptoms, 205
  functional dysautonomia, 165–172, 167f
    complex regional pain syndrome, 170–172
    diet-induced thiamine deficiency, 168–170
    family histories in complicated cases, 172
    gastrointestinal dysmotility, 165–168
    hypopyrexia, 165–168
    night terrors, 165–168
    pandysautonomia, 168–170
    postural orthostatic tachycardia syndrome, 168–170
    reflex sympathetic dystrophy, 170–172
  sudden infant death syndrome (SIDS), 232b–233b
  thiamine responsive dysautonomias, 172–200
    in adults, 200–205
    pediatric cases of, 172–200
Dysautonomic responses, 242b–243b

# E
Edema, 4
Electrocardiogram, 4
Electron carriers, 69
Electron transport chain (ETC), 69
Energy metabolism, 268–274, 313–314
  chemistry, 311–313
  iatrogenesis, 314–316
  malnutrition, 307–309
  medically unexplained symptoms, 309–311, 314–316
  negative labs, 317–318
  thiamine, 318–320
Enteric nervous system, 29
Enuresis, 182b
Environmental stressors, 264, 282–285
  dysautonomia, 284–285
  mitral valve prolapse, 284–285
  neurosis, 284–285
  pharmaceutical stressors, 285–288
Eosinophilic esophagitis (EoE), 49, 241–243, 242b–243b
Epigastric pain, 176b–177b
Epinephrine, 37–38
Epistaxis, 180b
Erythrocyte transketolase activity (ETKA), 220
ETC. *See* Electron transport chain (ETC)
ETKA. *See* Erythrocyte transketolase activity (ETKA)

# F
Failure to thrive, thiamine-deficient infants, 172–175, 173b–174b
Familial dysautonomia
  molecular components, 206–207
  symptoms, 205
Fatigue, 129–130, 176b–177b, 203–205, 203b–204b, 279b
Fatty liver, 273b
Functional dysautonomia, 165–172, 167f, 194b–195b. *See also* Dysautonomia
  complex regional pain syndrome, 170–172
  diet-induced thiamine deficiency, 168–170
  family histories, in complicated cases, 172
  gastrointestinal dysmotility, 165–168
  hypopyrexia, 165–168
  night terrors, 165–168
  pandysautonomia, 168–170
  postural orthostatic tachycardia syndrome, 168–170
  reflex sympathetic dystrophy, 170–172

# G
Gait and balance, 128
Gastrointestinal beriberi, 3–4

Gastrointestinal dysmotility syndromes, 5, 49, 165–168
Genetic stressors, 264, 276–297, 295t–296t
　alpha-1 antitrypsin (AAT), 276–277
　disturbances of energy metabolism, 288–294
　environmental stressors, 282–285
　familial genetic liabilities and thiamine, 277–282, 280t
Glutamic acid, 121
Glyoxalases, 136
Goose bumps, 45
Goose skin, 45

## H

HACL1 enzyme, 217–218
Hashimoto's thyroiditis, 202b–203b, 286b–287b
Headaches, 244b–245b, 278b
Herpangina infection, 246b–248b
Heterozygous AAT deficiency, 278b–279b
Hexose monophosphate shunt (HMPS), 73–74, 111
High-calorie malnutrition, 79–80
　adaptive mechanisms, energy homeostasis, 218–220
　autism spectrum disorders, 220–222
　cardiovascular disease, 216–218
　mitochondrial stress, 215–216
　obesity, 216–218
　sudden infant death syndrome (SIDS), 227b–230b
　sugar and thiamine, 220–222
　thiamine, 241–253
　　angioedema, 243–245
　　dermatitis, 243–245
　　eosinophilic esophagitis (EoE), 241–243
　　in hypoxia and ragged red fibers, 235–237
　　immunity and autoimmunity, 246–253
　　in menstrual and reproductive disorders, 237–239
　　in neurodegenerative disorders, 239–240
　　in obstetrics, 240–241
　　repeat infections, 246–253
　　in sudden infant death syndrome, 222–235
　　urticaria, 243–245
　　type 2 diabetes, 216–218
High-dose thiamine therapy, 131b
Horizontal nystagmus, 6
Human papillomavirus (HPV) vaccine, 266
5-Hydroxytryptamine (5-HT), 40
Hyperactive stress response, 270–271
Hyperactivity, 181–183, 182b–183b, 193b–194b
Hyperexcitable deep tendon reflexes, 288
Hyperglycemia, 219
Hypersomnia, 129–130
Hyperuricuria, 119–120
Hypoactive stress response
　hyperactive stress response, 270–271
　sick brain syndrome, 269b–270b
　stress responsiveness, genetic variation, 270
　unbalanced/oscillating responses, 271
Hypophagia, 173b–174b
Hypopyrexia, 165–168
Hypothalamus, 32–33
Hypothermia, 182b
Hypoxia, 235–237
Hypoxia inducible factor (HIF), 66
Hypoxias, 187–192

## I

Infantile beriberi, 6–7
Infantile myoclonus, 196b
Intermittent ataxia, 77b
Intermittent cerebellar ataxia, 141–146

## J

Juvenile beriberi, 7

## K

Kakke, 1–6

## L

Lactate, 68–69
Lactic acidosis, 115b
Leg disease, 1–2
Leigh's disease, 113–114, 236

Lesch–Nyhan syndrome, 119–120
Life-threatening croup, 195b

# M
Malnutrition, 2–3, 80, 307–309
Mass resonance spectrometry (MRS), 115
Medically unexplained symptoms, 309–311, 314–316
MELAS. *See* Mitochondrial encephalomyopathy, lactic acidosis, and stroke-like episodes (MELAS)
Mendelian characteristics, 264
Menstrual cycle, 237–239
Metabolic flexibility, 217
Metabolic instability, 193b
Metabolic mismatches, 274–276
Metformin, 88, 218
Methionine, 121
Methylation, 148–149
Methylglyoxal, 136
Mitochondria, 15, 90–92
  from diet, 77–79
  diet to ATP, 67–70
    acetyl-CoA synthesis, 68
    alpha oxidation, 68
    beta oxidation, 68
    electron carriers, 69
    electron transport chain (ETC), 69
    lactate, 68–69
    redox homeostasis, 69–70
  macronutrients, 64–67
  micronutrients, 64–67, 67f
  mitochondrial damage, 79–89
  mitochondrial energetics, 63–64
  mitochondrial function, 70–77
  mitochondrial genetics, 62–63
  modern thiamine deficiency, 79–89
  primary mitochondrial disorders, 61–62
  rethinking nutrition, 93
  secondary mitochondrial disorders, 61–62
  thiamine chemistry, 70–77
  thiamine deficiency in clinical care, 90–92
Mitochondrial basics, 64–67
Mitochondrial cocktail, 236–237
Mitochondrial damage, 79–89, 315–316
Mitochondrial DNA (mtDNA), 60, 62
Mitochondrial dysfunction, 311
Mitochondrial encephalomyopathy, lactic acidosis, and stroke-like episodes (MELAS), 236–237
Mitochondrial energetics, 63–64
Mitochondrial functioning
  essential nutrients, 67–70
    acetyl-CoA synthesis, 68
    alpha oxidation, 68
    beta oxidation, 68
    electron carriers, 69
    electron transport chain (ETC), 69
    lactate, 68–69
    redox homeostasis, 69–70
  thiamine chemistry, 70–77
Mitochondrial genetics, 62–63
Mitochondrial stress, 215–216
Mitral valve prolapse (MVP), 170–171, 238–239, 284–285
Modern nutrient deficiency, 80–81
mtDNA. *See* Mitochondrial DNA (mtDNA)
mtDNA damage, 63–64
Multinutrient deficiencies, 193b–194b
Muscle cramps, 204b
Muscle weakness, 48–49

# N
NAFLD. *See* Nonalcoholic fatty liver disease (NAFLD)
Naked/empty calories, 81–83, 82b
Naturally occurring thiamine inhibitors, 83–84
Nervous system disruption, 5–6
Neuritic beriberi, 3–4
Neurodegenerative disorders, 239–240
Neuropathy, 48–49
Neurosis, 284–285
Neurotransmission, 35–41
Night terrors, 165–168, 181–183, 182b–183b
Nitrogen balance, 121
Nocturnal sweating, 278b–279b
Nonalcoholic fatty liver disease (NAFLD), 218
Noradrenaline, 41–42

Norepinephrine, 37–38
Nuclear DNA (nDNA), 60
Nutritional liabilities, 264–265

## O

Obesity, 216–218, 307–309
Occasional hypogastric pain, 204b
Oligoaminoaciduria, 22
Orexin/hypocretin neurons, 130
Oxidation, 9–10
Oxidative metabolism, 21–22, 308–309
Oxidative stress, 215–216

## P

Pandysautonomia, 168–170
Panic attack, 12
Panic disorder (PD), 51–52
Paradox, 22, 138–139
Parasympathetic tract, 29
Paresthesia, 48b
Parkinson's disease, 239–240
Paroxysmal abdominal pain, 168
Pentose phosphate cycle, 73–74
Peripheral neuropathy, 6, 48b
Pharmaceutically induced electron transport inhibition, 87f
Pharmaceutically induced mitochondrial uncoupling, 86f
Pharmaceutical stressors, 285–288
Pigeons, 3
Piloerection, 46b, 182b
Polished rice, 2–3
Polyneuritis, 3
Poor visual acuity, 193b–194b
Postural orthostatic tachycardia syndrome (POTS), 47, 79, 168–170, 202b–203b, 267, 267t, 286b–287b
 thiamine deficiency post-gardasil vaccine, 48b
Prader-Willi syndrome, 167–168
Prefrontal cortex (PFC), 34
Prematurity, 175b
Pressure dysregulation, 46–48
Primary mitochondrial disorders, 61–62
Progressive autonomic instability, 201b
Pseudohypoxia, 9–10, 66, 235–236
Psychiatric symptoms, 273b
Psychosis, 271b

Pulse rate, 4
Purkinje cells, 127–128
Pyridoxal 5'-phosphate (PLP), 75
Pyridoxine, 196–200, 196b, 198f–199f
Pyruvate dehydrogenase complex (PDHC), 73–74
Pyruvate dehydrogenase deficiency (PDD), 140–141
 intermittent cerebellar ataxia, 141–146
  Bender-Gestalt test, 144f
  cognitive testing, 144
  ion exchange in urine amino acids, 142f–143f
  long-term progress, 145
Pyruvate metabolism, 110–111

## Q

Quinolinic acid, 199

## R

Ragged red fibers, 235–237
Rapid eye movement sleep behavior disorder (RBD), 239
Reactive oxygen species (ROS), 69–70, 217–218
Reading difficulties, 182b–183b
Recommended daily allowance (RDA), 130–137
Recurrent abdominal pain, 277b
Recurrent episodes of diaphoresis, 191b–192b
Recurrent febrile asthma, 279b
Recurrent febrile lymphadenopathy, 183–187, 185t
Recurrent fevers, 184b
 and cervical lymphadenopathy, 184b–185b
Recurrent urticaria, 244b
Redox homeostasis, 69–70
Reduced visual acuity, 6
Reflex, 265–266
Reflex sympathetic dystrophy, 151, 170–172
Repeat fevers of unknown etiology, 186b
Repeat flu-like symptoms, 204b
Reproductive disorders, 237–239
Reye's syndrome, 123–126, 124f–125f, 187b–190b, 190f–191f

Reynaud's disease, 283b
Rheumatoid arthritis, 248b–249b, 251t

## S

Secondary mitochondrial disorders, 61–62
Serotonin, 40
Serotonin reuptake inhibitors (SSRIs), 40
Severe asthma, 281b
Sham rage, 33
Shoshin beriberi, 289b–294b, 291f, 293f
Sick brain syndrome, 269b–270b
Sickness behaviors, 129–130
SIDS. *See* Sudden infant death syndrome (SIDS)
Single-nucleotide polymorphisms (SNPs), 267
SLC19A2 gene, 78
Sleep irregularities, 177b–178b
Sleepwalking, 181–183, 182b–183b
Slowed growth, 242b–243b
Solute carriers (SLCs), 77–78
Somatic spinal reflex, 31
Stiffness, 244b–245b
Stress, 265–268, 274–276
Stress factor, 266
Stressors, 265–268, 274–276
Stress response
  ATP, 268
  energy equation, 272–274
  hypoactive stress response
    hyperactive stress response, 270–271
    sick brain syndrome, 269b–270b
    stress responsiveness, genetic variation, 270
    unbalanced/oscillating responses, 271
Stress responsiveness, 270
Subacute necrotizing encephalomyelopathy (SNE), 113
Sudden infant death syndrome, 187–192
Sudden infant death syndrome (SIDS), 222–235, 227b–230b, 232b–233b
  dihydroxyphenylalanine (DOPA), 225
  with cyanosis, 231b
  hemodynamic features, 223–224
  orexin/hypocretin nuclei, 226
  urinary biogenic amines, 225, 225t
Suspected chromosomal abnormality, 173b
Sweating, 44–46
Swollen fingers, 244b–245b
Sympathetic tract, 29
Syncope, 278b

## T

Thiaminase I, 84
Thiaminases, 83–84
Thiamine, 70–77, 196b, 241–253, 318–320. *See also* Thiamine metabolism, evaluation/treatment of
  angioedema, 243–245
  ATP, 15
  and blood oxygenation, 10b
  in brain, 77
  in clinical care, 139–146
    intermittent cerebellar ataxia, 141–146
    pyruvate dehydrogenase deficiency, 140–141
  dermatitis, 243–245
  eosinophilic esophagitis (EoE), 241–243
  in hypoxia and ragged red fibers, 235–237
  immunity and autoimmunity, 246–253
  laboratory measures, 110–111
  Leigh's disease, 113–114
  with malnutrition, 2–3
  in menstrual and reproductive disorders, 237–239
  mitochondria, 15
  in nerve function, 75–77
  nervous system, 16–17
  in neurodegenerative disorders, 239–240
  in obstetrics, 240–241
  oxidative metabolism, 16
  repeat infections, 246–253
  in sudden infant death syndrome, 222–235
  thiamine monophosphate (TMP), 72
  thiamine pyrophosphate (TPP), 72–73
    pyruvate dehydrogenase complex (PDHC), 73–74
    TCA and ETC proteins, 74–75
  urticaria, 243–245
IV thiamine, 137–139
  additional nutrients, 138, 139t
  paradoxical reactions, 138–139

Thiamine deficiency, 107–108, 114–126, 202b–203b
  anorexia, 175–177
  blood/urine pyruvate, 114–115
  cerebral lactate doublets, 115–116
  creatinine, 116–120
  vs. dependency, 109–110
  in healthy humans, 163–164
  intermittent ataxia, 77b
  lactate, 115
  nonlaboratory methods, 126–130
    anorexia, 129–130
    asymmetrical pulse pressure, 127
    cerebellar functioning, 127–129
    fatigue, 129–130
    hypersomnia, 129–130
    orthostatic hyper/hypotension, 127
  in office, 109
  Reye's syndrome, 123–126
  solute carrier (SCL) mutations, 267t
  threshold and tipping points, 164–165
  uric acid, 116–120
  urinary amino acids, 120–123
  urinary creatine, 116–120
Thiamine deficiency post-gardasil vaccine, 48b
Thiamine deficiency syndromes, 8–12, 9t
Thiamine-deficient dysautonomias. *See* Dysautonomia
Thiamine-deficient lactic acidosis, 69b
Thiamine dependency, 109–110, 136–137
Thiamine derivatives, 132–133
Thiamine dosing, 131–132
Thiamine metabolism, evaluation/treatment of
  laboratory measures, 110–111
  measuring thiamine functionally, 111–114
    Leigh's disease, 113–114
    patterns of transketolase activity, 113
    research for TKA and TPPE, 112–113
    thiamine pyrophosphate (TPP) effect, 112
    transketolase activity (TKA), 111
  nutrient interactions, 146–152
    beriberi with methylation issues, 147–148

    nutrient-responsive complex regional pain syndrome, 151–152
    thiamine-responsive febrile lymphadenopathy, 149
    thiamine-responsive hypoglycemia with biotin, 147
    thiamine-responsive megaloblastic anemia, 148–149
  IV thiamine, 137–139
    additional nutrients, 138, 139t
    paradoxical reactions, 138–139
  thiamine deficiency, 107–108, 114–126
    blood/urine pyruvate, 114–115
    cerebral lactate doublets, 115–116
    creatinine, 116–120
    lactate, 115
    nonlaboratory methods, 126–130
    Reye's syndrome, 123–126
    uric acid, 116–120
    urinary amino acids, 120–123
    urinary creatine, 116–120
  thiamine status evaluation, 108–110
    acute/emergent care, 109
    thiamine deficiency in office, 109
    thiamine deficiency vs. dependency, 109–110
  thiamine therapy, 130–137
    thiamine dependency, 136–137
    thiamine derivatives, 132–133
    thiamine dosing, 131–132
    TTFD clinical evaluation, 133–136
Thiamine monophosphate (TMP), 72
Thiamine propyl disulfide (TPD), 132
Thiamine pyrophosphate (TPP), 16, 65–66, 71f, 72–73, 167–168
  pyruvate dehydrogenase complex (PDHC), 73–74
  TCA and ETC proteins, 74–75
Thiamine pyrophosphate effect (TPPE), 42, 112–113, 220, 222
Thiamine responsive dysautonomias
  in adults, 200–205
    cardiac irregularity and associated symptoms, 201–203, 202f
    fatigue, 203–205

pediatric cases of, 172–200
  anorexia and thiamine deficiency, 175–177
  attentional deficits, 181–183
  cyclic vomiting syndrome (CVS), 177–181
  failure to thrive, thiamine-deficient infants, 172–175
  hyperactivity, 181–183
  hypoxias, 187–192
  night terrors and sleepwalking, 181–183
  pyridoxine, 196–200, 199f
  reassessing complicated cases, 200
  recurrent febrile lymphadenopathy, 183–187, 185t
  slowed growth, thiamine-deficient children, 175
  thiamine and brain inflammation, 196–200
Thiamine status evaluation, 108–110
  acute/emergent care, 109
  thiamine deficiency in office, 109
  thiamine deficiency vs. dependency, 109–110
Thiamine sufficiency
  cattle research, 84–85
  environmental chemicals block thiamine uptake, 89
  mitochondrial damage, 85–88
  naked/empty calories, 81–83, 82b
  naturally occurring thiamine inhibitors, 83–84
  pharmacologically induced thiamine deficiency, 85–88
Thiamine tetrahydrofurfuryl disulfide (TTFD), 132–133, 310
  clinical evaluation, 133–136
    blood pressure in SHR rats, 134–136, 135f
    prolonged thiamine deficiency, 136
Thiamine therapy, 130–137
  thiamine dependency, 136–137
  thiamine derivatives, 132–133
  thiamine dosing, 131–132
  TTFD clinical evaluation, 133–136
Thiamine transporters, 77–79
Thiamine triphosphate (TTP), 16
TKA. See Transketolase activity (TKA)
TPPE. See Thiamine pyrophosphate effect (TPPE)
Transamination, 121
Transketolase activity (TKA), 111–113, 221
Transmethylation, 121–122
TTFD. See Thiamine tetrahydrofurfuryl disulfide (TTFD)
Twinkie case, 265–266
Type 2 diabetes, 216–218

# U

Ubiquinone, 69
Unbalanced/oscillating responses, 271
Uric acid, 116–120
Urinary amino acids, 120
  functional autonomic disturbances, 122–123
  thiamine deficiency, 122–123
  transamination, 121
  transmethylation, 121–122
Urinary creatine, 116–120
Urinary keto acids, 123
Urticaria, 243–245

# V

Vaccine-induced hypersomnia, 286b–287b
Vasomotor function, 5
Vertigo and ataxia, 6
Vitamin B6, 199–200
Vomiting, 173b–174b, 180b, 193b, 273b
  and epistaxis, 180b

# W

Warburg effect, 218–220
Wernicke's encephalopathy, 109
Wet beriberi, 7–8
White rice, 2
Whole blood HPLC, 111

Made in the USA
Columbia, SC
03 March 2019